ANNALS *of* THE NEW YORK ACADEMY OF SCIENCES

The New York Academy of Sciences
7 World Trade Center
250 Greenwich Street, 40th Floor
New York, NY 10007-2157

annals@nyas.org
www.nyas.org/annals

The New York Academy of Sciences

Published by Blackwell Publishing
On behalf of the New York Academy of Sciences

Boston, Massachusetts
2010

ANNALS *of* THE NEW YORK ACADEMY OF SCIENCES

VOLUME 1202

ISSUE

Cooley's Anemia: Ninth Symposium

ISSUE EDITORS

Elliott P. Vichinsky and Ellis J. Neufeld

This volume presents manuscripts stemming from the "Ninth Cooley's Anemia Symposium," held October 21–24, 2009 at the New York Academy of Sciences, and sponsored by the Cooley's Anemia Foundation and the New York Academy of Sciences.

TABLE OF CONTENTS

ix Preface to *Cooley's Anemia: Ninth Symposium*
Elliott P. Vichinsky and Ellis J. Neufeld

xi Clinical trials in thalassemia: insights from the patient community
Gina Cioffi

1 Pathogenesis and management of iron toxicity in thalassemia
Chaim Hershko

10 The role of antioxidants and iron chelators in the treatment of oxidative stress in thalassemia
Eitan Fibach and Eliezer A. Rachmilewitz

17 Thalassemia as a global health problem: recent progress toward its control in the developing countries
D.J. Weatherall

24 Iron metabolism and ineffective erythropoiesis in β-thalassemia mouse models
Pedro Ramos, Luca Melchiori, Sara Gardenghi, Nico Van-Roijen, Robert W. Grady, Yelena Ginzburg, and Stefano Rivella

31 Hepcidin in β-thalassemia
Elizabeta Nemeth

36 Therapy for β-globinopathies: a brief review and determinants for successful and safe correction
Ajay Perumbeti and Punam Malik

TABLE OF CONTENTS, CONTINUED

45 Humanized mouse models of Cooley's anemia: correct fetal-to-adult hemoglobin switching, disease onset, and disease pathology
Yongliang Huo, Sean C. McConnell, Shanrun Liu, Tingting Zhang, Rui Yang, Jinxiang Ren, and Thomas M. Ryan

52 Strategy for a multicenter phase I clinical trial to evaluate globin gene transfer in β-thalassemia
Michel Sadelain, Isabelle Rivière, Xiuyan Wang, Farid Boulad, Susan Prockop, Patricia Giardina, Aurelio Maggio, Renzo Galanello, Franco Locatelli, and Evangelia Yannaki

59 Hematopoietic stem cell mobilization strategies for gene therapy of beta thalassemia and sickle cell disease
Evangelia Yannaki and George Stamatoyannopoulos

64 Transcriptional silencing of fetal hemoglobin by BCL11A
Vijay G. Sankaran, Jian Xu, and Stuart H. Orkin

69 The challenge of obtaining therapeutic levels of genetically modified hematopoietic stem cells in β-thalassemia patients
Derek A. Persons

75 Deferiprone
Antonio Piga, Simona Roggero, Ilaria Salussolia, Davide Massano, Melania Serra, and Filomena Longo

79 Combined iron chelation therapy
Renzo Galanello, Annalisa Agus, Simona Campus, Fabrice Danjou, Patricia J. Giardina, and Robert W. Grady

87 Deferasirox—current knowledge and future challenges
John B. Porter

94 Monitoring the efficiency of iron chelation therapy: the potential of nontransferrin-bound iron
R.C. Hider, A.M.N. Silva, M. Podinovskaia, and Yongmin Ma

100 Critical appraisal of growth retardation and pubertal disturbances in thalassemia
Ratna Chatterjee and Rekha Bajoria

115 Magnetic resonance assessment of iron overload by separate measurement of tissue ferritin and hemosiderin iron
Ed X. Wu, Daniel Kim, Christina L. Tosti, Haiying Tang, Jens H. Jensen, Jerry S. Cheung, Li Feng, Wing-Yan Au, Shau-Yin Ha, Sujit S. Sheth, Truman R. Brown, and Gary M. Brittenham

TABLE OF CONTENTS, CONTINUED

123 Predicting pituitary iron and endocrine dysfunction
John C. Wood, Leila Noetzl, Aleya Hyderi, Mehrdad Joukar, Thomas Coates, and Steven Mittelman

129 Better survival and less cardiac morbidity in female patients with thalassemia major: a review of the literature
Maria Marsella, Alessia Pepe, and Caterina Borgna-Pignatti

134 A preclinical approach for gene therapy of β-thalassemia
Laura Breda, Dorothy A. Kleinert, Carla Casu, Laura Casula, Luca Cartegni, Eitan Fibach, Irene Mancini, Patricia J. Giardina, Roberto Gambari, and Stefano Rivella

141 The role of reduced intensity preparative regimens in patients with thalassemia given hematopoietic transplantation
Alice Bertaina, Maria Ester Bernardo, Angela Mastronuzzi, Giorgio La Nasa, and Franco Locatelli

149 Progress in hematopoietic stem cell transplantation as allogeneic cellular gene therapy in thalassemia
Antonella Isgrò, Javid Gaziev, Pietro Sodani, and Guido Lucarelli

155 Emerging insights in the management of hemoglobin E beta thalassemia
Nancy F. Olivieri, Vivekanandan Thayalsuthan, Angela O'Donnell, Anuja Premawardhena, Christopher Rigobon, Giulia Muraca, Christopher Fisher, and David J. Weatherall

158 Fetal globin gene inducers: novel agents and new potential
Susan P. Perrine, Serguei A. Castaneda, David H.K. Chui, Douglas V. Faller, Ronald J. Berenson, Noppadol Siritanaratku, and Suthat Fucharoen

165 Detection of the cardiovascular complications of thalassemia by echocardiography
John Malcolm Walker and Sunil Nair

173 Cardiovascular MRI in thalassemia major
John C. Wood and Leila Noetzli

180 Complexity of alpha thalassemia: growing health problem with new approaches to screening, diagnosis, and therapy
Elliott Vichinsky

188 Nutritional deficiencies in patients with thalassemia
Ellen B. Fung

197 Ferritin iron minerals are chelator targets, antioxidants, and coated, dietary iron
Elizabeth C. Theil

TABLE OF CONTENTS, CONTINUED

205 Pulmonary hypertension in thalassemia
Claudia R. Morris and Elliott P. Vichinsky

214 The natural history of thalassemia intermedia
Caterina Borgna-Pignatti, Maria Marsella, and Nicolò Zanforlin

221 Hepcidin and Hfe in iron overload in β-thalassemia
Sara Gardenghi, Pedro Ramos, Antonia Follenzi, Niva Rao, Eliezer A. Rachmilewitz, Patricia J. Giardina, Robert W. Grady, and Stefano Rivella

226 Fertility potential in thalassemia major women: current findings and future diagnostic tools
Sylvia T. Singer, Nancy Sweeters, Olivia Vega, Annie Higa, Elliott Vichinsky, and Marcelle Cedars

231 Redefining thalassemia as a hypercoagulable state
M. Domenica Cappellini, Irene Motta, Khaled M. Musallam, and Ali T. Taher

237 Treatment options for thalassemia patients with osteoporosis
Evangelos Terpos and Ersi Voskaridou

244 Health care transition in thalassemia: pediatric to adult-oriented care
Laurice Levine and Matthew Levine

248 Ninth Cooley's Anemia Symposium: summary and perspective
Arthur W. Nienhuis

Preface to *Cooley's Anemia: Ninth Symposium*

The Ninth Cooley's Anemia Symposium was held at the New York Academy of Sciences on October 21–24, 2009. This volume is dedicated to the leadership of the Cooley's Anemia Foundation and Sir David Weatherall, MD, FRS. The foundation was founded in 1954 by Frank Ficarra, the parent of two children with thalassemia, and has grown in the intervening decades to be the major voice for the thalassemia community in the United States. Sir David Weatherall was a leading speaker at the first symposium held at the New York Academy of Sciences in 1964 and has contributed to subsequent *Annals* volumes. In this volume, as a keynote speaker, he outlines the global health problem posed by thalassemia and international approaches to address it.

In addition to presentations at the symposium that shed light on the major advances in the understanding and treatment of thalassemia, the goal of this symposium was to provide dynamic educational interactions among basic scientists, clinical investigators, physicians, and patients. It is the hope of the thalassemia community that such interactions will result in improved quality of life for patients now and facilitate a cure in the near future.

This volume discusses advances in overcoming obstacles to successful gene therapy and the design and results of phase I clinical trials. Progress in stem cell transplantation using reduced intensity preparations, cord blood stem cells, and unrelated donors will expand access to transplants. Increased understanding of gamma-globin gene expression and the development of new therapeutic agents that induce fetal hemoglobin production suggest that transfusion independence may become possible for many patients. Potential therapeutic options resulting from discoveries in iron metabolism are being developed, including hepcidin agonists, Jak2 inhibitors, and peptides that accelerate iron release from ferritin. Prediction and prevention of future organ dysfunction from iron-induced tissue injury appear likely because of improved imaging technology and chelation therapy options. The symposium highlighted important clinical issues, including nutrition, fertility, pediatric–adult transition, pulmonary hypertension, cardiac disease, thrombosis, osteoporosis, growth, and the phenotypic diversity of thalassemia.

The ongoing efforts of the Cooley's Anemia Foundation were instrumental in making this symposium a successful one. We are especially grateful to Anthony Viola, national president of the Cooley's Anemia Foundation, as well as to the members of the executive and medical advisory boards. This meeting would not have occurred without the efforts of our colleagues on the organizing committee: Kathy Granger, Gina Cioffi, and Alan Cohen; as well as Marta Murcia, Sonya Dougal, and Melanie Koundourou. We would also like to thank Douglas Braaten, director and executive editor of the *Annals*, and Joseph Abrajano, assistant editor, for accomplishing the difficult task of editing the symposium presentations for inclusion in this volume. We are thankful to Susan Shurin, acting director of the National Heart, Lung, and Blood Institute; Elizabeth Nabel, past director of the NHLBI; and Griffin P. Rodgers, director of the National Institute of Diabetes and Digestive and Kidney Diseases, for their support for the symposium and their dedication to Cooley's anemia research.

doi: 10.1111/j.1749-6632.2010.05672.x

We also thank Erica Riray and Shanda Robertson for their administrative work to produce this volume in the *Annals* series. Finally, we would like to express our heartfelt admiration and thanks to the patients and the outstanding participants.

Elliott P. Vichinsky
Children's Hospital and Research Center
Oakland, California

Ellis J. Neufeld
Children's Hospital
Boston, Massachusetts

 Ann. N.Y. Acad. Sci. 1202 (2010) ix–x

Ann. N.Y. Acad. Sci. ISSN 0077-8923

ANNALS OF THE NEW YORK ACADEMY OF SCIENCES
Issue: *Cooley's Anemia: Ninth Symposium*

Clinical trials in thalassemia: insights from the patient community

There is a significant need for a wide range of clinical trials in the area of thalassemia and its related complications; however, the small U.S. thalassemia patient population ($n < 1{,}500$) limits trial enrollment and may deter investigators from initiating a U.S. based trial. Results from a survey conducted by the website for the Center for Information and Study on Clinical Research Participation (CISCRP) found that among people who suffer from severe chronic illness, only 6% participate in clinical trials.[1] Recognizing the problems of clinical trial recruitment in general and within the Thalassemia Clinical Research Network in particular, we sought insights from our patient population regarding trials that depend upon the participation of individuals with thalassemia.

Although once considered a pediatric disorder, advances in treatment have resulted in an increase in life expectancy for people born with thalassemia. As a result, many patients now live into their 30's and 40's and beyond, and the widespread adoption of chelation therapy and the advent of more recent, easier-to-administer chelation therapies may mean that life expectancy will increase even more. As the number of adult thalassemia patients increases, more patients are potentially available to participate in clinical trials; however, as adults, these patients have greater constraints placed upon the time they have available for trial participation in addition to limited eligibility due to secondary complications.

Moreover, changing immigration patterns create changes in the make-up of the thalassemia community. Recent decades have seen a greater influx of individuals from south Asia, southeast Asia, and China; many of the thalassemia patients from these communities have the α-thalassemia, rather than β-thalassemia variants.

Geographic factors also impact the thalassemia community. The Cooley's Anemia Foundation estimates that about half of U.S. patients are seen at a major thalassemia treatment center, and that about half are not. It is assumed that geographic inaccessibility is a major factor for many of those who are not affiliated with a major treatment center.

Patient perceptions of clinical trials

In general, awareness of the existence of clinical trials for thalassemia seems to be high among the community; it is assumed that awareness of specific clinical trials can vary significantly, but it is also assumed that patients affiliated with a major thalassemia treatment center have greater opportunity to be exposed to knowledge concerning specific trials, especially those in which their center is participating.

Many patients also are aware that clinical trials offered to the community are insufficiently enrolled. Patients have reported being approached for trials for which they are ineligible but for which they would have participated if possible.

The patient community understands that trials are vital and will lead to a better quality of life; however, there is some concern among the community about the safety of clinical trials, and this factor can have an impact upon trial participation.

doi: 10.1111/j.1749-6632.2010.05592.x

Patient critiques of clinical trials

Although many patients believe that clinical trials are vital to the thalassemia community and that trials will ultimately lead to a better quality of life, many also do not think that trials are designed to accommodate personal needs.

Individuals with transfusion-dependent thalassemia in particular must already dedicate a significant amount of time to regular hospital visits, often on a bi-weekly basis. They are in the unfortunate position of having to juggle a difficult, time-consuming therapy with all of the other demands of a normal life: work, school, family, social relationships, career development (networking, meetings, etc.), social/religious obligations, exercise, etc. In addition, because of the high incidence of complications related to thalassemia, many patients must spend additional time on treatments related to such complications as diabetes, low bone mass, and organ impairment. As a result, their time is precious and so the more time required of a particular clinical trial, the less likely a patient is to participate.

Transportation issues are also a factor. A visit to the hospital can involve any number of transportation-related expenditures, ranging from round-trip bus or subway fare to commuter train fare to parking and toll expenses. In some instances, patients may incur more expensive train or plane costs.

Overall, patients often believe that the demands placed upon them as adults, and in particular as working or college-enrolled adults, are often not taken into consideration when designing trials. In addition, many patients believe that the expertise which they have developed in regard to their disorder is discounted; they believe that greater patient input into trial design is crucial if researchers truly wish to recruit significant numbers of patients.

Patient motivators

Patients believe that there are a number of motivators that can influence an individual's willingness to enroll in a clinical trial. Financial incentives are an obvious choice, and may range from reimbursement of transportation expenses to compensation for time consumed by the trial. However, there are a number of other motivators which can play an equal, and in some instances greater, role in influencing patient enrollment. These include:

- *A sense of hope:* Trials that in some way promote the idea that there is hope for patients with thalassemia, or for treating certain aspects of thalassemia, have greater appeal to the population.
- *Assurances concerning safety:* Patients need to be assured that, to all reasonable extents, their participation in a trial will not jeopardize their health.
- *Demonstration of direct benefit:* Sometimes the purpose of a trial may be clear to investigators but may not be presented in terms that allow participants to see exactly how the trial may produce a benefit that translates directly to the community.
- *Report on success among patients:* Often, patients believe that they participate in a trial and then never hear about its ultimate outcome. Communicating results of a trial with the participants brings them full circle, gives them a sense of closure and encourages them to participate in future trials.

It is also essential to remember that in some cases, potential study outcomes can be quite important. Trials that seek to reduce transfusion requirements, provide information on potential health impact or predict improvement in quality of life can definitely sway a patient, as can those that investigate potential curative approaches for thalassemia.

Based upon information from the patient community, the Cooley's Anemia Foundation presents the following recommendations for increasing patient participation in thalassemia-based clinical trials:

1. Involve patients to a greater degree in the design of studies
   - Limit hospital stays to a maximum of three days
   - Consider transportation issues and ways to alleviate this burden
   - Recruit and conduct studies outside of TCRN sites
2. Utilize an appropriate mix of motivators
   - Financial incentives should be considered, especially for more involved studies that include hospital stays
   - Present a clear picture of the safety profile of the trial and be prepared to address patient concerns in this area
   - Point out aspects of the trial that are important to the patient population:
     - How it may provide a health/medical benefit now
     - How it may provide a health/medical benefit in the future
     - How it may impact positively upon quality of life issues
3. Keep the lines of communication open with the thalassemia patient community
4. Demonstrate respect for the knowledge and expertise of the thalassemia patient community, as well as for the real life demands and challenges they face

A key reminder to all involved in clinical trials comes from one patient with extensive participation in trials: "The best trials are where the PI is friendly before, during, and after participation. It is really bad when a PI shows interest in you just to enroll you then blows you off afterwards. These people should be banned from working with patients."

GINA CIOFFI, ESQ.
National Executive Director
Cooley's Anemia Foundation

Reference

1. Facts and Figures, Website for the Center for Information and Study on Clinical Research Participation (CISCRP).

Ann. N.Y. Acad. Sci. ISSN 0077-8923

ANNALS OF THE NEW YORK ACADEMY OF SCIENCES
Issue: *Cooley's Anemia: Ninth Symposium*

Pathogenesis and management of iron toxicity in thalassemia

Chaim Hershko

Department of Hematology, Shaare Zedek Medical Center, Jerusalem, Israel

Addresses for correspondence: Chaim Hershko, Department of Hematology, Shaare Zedek Medical Center, P.O. Box 3235, Jerusalem, Israel. hershko@szmc.org.il

In thalassemia major, iron overload is the joint outcome of multiple blood transfusions and an inappropriately increased iron absorption associated with ineffective erythropoiesis. Threshold values for iron toxicity are a liver iron concentration exceeding 440 mmoles/g dry weight, serum ferritin >2500 ng/mL, DFO urinary iron excretion >20 mg/day, and transferrin saturation >75%. The outpouring of catabolic iron that exceeds the iron-carrying capacity of transferrin results in the emergence of non-transferrin-bound iron (NTBI). NTBI is cleared preferentially by the liver and myocardium at a rate exceeding 200 times that of transferrin iron. NTBI catalyzes the formation of free radicals, resulting in oxidative stress and damage to mitochondria, lysosomes, lipid membranes, proteins, and DNA. The long-term consequences of iron toxicity, including cirrhosis, myocardiopathy, and endocrine disorders, are preventable and mostly reversible by effective iron chelation therapy. Recent technologic advances in the documentation of organ-specific siderosis and the improved efficiency of iron chelating programs resulted in a spectacular improvement in the prevention of iron-induced end-organ failure and improved survival in thalassemic patients.

Keywords: thalassemia major; iron; erythropoiesis

Mechanism of iron accumulation

Normal iron homeostasis fails to prevent the harmful accumulation of iron in two major disease categories: in inherited hemochromatosis syndromes where abnormal hepcidin regulation results in increased intestinal iron absorption and in iron loading anemias such as thalassemia major (TM) where transfusional iron overload is aggravated by increased iron absorption, caused by increased rates of ineffective erythropoiesis (Fig. 1).[1,2]

The rate of intestinal iron loading is variable, depending on the underlying genetic basis but is generally a fraction of the rate seen with transfusional iron loading. Humans cannot increase iron excretion to compensate for iron overload. Consequently, excess iron must be removed therapeutically. The most simple and effective method for removing, or preventing the accumulation of excess iron in hereditary hemochromatosis is by repeated phlebotomies. However, in iron loading anemias, phlebotomies are impractical and alternative methods, such as the use of iron chelators enhancing urinary or fecal iron excretion, have been developed.

With regular blood transfusions, iron stores increase to many times normal unless chelation treatment is given. Apprimately 200 mg of iron is present in each unit of donated blood or about 1.08 mg of iron per 1 mL of pure red blood cells. The total amount of iron transfused can be calculated by the volume of each unit transfused and the sum of blood transfusions. Mean transfusional loading in TM is 0.4 mg/kg/day but this varies considerably with 20% of patients <0.3, about 60% 0.3–0.5, and a further 20% >0.5 mg/kg/day.

Chelatable iron, NTBI, and iron toxicity

In health, iron is kept nontoxic by binding to molecules such as transferrin but in iron overload, the capacity to bind iron is exceeded both within cells and in the plasma compartment. This free iron will cause damage to many tissues in the body and will be fatal unless treated by iron chelation therapy.

doi: 10.1111/j.1749-6632.2010.05544.x

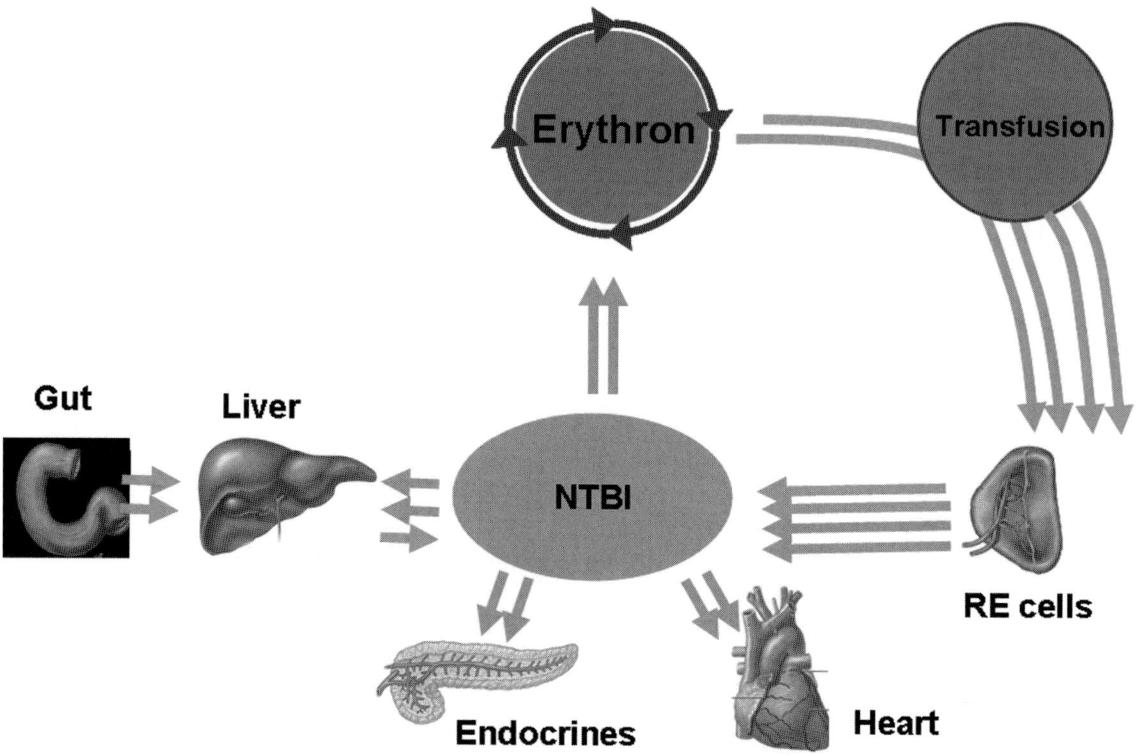

Figure 1. Iron balance in thalassemia major. Iron overload is the joint product of repeated blood transfusions and inappropriately increased iron absorption caused by ineffective erythropoiesis and anemia. Excess iron acquired by hyperabsorption is filtered through the liver via the portal system, and predominant hepatic parenchymal siderosis is typical of all conditions with increased iron absoption such as hereditary hemochromatosis and untransfused thalassemia intermedia. The first station in the accumulation of transfusional hemosiderosis is the RE system (spleen). Subsequently, RE iron is recycled to parenchymatous organs. With increasing severity of iron overload, the iron binding capacity of circulating transferrin is exceeded, resulting in the emergence of NTBI. The rate of NTBI iron uptake by the heart, liver, and other organs is many times faster than of transferrin iron, resulting in accelerated rates of iron deposition and cellular damage. Green arrows: transferrin iron. Brown arrows: NTBI.

Repeated blood transfusions lead to increasing saturation of transferrin and ultimately to the presence of iron species in the plasma that are not bound to transferrin, the so called non-transferrin-bound iron (NTBI).[3] These species are likely to be heterogenous, consisting of iron citrate monomers, oligomers, and polymers, as well as protein bound forms.[4] Some NTBI species are taken up by the myocardium and endocrine tissues through L-type voltage dependent calcium channels[5] that are not present on all tissues and this is likely to explain the pattern of tissue iron deposition in transfusional iron overload.

NTBI is a powerful catalyst for the formation of hydroxyl radicals from reduced forms of O_2. Under normal conditions mitochondria, microsomes, and peroxisomes produce significant amounts of reactive oxygen species (ROS). The cellular concentration of ROS is kept fairly constant by activities that convert ROS into nontoxic by-products. In addition to cellular or plasma antioxidants, the modulation of iron availability is the main mechanism for keeping ROS levels under strict control allowing the physiologic roles of the relatively safe O_2^-, and H_2O_2 to take place while preventing excessive production of the highly reactive $OH^·$ by Fenton chemistry.[6] ROS are capable of causing oxidative damage to macromolecules leading to lipid peroxidation, oxidation of amino acid side chains (especially cysteine), formation of protein–protein cross-links, oxidation of polypeptide backbones resulting in protein fragmentation, DNA damage, and DNA strand breaks[7] (Table 1).

The accelerated production of ROS generated in chronic and acute inflammatory conditions or under environmental stress is cytotoxic.

Table 1. Damage caused by ROS

Lipid peroxidation
Oxidation of amino acid side chains (especially cysteine)
Formation of protein–protein cross-links
Oxidation of polypeptide backbones leading to protein fragmentation
DNA damage and DNA strand breaks

Iron-loading results in increased generation of toxic hydroxyl radicals, as demonstrated *in vivo* in rats with chronic dietary iron overload using an electron spin resonance spin-trapping method. A number of possible mechanisms may explain the subsequent loss of respiratory enzyme activity in iron-loaded cells: (a) Free radicals may interact with lipid components of the mitochondrial membrane such as cardiolipin, which are particularly rich in polyunsaturated fatty acids and therefore very susceptible to peroxidative damage. Loss of cardiolipin and other vital lipid constituents of the mitochondrial membrane may impair respiratory chain assembly and activity; (b) Peroxidation of polyunsaturated fatty acids results in the formation of highly reactive aldehydes, such as malonyl-dialdehyde and 4-hydroxynonenal. These reactive aldehydes form covalent links with proteins, or protein adducts,[8] involving mainly the amino group of lysine residues and sulfhydryl groups, resulting in altered enzyme activity. Lastly, (c) the direct binding of Fe(II) to a metal-binding site on the respiratory enzyme and its reaction with H_2O_2 yields active oxygen species leading to the conversion of some amino acid residues to carbonyl derivatives, loss of catalytic activity, and increased susceptibility to proteolytic degradation. A vicious circle may be created by the oxidative inactivation of enzymes participating in the mitochondrial respiratory chain wherein loss of enzyme activity may lead to incomplete reduction of molecular oxygen and increased formation of free radicals.[9]

In thalassemia, transfusional iron loading begins within a few months of birth. Untreated transfusional iron overload in TM is fatal in the second decade of life, usually from cardiac failure or arrhythmia. Infection is the second commonest cause of death in thalassemic patients. Iron overload also causes anterior pituitary damage with hypogonadism and poor growth. Other endocrine complications, namely diabetes, hypothyroidism, and hypoparathyroidism, are also important, and their frequency has been steadily decreasing since the introduction of DFO chelation therapy in the late 1970s. Liver disease with fibrosis and eventually cirrhosis is also a serious complication. Hepatoma from the effects of iron overload with or without the additional risks from hepatitis is increasingly seen,[10] as chelated patients may now live beyond the 5th and 6th decades of life.

Excess iron is mostly deposited in reticuloendothelial (RE) cells (macrophages) in the spleen, hepatic Kupffer cells, and bone marrow, and in parenchymal tissues, such as the myocardium, liver, and endocrine organs. In contrast to RE cells in which iron accumulation is relatively harmless, parenchymal siderosis may result in significant organ damage.

Experimental and clinical observations indicate that urinary excretion of chelated iron is derived mainly from RE cells. Studies with DFO in hypertransfused rats have shown that in contrast to hepatocellular radioiron excretion, which is confined entirely to the bile, most of the radioiron excretion derived from RE cells is recovered in the urine. Moreover, when water-soluble synthetic chelators that do not enter cells easily, such as DTPA, are employed in the same experimental model, there is no enhancement at all of hepatocellular iron excretion, but the enhancement of urinary RE radioiron excretion is similar, or higher than that observed previously with DFO.[11] Hence, DFO obtains iron for chelation by one of two alternative mechanisms; (a) *in situ* interaction with hepatocellular iron and subsequent biliary excretion, and; (b) chelation of iron derived from RBC catabolism in the RE system directly or following its release into the plasma in the form of NTBI with subsequent urinary excretion. Iron chelated from myocardial cells, although critically important, represents only a tiny fraction of total excretion. Such iron, once mobilized into the plasma, will be excreted in the urine.

Beneficial effects of iron chelation

The primary objective of chelation therapy is to maintain body iron at safe levels at all times. Iron stored as ferritin or hemosierin is not chelated directly at clinically useful rates so that once accumulated, iron removal is slow and inefficient, relying on the tiny fraction of "labile iron" that is available for chelation at any moment. Chelation with DFO has traditionally been started only after 2–3 years of transfusion or when ferritin exceeds 1000 g/L, to avoid unwanted over-chelation at low levels of body iron. While the slow process of decreasing tissue iron to safe levels is being achieved, a second goal is to make iron as safe as possible by binding the toxic labile iron pools responsible for causing tissue damage. Plasma nontransferin iron and labile iron rebound rapidly after a chelator is cleared from plasma[12,13] so that in principle, the continuous presence of a chelator is desirable. Continuous chelation therapy also has the potential to minimize the uptake of NTBI species into organs such as heart and endocrine tissues.

Design of iron chelators

Iron(III) has six coordination sites that can be accommodated by one large molecule such as deferoxamine (DFO) (hexadentate chelation, Fig. 2). Such molecules tend to have high stability once bound to iron(III) but unfortunately it has not been possible to design hexadentate chelators that are small enough to allow efficient oral absorption. Smaller molecules can be absorbed from the gut more effectively and can bind iron(III) in either a 2:1 ratio with each molecule providing three binding sites (tridentate chelation, e.g., deferasirox, DFS) or a 3:1 ratio with each molecule providing two sites (bidentate chelation, e.g., deferiprone, DFP).

Chelatable iron is encountered both within cells and within the plasma compartment. Access of chelators to intracellular pools is affected by their size, charge, lipid solubility, iron coordination structure, and metabolism.[14] Thus, in addition to being absorbed more rapidly from the GI tract, small, neutrally charged bidentate molecules such as DFP are able to access intracellular iron pools more rapidly than DFO.[15] It is important that the binding of iron to a chelator prevents the further redox cycling of iron. The chelator should also not inhibit essential metalloenzymes such as ribonucleotide reductase within cells.[16] In practice, all chelators exhibit some affinity for other metals such as zinc, copper, and aluminum but clinically available chelators do not appear to be limited in their use by such metal binding. The success of iron chelators is also affected by their pharmacokinetic and pharmacodynamic

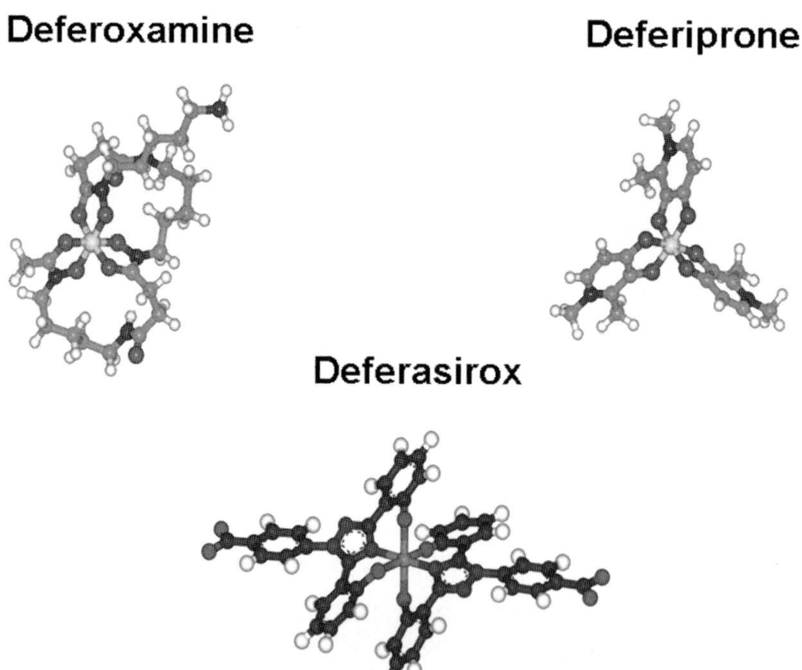

Figure 2. The three leading iron chelating drugs for clinical use. Deferoxamine is a hexadentate drug and a single molecule is able to cover all six coordination sites of iron. By comparison, deferiprone is bidentate requiring three molecules and deferasirox is tridentate, requiring two molecules to cover all six coordination sites.

interactions. Depending on the rate of absorption, elimination, and metabolism, plasma and cellular concentrations of chelators and their iron complexes differ considerably. These considerations will also have a bearing on the balance between cellular iron uptake and iron removal and hence the success of chelation therapy.

In order to identify safe and effective compounds that are orally active, more than one thousand candidate compounds have been screened in animal models. However, only three compounds were shown to be effective in clinical use over a sustained period, namely DFO, deferiprone (DFP), and deferasirox (DFS). A comparison of molecular weights, chelating properties, recommended daily dose, method of delivery, and other properties of these three leading chelators is presented in Table 2.

Clinical results of iron chelation therapy

The clinical aspects of iron chelation will be covered extensively by other speakers in this symposium. Therefore, in the text that follows I shall limit myself only to the highlights of the three major iron chelating drugs in current use.

Deferoxamine

Because of its proven efficacy and the extensive experience with its long-term use in many thousands of patients, deferoxamine (DFO) is still considered the gold standard of iron chelation therapy. DFO is a hexadentate chelator (Fig. 2), binding iron at a 1:1 molar ratio and preventing its participation in toxic reactions. DFO treatment should be started when serum ferritin levels exceed 1000 μg/L which usually occurs after the first 10 or 20 transfusions. DFO is infused via a thin s.c. needle inserted to the arm or abdomen nightly, connected to a portable pump over 8–12 h, 5–7 times per week at a daily dose of 20–60 mg/kg. In most patients, a urinary iron excretion of 0.5 mg/kg/day is usually sufficient to ensure negative iron balance.

The introduction of DFO for iron chelation therapy of transfusional siderosis has changed the life expectancy and life quality of patients with TM. Its long-term efficacy has been extensively documented in large multicenter trials in Italy and elsewhere. Only 70% of patients born before 1970 and hence prior to the modern era of iron chelation survived to age 20 years compared with 89% of patients born after 1970 and therefore receiving effective chelation from an early age.[17] In a report on thalassemic patients treated by DFO at a single institution, survival at 40 years was 83% and in compliant patients born after 1975 survival at 25 years was 100%.[18] The cohort-of-birth related improvement in survival was reflected in an inverse,

Table 2. Comparison of the three leading iron chelating drugs

Compound	Deferoxamine	Deferiprone	Deferasirox
Molecular weight (Da)	657	139	373
Chelating properties	Hexadentate	Bidentate	Tridentate
Iron binding affinity (pM)	26.6	19.9	22.5
Chelation efficiency (%)	13	7	27
Recommended dose mg/kg/day	30–50	75–100	20–40
Delivery	s.c. or i.v. 8–12 h 5 days/week	Oral three times daily	Oral, once daily
Half-life	20–30 min	3–4 h	12–16 h
Lipid solubility	Low	Intermediate	High
Excretion	Urinary and fecal	Urinary	Fecal
Peak plasma levels (μM)	5–10	90–450	80
Adverse effects	Ocular, auditory toxicity, growth retardation, local reactions, allergy	Gastrointestinal upset, arthralgia, agranulocytosis/neutropenia	Gastrointestinal upset, rash, ocular, auditory toxicity, mild reversible increase in creatinine

mirror-like decrease in cardiac mortality, supporting the assumption that prevention of cardiac mortality is the most important beneficial effect of DFO therapy. The strongest direct evidence supporting the beneficial effect of DFO on hemosiderotic heart disease is the reversal of established myocardiopathy in some far-advanced cases.

Compliance with the rigorous requirements of daily subcutaneous DFO infusions is still a serious limiting factor in treatment outcome. In the United Kingdom, survival in the year 2000 among thalassemic patients by the age of 35 years was only 50%[19] and mortality was largely attributed to poor compliance. All patients noncompliant with DFO treatment remained at risk of lethal cardiac complications.[18] This is the rationale behind the intensive efforts to develop alternative, orally effective iron chelators that would be more convenient for use and could improve compliance.

Deferiprone

Urinary iron excretion with DFP is roughly equal to DFO and is probably derived from the same chelatable pool with one exception: DFP readily enters cells[20] because of its smaller size (m.w. 139 v.s. 560) and higher lipophilicity compared with DFO. Thus, DFP may access intracellular chelatable iron more effectively than DFO. On the other hand DFP, unlike DFO does not enhance biliary iron excretion, likely because of rapid glucuronidation and inactivation within hepatocytes.

The cardioprotective effect of DFP is the most remarkable advantage of this compound. Long-term, prospective trials are now available comparing the ability of chelation therapy with either deferoxamine or DFP to prevent heart disease. In a prospective nonrandomized study, 54 DFP-treated patients were compared with 75 DFO-treated patients for cardiac complications and survival.[21] By the end of the six-year follow-up period three patients died, all in the DFO group, despite attempted rescue by intensified i.v. therapy. Worsening of pre-existing cardiac disease or new onset of cardiac abnormalities was observed in 4% of the DFP group compared with 20% of the DFO-treated patients. The authors concluded that these findings suggest long-term DFP treatment provides better protection against the cardiotoxicity of iron than DFO.

Two subsequent studies attempted to evaluate the effect of DFP on cardiac mortality. The first of these involved all thalassemic patients treated at seven Italian hospitals[22] born between 1970 and 1993 who did not experience cardiac complications prior to 1995. There were 359 patients treated by DFO only, and 157 receiving DFP for a median duration of 4.3 years between 1995 and the end of 2003. There were 52 cardiac events including 10 cardiac deaths among patients treated with DFO. By contrast, no cardiac event occurred in any of the patients during DFP treatment or within 18 months after DFP. This study, although retrospective, was subjected to exceptionally detailed and meticulous statistical analysis. The estimated hazard of a cardiac event on DFP was less than one-tenth that in patients on DFO. However, the dropout rate on DFP was high (46 patients or 31%) including 21 patients with increasing ferritins or liver iron, neutropenia in 8, and agranulocytosis in 1 patient.

Further evidence supporting the cardioprotective effect of DFP was produced following the introduction of the T2* method for estimating cardiac iron concentrations. In a study of 61 thalassemic patients with moderate cardiac siderosis (T2* 8–20 ms)[23] patients were randomized to continue on DFO 43 mg/kg/day or DFP 92 mg/kg/day. After 1 year of treatment, the improvement in T2* and increase in left ventricular ejection fraction were significantly greater for DFP than for DFO. The authors concluded that DFP monotherapy was significantly more effective than DFO in improving asymptomatic myocardial siderosis in beta-TM.

Deferasirox

DFS is a synthetic chelator with a plasma half-life of 11–19 h allowing its use by once-daily oral dosing. At a daily dosing of 20 mg/kg, peak plasma levels reach a mean of 80 μM with trough values of 20 μM (Table 2).[24] The ability of DFS to eliminate NTBI from the circulation is outstanding.[39,40]

In a randomized prospective study involving 586 thalassemic patients in whom the long-term effects of DFS were compared with DFO.[25] At DFS dose ranges of 20–30 mg/kg/day both drugs were equally effective as judged by LIC and ferritin measurements. These results agree very well with the results of previous studies. A question of vital importance is the effect of DFS on cardiac siderosis and the prevention of cardiac complications. *In vitro*[26,27] and animal studies[28] suggested that DFS would be effective at accessing myocardial iron. The efficacy of deferasirox in reducing or preventing cardiac iron overload was assessed in a recent study in 192 patients with beta-thalassemia in a 1-year prospective, multicenter trial (29). One hundred fourteen of these patients had myocardial T2* ranging from 5 to 20 ms indicating cardiac siderosis, and serum ferritin more than 2500 ng/mL. Myocardial T2 improved from a baseline of 11.2 ms to 12.9 ms ($P < 0.001$). In the prevention arm, baseline myocardial T2* was unchanged from 32.0 ms to 32.5 ms ($P = 0.57$). This prospective study suggests that deferasirox is effective in removing and preventing myocardial iron accumulation.

In general, DFS is well tolerated.[25,38] Adverse events were generally mild including transient gastrointestinal events in 15%, skin rash in 11% and mild, dose-dependent increases in serum creatinine in 38% of patients which generally remained within the normal range and did not exceed two times the upper limit of normal. Increases in creatinine typically occurred within a few weeks of starting or increasing therapy, were not progressive and reversible or stabilized with dose adjustment when necessary. Follow-up data in the five core phase II/III studies is now at a median of 3.5 years with no evidence of new or progressive toxicities.[30] It is too early yet to allow any statements on the impact of DFS on survival. Recommended patient monitoring includes monthly creatinine and liver function and annual auditory and ophthalmic examinations, including slit-lamp examination and fundoscopy.

Combined chelation therapy

Combined chelation treatment is gaining increasing popularity, in particular in mediterranean countries.[31,32,33,37] Although at inception its rationale was a shuttle-and-sink hypothesis, there is no compelling evidence that the simultaneous presence of both chelators is necessary to achieve increased chelation. A simple additive effect resulting from the increased exposure time to chelation is quite likely. Although maximal exposure time to chelation could be achieved by alternating DFO every night and DFP every day, in practice many other regimes have been used. The choice of combination regime may vary depending on what the reason for adding a second drug is. If the primary aim is to identify a regime that the patient is most likely to comply with in an otherwise low risk situation, the choice of combination may differ from someone who has extreme levels of iron overload or already has significant cardiac problems.

The effects of combined treatment on heart and on survival have been reported in a number of prospective randomized as well as nonrandomized observational studies. In an important randomized controlled study involving 65 patients with moderate heart iron loading (T2* 8–20 ms), myocardial T2* changes with combined DFP 75 mg/kg 7 days a week plus desferrioxamine 5 days were compared with patients who remained on standard desferrioxamine five times a week[34] T2* improved in both groups but was significantly greater (6 ms) with combined treatment than with desferrioxamine monotherapy (3 ms). In another observational study in 79 patients with severe iron overload who were previously noncompliant with s.c. DFO, combined treatment resulted in significant improvements in cardiac T2*.[35]

In thalassaemia major patients from Cyprus, 539 patients born after 1960 and on whom accurate clinical data were available were followed over the period from 1980 to 2004. Overall there were 58 deaths, 53% of which were due to cardiac causes.[36] There was a significant trend of increasing cardiac mortality between 1980 and 2000 and a decline after 2000, which the authors suggested to be due to the introduction of a combined DFP–deferoxamine therapy at this time. There were no deaths reported in patients treated with combined therapy between 2000 and 2004 using a regime similar to that employed in Italy.[35] Longer follow up to the present time appears to confirm these favorable estimates of decreased cardiac mortality in thalassemia.

Formal safety data on combined treatment are limited. In general, alternating regimes are less likely to be associated with increased toxicity compared with regimes where chelation is simultaneous or overlapping.

Conclusions

Iron overload in thalassemia is the joint outcome of multiple blood transfusions and inappropriately increased iron absorption associated with ineffective erythropoiesis. The massive release of catabolic iron from the RE system, combined with the accumulation of iron over many years of transfusional siderosis, results in complete saturation of the iron-carrying capacity of transferrin and the emergence of NTBI. NTBI is cleared preferentially by the liver and myocardium at a rate exceeding 200 times that of transferrin iron. NTBI catalyzes the formation of free radicals, resulting in oxidative stress and damage to mitochondria, lysosomes, lipid membranes, proteins, and DNA. However, the long-term consequences of iron toxicity, including cirrhosis, myocardiopathy, and endocrine disorders, are preventable and mostly reversible by effective iron chelation therapy. Recent technologic advances in the documentation of organ-specific siderosis and the improved efficiency of iron chelating programs resulted in a spectacular improvement in the prevention of iron-induced end-organ failure and improved survival in thalassemic patients.

Conflicts of interest

The author received honoraria from Novartis Switzerland and Apotex Canada.

References

1. Finch, C.A., K. Deubelbeiss, J.D. Cook, *et al.* 1970. Ferrokinetics in man. *Medicine (Baltimore)* **49:** 17–53.
2. Tanno, T., N.V. Bhanu, P.A. Oneal, *et al.* 2007. High levels of GDF15 in thalassemia suppress expression of the iron regulatory protein hepcidin. *Nature Med.* **13:** 1096–1101.
3. Hershko, C., G. Graham, G. Bates & E. Rachmilewitz. 1978. Non-specific serum iron in thalassaemia; an abnormal serum fraction of potential toxicity. *Br. J. Haematol.* **40:** 255–263.
4. Evans, R.W., R. Rafique, A. Zarea, *et al.* 2008. Nature of non-transferrin-bound iron: studies on iron citrate complexes and thalassemic sera. *J. Biol. Inorg. Chem.* **13:** 57–74.
5. Oudit, G.Y., H. Sun, M.G. Trivieri, *et al.* 2003. L-Type Ca2+ channels provide a major pathway for iron entry into cardiomyocytes in iron-overload cardiomyopathy. *Nature Med.* **9:** 1187–1194.
6. Halliwell, B. & J.M. Gutteridge. 1992. Biologically relevant metal ion-dependent hydroxyl radical generation. An update. *FEBS Lett.* **307:** 108–112.
7. Cadenas, E. 1989. Biochemistry of oxygen toxicity. *Annu. Rev. Biochem.* **58:** 79–110.
8. Houglum, K., M. Filip, J.L. Witztum & M. Choikier. 1990. Malondialdehyde and 4-hydroxynonenal protein adducts in plasma and liver of rats with iron overload. *J. Clin. Invest.* **86:** 1991–1998.
9. Pitkainen, S. & B.H. Robinson. 1996. Mitochondrial complex I deficiency leads to increased production of superoxide radicals and induction of superoxide dismutase. *J. Clin. Invest.* **98:** 345–351.
10. Borgna-Pignatti, C., S. Rugolotto, P. De Stefano, *et al.* 2004. Survival and complications in patients with thalassemia major treated with transfusion and deferoxamine. *Haematologica* **89:** 1187–1193.
11. Hershko, C. & D. Weatherall. 1988. Iron chelating therapy. *CRC Crit. Rev. Clin. Lab. Sci.* **26:** 303–345.
12. Cabantchik, Z.I., W. Breuer, G. Zanninelli & P. Cianciulli. 2005. LPI-labile plasma iron in iron overload. *Best Pract. Res. Clin. Haematol.* **18:** 277–287.
13. Porter, J.B., R.D. Abeysinghe, L. Marshall, *et al.* 1996. Kinetics of removal and reappearance of non-transferrin-bound plasma iron with deferoxamine therapy. *Blood* **88:** 705–713.
14. Porter, J.B., S. Singh, K.P. Hoyes, *et al.* 1994. Lessons from preclinical and clinical studies with 1,2-diethyl-3-hydroxypyridin-4-one, CP94 and related compounds. *Adv. Exp. Med. Biol.* **356:** 361–370.
15. Glickstein, H., R.B. El, M. Shvartsman & Z.I. Cabantchik. 2005. Intracellular labile iron pools as direct targets of iron chelators: a fluorescence study of chelator action in living cells. *Blood* **106:** 3242–3250.
16. Cooper, C.E., G.R. Lynagh, K.P. Hoyes, *et al.* 1996. The relationship of intracellular iron chelation to the inhibition and regeneration of human ribonucleotide reductase. *J. Biol. Chem.* **271:** 20291–20299.
17. Gabutti, V. & C. Borgna-Pignatti. 1994. Clinical manifestations and therapy of transfusional haemosiderosis. *Bailliere's Clin. Haematol.* **7:** 919–940.
18. Davis, B.A., C. O'Sullivan, P.H. Jarritt, *et al.* 2004. Value of sequential monitoring of left ventricular ejection fraction in the management of thalassemia major. *Blood* **104:** 263–269.
19. Modell, B., M. Khan & M. Darlison, 2000. Survival in beta-thalassaemia major in the UK: data from the UK Thalassaemia Register. *Lancet* **355:** 2051–2052.
20. Hershko, C., G. Link, A. Pinson, *et al.* 1991. Iron mobilization from myocardial cells by 3-hydroxypyridin-4-one chelators: studies in rat heart cells in culture. *Blood* **77:** 2049–2053.
21. Piga, A., C. Gaglioti, E. Fogliacco, *et al.* 2003. Comparative effects of deferiprone and deferoxamine on survival and cardiac disease in patients with thalassemia major: a retrospective analysis. *Haematologica.* **88:** 489–496.
22. Borgna-Pignatti, C., M.D. Cappellini, P. De Stefano, *et al.* 2006. Cardiac morbidity and mortality in deferoxamine- or deferiprone-treated patients with thalassemia major. *Blood* **107:** 3733–3737.
23. Pennell, D.J., V. Berdoukas, M. Karagiorga, *et al.* 2006. Randomized controlled trial of deferiprone or deferoxamine in beta-thalassemia major patients with asymptomatic myocardial siderosis. *Blood* **107:** 3738–3744.
24. Nisbet-Brown, E., N.F. Olivieri, P.J. Giardina, *et al.* 2003. Effectiveness and safety of ICL670 in iron-loaded patients with thalassaemia: a randomised, double-blind, placebo-controlled, dose-escalation trial. *Lancet* **361:** 1597–1602.
25. Cappellini, M.D., A. Cohen, A. Piga, *et al.* 2006. A phase 3 study of deferasirox (ICL670), a once-daily oral iron chelator, in patients with beta-thalassemia. *Blood* **107:** 3455–3462.
26. Glickstein, H, R.B. El, G. Link, *et al.* 2006. Action of chelators in iron-loaded cardiac cells: accessibility to intracellular labile iron and functional consequences. *Blood* **108:** 3195–3203.
27. Hershko, C., A.M. Konijn, H.P. Nick, *et al.* 2001. ICL670A: a new synthetic oral chelator: evaluation in hypertransfused rats with selective radioiron probes of hepatocellular and reticuloendothelial iron stores and in iron-loaded rat heart cells in culture. *Blood* **97:** 1115–1122.

28. Wood, J.C., M. Otto-Duessel, M. Aguilar, *et al.* 2005. Cardiac iron determines cardiac T2*, T2, and T1 in the gerbil model of iron cardiomyopathy. *Circulation* **112:** 535–543.
29. Pennell, D.J., J.B. Porter, M.D. Cappellini, *et al.* 2010. Efficacy of deferasirox in reducing and preventing cardiac iron overload in beta-thalassemia. *Blood* **115:** 2364–2371.
30. Cappellini, M.D., J.D. Porter, A. El-Beshlawy, *et al.* 2010. Tailoring iron chelation by iron intake and serum ferritin: the prospective EPIC study of deferasirox in 1744 patients with transfusion-dependent anemias. *Haematologica* **95:** 557–566.
31. Hoffbrand, A.V., A. Cohen & C. Hershko. 2003. Role of deferiprone in chelation therapy for transfusional iron overload. *Blood* **102:** 17–24.
32. Hershko, C., G. Link, A. Konijn & Z.I. Cabantchik. 2005. Objectives and mechanism of iron chelation therapy. *Ann. N. Y. Acad. Sci.* **1054:** 124–135.
33. Wonke, B., C. Wright & A.V. Hoffbrand. 1998. Combined therapy with deferiprone and desferrioxamine. *Br. J. Haematol.* **103:** 361–364.
34. Tanner, M.A., R. Galanello, C. Dessi, *et al.* 2007. A randomized, placebo-controlled, double-blind trial of the effect of combined therapy with deferoxamine and deferiprone on myocardial iron in thalassemia major using cardiovascular magnetic resonance. *Circulation* **115:** 1876–1884.
35. Origa, R., P. Bina, A. Agus, *et al.* 2005. Combined therapy with deferiprone and desferrioxamine in thalassemia major. *Haematologica* **90:** 1309–1314.
36. Telfer, P., P.G. Coen, S. Christou, *et al.* 2006. Survival of medically treated thalassemia patients in Cyprus. Trends and risk factors over the period 1980–2004. *Haematologica* **91:** 1187–1192.
37. Maggio, A., A. Vitrano, M. Capra, *et al.* 2009. Long-term sequential deferiprone-deferoxamine versus deferiprone alone for thalassaemia major patients: a randomized clinical trial. *Br. J. Haematol.* **145:** 245–254.
38. Taher, A., A. El-Beshlawy, M.S. Elalfy, *et al.* 2009. Efficacy and safety of deferasirox, an oral iron chelator, in heavily iron-overloaded patients with beta-thalassaemia: the ESCALATOR study. *Eur. J. Haematol.* **82:** 458–465.
39. Daar, S., A. Pathare, H. Nick, *et al.* 2009. Reduction in labile plasma iron during treatment with deferasirox, a once-daily oral iron chelator, in heavily iron-overloaded patients with beta-thalassaemia. *Eur. J. Haematol.* **82:** 454–457.
40. Zanninelli, G., W. Breuer & Z.I. Cabantchik. 2009. Daily labile plasma iron as an indicator of chelator activity in Thalassaemia major patients. *Br. J. Haematol.* **147:** 744–751.

Ann. N.Y. Acad. Sci. ISSN 0077-8923

ANNALS OF THE NEW YORK ACADEMY OF SCIENCES
Issue: *Cooley's Anemia: Ninth Symposium*

The role of antioxidants and iron chelators in the treatment of oxidative stress in thalassemia

Eitan Fibach[1] and Eliezer A. Rachmilewitz[2]

[1]Department of Hematology, Hadassah-Hebrew University Medical Center, Ein-Kerem, Jerusalem, Israel. [2]Department of Hematology, The Edith Wolfson Medical Center, Holon, Israel

Address for correspondence: Professor E. Fibach, Department of Hematology, Hadassah-Hebrew University Medical Center, Jerusalem 91120, Israel. Fibach@yahoo.com

On the basis of all the presented data, one can conclude that oxidative stress plays a major role in the pathophysiology of thalassemia and other congenital and acquired hemolytic anemias. Free extracellular (labile plasma iron, LPI) and intracellular (labile iron pool, LIP) iron species that have been identified in thalassemic blood cells are responsible for generation of oxidative stress by catalyzing formation of oxygen radicals over the antioxidant capacity of the cell. Consequently, there is a rationale for iron chelation to eliminate the free-iron species, which in this respect, act like antioxidants. In addition, antioxidants such as vitamin E and polyphenols are also capable of ameliorating increased oxidative stress parameters and, given together with iron chelators, may provide a substantial improvement in the pathophysiology of hemolytic anemias and particularly in thalassemia.

Keywords: thalassemia; oxidative stress; antioxidants; iron overload, iron chelators

Introduction

The primary etiology of thalassemia is mutations in the globin genes, resulting in absence or reduced production of one of the globin polypeptides.[1] The remaining subunit is unstable, transforms to hemichrome with the final outcome of dissociation of heme from globin and iron from heme.[2] The cellular damage is mainly mediated by the state of oxidative stress and the effect of free oxygen radicals on various cell components. Oxidative stress was documented in various types of thalassemia as well as in other hereditary and acquired hemolytic anemias.[3] The main cause of oxidative stress in thalassemia is iron overload, which results from increased iron absorption in the gastrointestinal tract and multiple blood transfusions as well as from intracellular denaturation of hemoglobin (Hb) subunits and eventual release of iron from heme.[2] When the access incoming iron surpasses the binding potential of transferrin, it accumulates as a nontrasferrin bound iron (NTBI) and its redox-active active form labile plasma iron (LPI) in the plasma and as labile iron pool (LIP) in the cells.[4] The free-iron species participate in chemical reactions that generate oxygen radicals that affect various cell components, particularly the cell membrane, damaging vital organs (heart, liver, and the endocrine system) as well as the hematopoietic system where the final outcome is hemolysis and ineffective erythropoiesis. The former is due to short survival of mature red blood cells (RBCs) as a result of enhanced susceptibility to undergo extravascular phagocytosis by macrophages in the spleen and the marrow. The latter is due to enhanced apoptosis of developing erythroid precursors in the bone marrow and extramedullary sites, with the end result of severe chronic anemia. The use of iron chelators and antioxidants, either separately or in combination, is therefore of significant importance for treatment of thalassemia and other diseases associated with iron overload and oxidative stress.

Oxidative status in thalassemia

The oxidative status of cells is determined by the balance between pro-oxidants and antioxidants. The pro-oxidants, referred to as reactive oxygen species (ROS), are classified into radicals and nonradicals.

doi: 10.1111/j.1749-6632.2010.05577.x

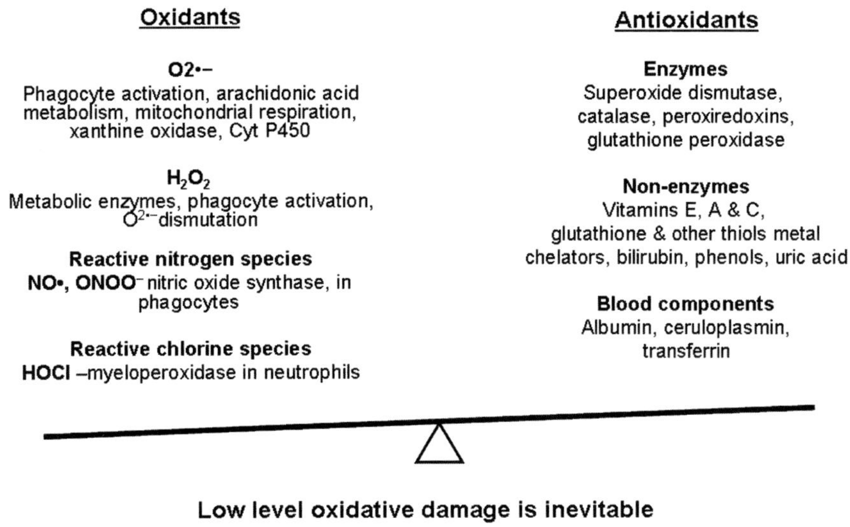

Figure 1. The oxidant/antioxidant balance.

Radicals are defined as molecules or molecular fragments containing at least one unpaired electron in the shells around the nucleus [depicted as a superscripted dot ($R^{\bullet}$)]. The presence of unpaired electrons usually confers a considerable degree of reactivity upon a free radical.[5] Radicals in biological systems include superoxide ion radical ($O_2^{\bullet -}$), hydroxyl radical ($OH^{\bullet}$), peroxyl ($ROO^{\bullet}$), alkoxyl radicals ($RO^{\bullet}$) and a single oxygen ($^1O_2$). The non-radical ROS include the hypochlorous acid (HClO), hydrogen peroxide (H_2O_2), organic peroxides, aldehydes, ozone (O_3), and O_2.

The generation of ROS occurs in most cells mainly during energy production. Approximately 2% of the total mitochondrial O_2 consumption results in $O_2^{\cdot -}$ production.[3] Although $O_2^{\bullet -}$ is not particularly reactive, it can act as a reductant toward divalent metal ions, and can react with itself by spontaneous or enzymatic (e.g., superoxide dismutase, SOD) dismutation to form H_2O_2. The latter is a mild oxidant, but in the presence of divalent metals (e.g., iron) it can generate the reactive hydroxyl radical. In addition to mitochondrial production, ROS are generated by enzymatic reactions; for example, NADPH oxidases produce ROS by reduction of O_2 to O_2^- that is rapidly converted to H_2O_2 (Fig. 1).

The ROS radicals react immediately with other molecules in their vicinity and therefore are short-lived. The toxicity of ROS depends on their reactivity and lifespan. Longer lifespan permits them to diffuse, interact with sensitive biological substrates and cause damage to various organelles. Thus, the highly reactive, but short-lived, $OH^{\bullet}$ damages only targets adjacent to its site of production.

Labile or "free" iron can convert relatively stable oxidants into powerful radicals. Iron concealed in proteins, as in catalytic sites of enzymes or stored in ferritin, is not exposed to oxygen radicals and cannot participate in this chemistry. At physiological pH, most of the iron is bound to biological chelates in its oxidized form, Fe^{+3}. In order to take part in the generation of $OH^{\bullet}$ (Haber–Weiss reaction), the iron must undergo reduction into its reduced form, Fe^{+2}, by superoxide radicals (Fenton reaction). Fe^{+2} can interact with H_2O_2, produced from the spontaneous or enzymatic dismutation of superoxide radicals, to yield $OH^{\bullet}$. The final result of these two reactions is the production of hydroxyl radicals:

$$Fe^{3+} + {}^{\bullet}O_2^- \rightarrow Fe^{2+} + O_2$$

$$Fe^{2+} + H_2O_2 \rightarrow Fe^{3+} + OH^- + {}^{\bullet}OH \text{ (Fenton reaction)}$$

$$\text{Net reaction: } {}^{\bullet}O_2^- + H_2O_2 \rightarrow {}^{\bullet}OH + HO^- + O_2$$

Free radicals can interact and damage various cellular components, including DNA, proteins, and lipids. Peroxidation of membrane lipids represents a primary consequence of cellular oxidative stress. Lipid peroxidation refers to the addition of oxygen to unsaturated fatty acids to form organic hydroperoxides (ROOH). Organic $ROO^{\bullet}$ and O_2-dependent peroxidation of lipids occurs during the initiation of the radicals that can also produce alkoxyl radicals (RO•) in metal-catalyzed reactions. The oxidation of phospholipids in the plasma membrane and internal organelle membranes such as the mitochondria interferes with their function. Moreover, lipid peroxidation yields additional reactive species, (e.g., 4-hydroxynonenal and malonaldehyde), which may contribute to toxicity.[6]

To protect against the deleterious effects of ROS, cells maintain an effective antioxidant system consisting of water- or lipid-soluble antioxidants and enzymes that remove ROS by metabolic conversion.[7] The major cellular antioxidant is the reduced thiol glutathione (GSH), which maintains sulfhydryl buffering capacity. The mitochondrial, cytoplasmic, and extracellular superoxide dismutases (SODs) catalyze the conversion of O_2^- to H_2O_2, which in turn is converted to water and O_2 by catalase. Glutathione peroxidases degrade organic peroxides at the expense of GSH. The GSH/GSH reductase and thioredoxin/thioredoxin reductase systems regenerate cellular GSH or reduced thioredoxin, respectively, at the expense of nicotinamide adenine dinucleotide phosphate (NADPH).[7] In addition, secondary antioxidant repair defenses remove or replace oxidative modified molecules. These include proteases that degrade oxidative-modified proteins as well as DNA repair or lipid repair enzymes.[3]

Antioxidants are defined on the basis of their capacity to prevent the pro-oxidation processes of ROS and their damage. A host of plant-derived flavonoid and polyphenolic compounds constitutes a dietary source of antioxidants. Among these include water-soluble (e.g., ascorbate) or lipid-phase antioxidants (e.g., vitamin E).[3]

Iron overload in thalassemia

Iron overload in thalassemia results from enhanced absorption of iron from the gastrointestinal track[8] and from multiple blood transfusions. Iron absorption is regulated by hepcidin. Following its production in the liver,[9] hepcidin is secreted into the circulation[10] and binds to ferroprotein, an iron exporter on the surface of absorptive enterocytes, as well as macrophages, hepatocytes, and placenta cells. This binding induces ferroprotein to be internalized and degraded; decreasing consequently the export of iron from these cells.[11] Hepcidin production is regulated by the iron status; normally, iron loading increases its expression[12] resulting in reduced intestinal iron absorption.

In thalassemia, however, in spite the state of iron overload, hepcidin levels are low. Thus, in a mouse model that mimics human β-thalassemia, hepcidin mRNA levels were lower in the livers of homozygous mice than in heterozygous mice and both had lower levels when compared to normal mice.[13] The low levels of hepcidin in thalassemia could be explained by the enhanced erythropoietic activity, which increases the demand for iron. In fact, under conditions of hemolysis, bleeding, hypoxia, and administration of erythropoietin, the expression of hepcidin in mice livers was decreased.[14] This may be mediated by overexpression of the growth differentiation factor 15, a member of the transforming growth factor-beta superfamily, which arises from an expanded erythroid compartment and contributes to iron overload in thalassemia by inhibiting hepcidin expression.[15]

To check whether suppression of hepcidin expression was caused by a serum factor, the influence of human thalassemic sera on hepcidin expression by a human hepatic cell line HepG2 was tested. The results showed that hepcidin expression was markedly decreased in the presence of thalassemic sera compared with sera from healthy individuals. In contrast, in sera from patients with hemochromatosis with iron overload, as expected, increased hepcidin expression was found in the hepatic cells.[16]

Most of the iron in the plasma is bound to transferrin that serves as a carrier protein that mediates the uptake of iron by cells through their surface transferrin receptors. However, in pathological conditions associated with iron overload, when the plasma iron levels exceed the binding capacity of trasferrin, it accumulates as NTBI. A fraction of NTBI is the LPI that can be engaged in redox recycling. This chemically ill-defined iron form can be taken up by cells, including mature RBCs and developing erythroid precursors (Prus and Fibach, manuscript submitted) via several pathways and be responsible in part for the major intracellular pathological consequences of iron overload (Fig. 2).

In erythroid cells, while most of the iron is in the form of Hb, some iron is in the form of redox-active labile iron. We have previously reported that in thalassemia the LIP is increased in mature RBCs and in erythroid precursors.[17] This may be the results of

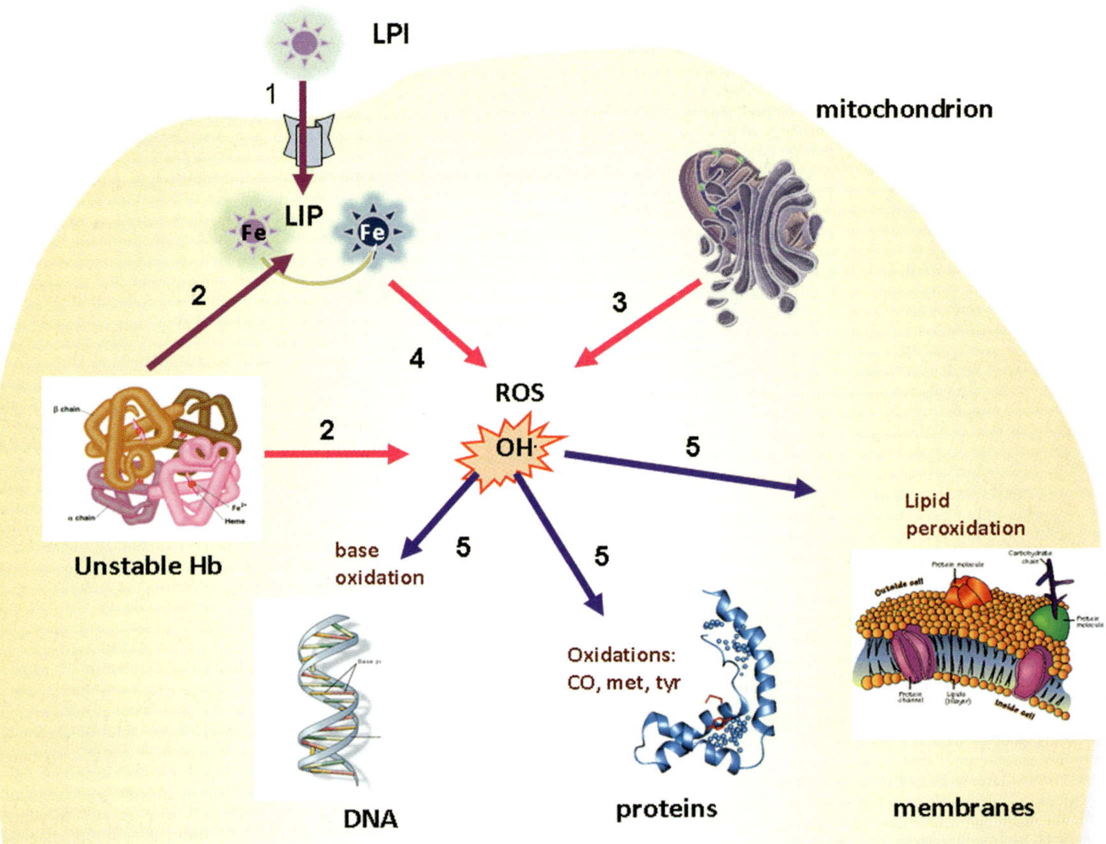

Figure 2. The role of free-iron species in generation of oxidative stress and cell damage in thalassemia. (1) The labile plasma iron (LPI), present in blood of iron overloaded thalassemic patients, enters into cells and accumulates as the labile iron pool (LIP). (2) Unstable Hb contributes to LIP accumulation and reactive oxygen species (ROS) generation in erythroid cells. (3) Normally, most cellular ROS is generated during energy production in the mitochondria, but (4) in thalassemia, the increased LIP accelerates ROS generation. (5) ROS, and particularly the highly reactive OH$^{\bullet}$ radicals, modify cellular DNA, proteins, and lipids.

abnormal iron turnover in the developing precursors owing to increased uptake of iron from iron-overloaded plasma, diminished utilization because of reduced Hb production, and owing to degradation of unstable Hb subunits. In addition, mature RBCs may take up LPI from the plasma and include iron in their LIP (Prus and Fibach, manuscript submitted). The increased LIP in these cells causes generation of access ROS that overwhelms their antioxidant capacity, leading to oxidative stress and consequently to damage of several cell components.

In thalassemia as well as in other hereditary and acquired anemias, the outcome is ineffective erythropoiesis because of enhanced apoptosis of erythroid precursors and short lifespan of mature RBCs. Changes in the cell membranes are responsible for both effects. For example, oxidative stress induces externalization of phosphatidylserine (PS) on the surface of erythroid cells causing their accelerated phagocytosis by macrophages.[18] Oxidative stress-mediated enhanced externalization of PS occurs also in platelets. Since PS is a procoagulant factor, its enhanced exposure on RBCs and platelets may be responsible for the high incidence of thromboembolic complications in thalassemic patients, particularly in β-thalassemia intermedia.[19]

Flow cytometry measurements of LIP and oxidative stress

In order to study the LIP and oxidative stress parameters in blood cells of thalassemic patients, we have adapted flow cytometry methodology.[20,21] This methodology provides several advantages: (1) It is a widely available technology in hematology laboratories and is used for various diagnostic applications. (2) Only fluorescence associated with cells is measured, but not soluble or particulate fluorescence. (3) Single cells are measured. (4) Various subpopulations can be identified (based on size, granularity, and expression of surface antigens) and measured simultaneously. (5) Since a large number of cells are analyzed, the results are statistically sound even for relatively small (<1%) subpopulations. (6) The mean value of each subpopulation is calculated simultaneously and separately; thus avoiding the bias inherent in biochemical methods that produce mean values of the entire population or requires isolation of the studied population. This is especially valid when a mixed population (e.g., blood cells) is studied. (7) The procedure can be automated to allow "high-throughput analysis," for example, for screening of antioxidants in large libraries of pure compounds or plant extracts. Although the flow data are expressed in arbitrary fluorescence units rather than weight or molar concentrations, they are useful for comparative purposes.

The methodology is based on measuring changes in cell fluorescence following loading with various markers. ROS generation and LIP content can be measured by loading cells with 2′-7-dichlorofluorescin diacetate and calcein acetomethoxy l ester, respectively. Both lipophilic compounds readily diffuse across the cell membrane and become deacetylated by intracellular esterases into polar derivatives (dichlorofluorescin and calcein, respectively) that are trapped inside the cells. When oxidized by ROS, a green fluorescent product, dichlorofluorescein, is produced.[22] The intensity of the fluorescence is proportional to the cellular concentration of ROS. Calcein is highly fluorescent, but its fluorescence is stochiometrically quenched by LIP and can be recovered by a cell-permeable iron chelator, such as salicylaldehyde isonicotinoyl hydrazone or deferiprone (DFP), which binds and removes iron from its complex with calcein. The increased calcein-fluorescence after treatment with the chelator measures the intracellular LIP.

Oxidative stress parameters that can be studied by flow cytometry include measurements of the intracellular content of the antioxidant GSH using mercury orange,[20] membrane lipid peroxidation by staining with fluor-DHPE,[20] and externalization of PS moieties, a marker of lipid membrane damage, by fluorochrome-conjugated annexin-V.[23]

This methodology enables the study of the effects of antioxidants and iron chelators both *in vivo* and *in vitro*. Since blood cells circulate throughout the body and they are readily accessible for analysis, they may represent the states of oxidative stress and iron overload in other cells and tissues.

Iron chelation and antioxidant treatments

The fact that iron plays a major role in the pathophysiology of thalassemia mainly through generation of oxidative stress suggests the potential of iron chelators and antioxidants separately or in combination for treatment.

Iron chelation. Three iron chelators are currently in clinical use for treatment of thalassemia. The most widely used chelator is deferoxiamine (DFO) that was demonstrated to significantly reduce the morbidity and mortality of these patients by preventing or reducing the damage to key organs such as the heart, liver, and endocrine glands. Although the side effects are minimal, the major disadvantage of DFO is its mode of administration that is either parenteral or through a portable infusion pump on a daily basis. Consequently, two oral chelators have been developed—DFP and deferasirox (DFR); their application improved compliance and quality of life.[24] Moreover, DFP is capable of mobilizing iron from tissues into the circulation where it binds to DFO and is excreted in the kidneys. This combination of chelators, known as the "shuttle hypothesis," was also able to remove LIP and to decrease LPI. By removing intra- and extracellular-iron species that generate free oxygen radicals, iron chelators act as antioxidants.[25] In fact, the antioxidant effect of treatment with DFR was demonstrated in multitransfused patients with myelodysplastic syndrome where amelioration of oxidative stress parameters was achieved after three months.[26]

Antioxidants

Vitamin E. In thalassemia and sickle cell disease, as well as other hemolytic anemias, hydrophilic and hydrophobic antioxidants are depleted because of the increased need to neutralize the oxidative stress.[27] With the exception of a compensatory increase in glutathione peroxidase activity found in thalassemia, all other parameters reviewed were significantly depressed. Since vitamin E is frequently deficient in homozygous β-thalassemia patients,[28] its supplementation was studied extensively. The results showed that in heterozygotes pateints, high dose of oral vitamin E decreased lipid peroxidation in RBCs and increased their survival.[29] Other studies showed improvement in the plasma antioxidant/oxidant balance, in the oxidation of low-density lipoproteins[30] and in the impaired osmotic fragility of RBCs.[31] Parenteral administration of vitamin E was more effective than oral administration.[32] Most of these studies, however, did not show a significant improvement in clinical parameters, that is, Hb concentration and transfusion requirement.

Curcumin. Curcumin, a natural herb used as food additive, contains polyphenol compounds. An extract derived from dried rhizomes of curcumin was given to patients with β-thalassemia/HbE disease on the basis that the β-diketone group and the hydroxyl/methoxy groups on phenyl rings are inducing antioxidant and iron chelating properties.[33] It showed a decrease in iron-catalysed lipid peroxidation *in vitro*.[34] The results in patients treated with curcumin for one year demonstrated a significant decrease in oxidative parameters concomitant with a decrease in methemoglobin and NTBI. These changes lasted as long as curcumin was administered. However, there were no changes in Hb levels throughout the period of treatment.[35]

Fermented papaya preparation

FPP, a natural health food product obtained by biofermentation of *Carica papaya*, has been shown to limit oxidative stress both *in vivo* and *in vitro*.[36] Administration of FPP to patients with β-thalassemia major and intermedia and to patients with β-thalassemia/HbE disease for 3 months yielded decrease in ROS generation, in membrane lipid peroxidation, and in externalization of PS residues concomitant with an increase in GSH. However, there were no changes in hematological parameters such as RBCs and Hb.[37]

The conclusion from these studies is that although all the antioxidants were able to ameliorate significantly parameters of oxidative stress in patients with thalassemia major, intermedia, and β-thalassemia/HbE disease, they were not capable of inducing changes in hematological parameters. Since the turnover of the erythron takes more than 100 days, it is possible that longer duration of this kind of treatment is required to obtain an increase in the number of RBCs and the Hb levels. Taken together, one must also bear in mind that the amount of ROS is a key issue, since they are essential for cell functioning,[38] such as gene transcription,[39] signal transduction, and cell proliferation. Therefore, antioxidant therapy should be designed carefully, considering the high reactivity of ROS, their short lifespan, their continuous production in close proximity to biological targets, and their ability to be modified into more reactive species. Their ability to selectively affect cell components, such as lipids and proteins, as well as the relationship between iron forms with redox potential and oxidative stress suggest that the use of a combination of different antioxidants and iron chelators might yield better results.

Conflicts of interest

The authors declare no conflicts of interest.

References

1. Gu, X. & Y. Zeng. 2002. A review of the molecular diagnosis of thalassemia. *Hematology* **7:** 203–209.
2. Rund, D. & E. Rachmilewitz. 2005. Beta-thalassemia. *N Engl. J. Med.* **353:** 1135–1146.
3. Fibach, E. & E. Rachmilewitz. 2008. The role of oxidative stress in hemolytic anemia. *Curr. Mol. Med.* **8:** 609–619.
4. Rachmilewitz, E.A., O. Weizer-Stern, K. Adamsky, *et al.* 2005. Role of iron in inducing oxidative stress in thalassemia: Can it be prevented by inhibition of absorption and by antioxidants? *Ann. N.Y. Acad. Sci.* **1054:** 118–123.
5. Halliwell, B. & J. Gutteridge. 1999. *Free Radicals in Biology and Medicine* (3rd ed.). Oxford University Press. Midsomer Norton, Avon, England.
6. Awasthi, Y.C., Y. Yang, N.K. Tiwari, *et al.* 2004. Regulation of 4-hydroxynonenal-mediated signaling by glutathione S-transferases. *Free Radic. Biol. Med.* **37:** 607–619.
7. Jones, D.P., J.L. Carlson, V.C. Mody, *et al.* 2000. Redox state of glutathione in human plasma. *Free Radic. Biol. Med.* **28:** 625–635.
8. Kushner, J.P., J.P. Porter & N.F. Olivieri. 2001. Secondary iron overload. *Hematol. Am. Soc. Hematol. Educ. Program.* 47–61.
9. Park, C.H., E.V. Valore, A.J. Waring & T. Ganz. 2001. Hepcidin, a urinary antimicrobial peptide synthesized in the liver. *J. Biol. Chem.* **276:** 7806–7810.
10. Ganz, T. 2003. Hepcidin, a key regulator of iron metabolism and mediator of anemia of inflammation. *Blood* **102:** 783–788.
11. Nemeth, E., M.S. Tuttle, J. Powelson, *et al.* 2004. Hepcidin regulates cellular iron efflux by binding to ferroportin and inducing its internalization. *Science* **306:** 2090–2093.
12. Pigeon, C., G. Ilyin, B. Courselaud, *et al.* 2001. A new mouse liver-specific gene, encoding a protein homologous to

human antimicrobial peptide hepcidin, is overexpressed during iron overload. *J. Biol. Chem.* **276:** 7811–7819.

13. Adamsky, K., O. Weizer, N. Amariglio, *et al.* 2004. Decreased hepcidin mRNA expression in thalassemic mice. *Br. J. Haematol.* **124:** 123–124.
14. Nicolas, G., L. Viatte, M. Bennoun, *et al.* 2002. Hepcidin, a new iron regulatory peptide. *Blood Cells Mol. Dis.* **29:** 327–335.
15. Tanno, T., N.V. Bhanu, P.A. Oneal, *et al.* 2007. High levels of GDF15 in thalassemia suppress expression of the iron regulatory protein hepcidin. *Nat. Med.* **13:** 1096–1101.
16. Weizer-Stern, O., K. Adamsky, N. Amariglio, *et al.* 2006. Downregulation of hepcidin and haemojuvelin expression in the hepatocyte cell-line HepG2 induced by thalassaemic sera. *Br. J. Haematol.* **135:** 129–138.
17. Prus, E. & E. Fibach. 2008. The labile iron pool in human erythroid cells. *Br. J. Haematol.* **142:** 301–307.
18. Freikman, I., J. Amer, J.S. Cohen, *et al.* 2008. Oxidative stress causes membrane phospholipid rearrangement and shedding from RBC membranes–an NMR study. *Biochim. Biophys. Acta.* **1778:** 2388–2394.
19. Taher, A., H. Isma'eel, G. Mehio, *et al.* 2006. Prevalence of thromboembolic events among 8,860 patients with thalassaemia major and intermedia in the Mediterranean area and Iran. *Thromb. Haemost.* **96:** 488–491.
20. Amer, J., A. Goldfarb & E. Fibach. 2004. Flow cytometric analysis of the oxidative status of normal and thalassemic red blood cells. *Cytometry* **60:** 73–80.
21. Prus, E. & E. Fibach. 2008. Flow cytometry measurement of the labile iron pool in human hematopoietic cells. *Cytometry A.* **73:** 22–27.
22. Keston, A.S. & R. Brandt. 1965. The fluorometric analysis of ultramicro quantities of hydrogen peroxide. *Anal. Biochem.* **11:** 1–5.
23. Freikman, I., J. Amer, I. Ringel & E. Fibach. 2009. A flow cytometry approach for quantitative analysis of cellular phosphatidylserine distribution and shedding. *Anal. Biochem.* **393:** 111–116.
24. Odame & D. Rund. 2008. Evidence-based treatment of Thalassemia Major. In *Evidence-Bases Hematology*. A. Mark, J.G. Crowther, J. Ginsberg, H.J. Schunemann, R.M. Meyer & R. Lottenberg, Eds. Blackwell Publishing. Hoboken, New Jersey.
25. Prus, E. & E. Fibach. 2009. Effect of iron chelators on labile iron and oxidative status of thalassaemic erythroid cells. *Acta Haematol.* **123:** 14–20.
26. Ghoti, H., E. Fibach, D. Merkel, *et al.* 2010. Changes in parameters of oxidative stress and free iron biomarkers during treatment with deferasirox in iron-overloaded patients with myelodysplastic syndromes. *Haematologica.* In press. doi:10.3324/haematol.2010.024992.
27. Chan, A.C., C.K. Chow & D. Chiu. 1999. Interaction of antioxidants and their implication in genetic anemia. *Proc. Soc. Exp. Biol. Med.* **222:** 274–282.
28. Modell, B., M. Khan & M. Darlison. 2000. Survival in beta-thalassaemia major in the UK: data from the UK Thalassaemia Register. *Lancet* **355:** 2051–2052.
29. Miniero, R., E. Canducci, D. Ghigo, *et al.* 1982. Vitamin E in beta-thalassemia. *Acta Vitaminol. Enzymol.* **4:** 21–25.
30. Tesoriere, L., D. D'Arpa, D. Butera, *et al.* 2001. Oral supplements of vitamin E improve measures of oxidative stress in plasma and reduce oxidative damage to LDL and erythrocytes in beta-thalassemia intermedia patients. *Free Radic. Res.* **34:** 529–540.
31. Kahane, I. & E.A. Rachmilewitz. 1976. Alterations in the red blood cell membrane and the effect of vitamin E on osmotic fragility in beta-thalassemia major. *Isr. J. Med. Sci.* **12:** 11–15.
32. Giardini, O., A. Cantani, A. Donfrancesco, *et al.* 1985. Biochemical and clinical effects of vitamin E administration in homozygous beta-thalassemia. *Acta Vitaminol. Enzymol.* **7:** 55–60.
33. Kalpravidh, R., N. Siritanaratkul, P. Insain, *et al.* 2010. Improvement in oxidative stress and antioxidant parameters in beta-thalassemia/Hb E patients treated with curcuminoid. *Clin. Biochem.* **43:** 423–429.
34. Grinberg, L., O. Shalev, H. Tonnesen & E. Rachmilewitz. 1996. Studies on curcumin and curcuminoids: XXVI. Antioxidant effects of curcumin on the red blood cell membrane. *Int. J. Pharmaceutics* **132:** 251–257.
35. Srichairatanakool, S., C. Thephinlap, C. Phisalaphong, *et al.* 2007. Curcumin contributes to in vitro removal of non-transferrin bound iron by deferiprone and desferrioxamine in thalassemic plasma. *Med. Chem.* **3:** 469–474.
36. Amer, J., A. Goldfarb, E.A. Rachmilewitz & E. Fibach. 2008. Fermented papaya preparation as redox regulator in blood cells of beta-thalassemic mice and patients. *Phytother. Res.* **22:** 820–828.
37. Fibach, E., E. Tan, S. Jamuar, *et al.* 2010. Amelioration of oxidative stress in RBC from patients with beta thalassemia major and intermedia and E-beta thalassemia following administration of fermented papaya preparation. *Phytotherapy Res.* In press. doi: 10.1002/ptr.3116.
38. Droge, W. 2002. Free radicals in the physiological control of cell function. *Physiol. Rev.* **82:** 47–95.
39. Engelhardt, J.F. 1999. Redox-mediated gene therapies for environmental injury: approaches and concepts. *Antioxid. Redox Signal.* **1:** 5–27.

Ann. N.Y. Acad. Sci. ISSN 0077-8923

ANNALS OF THE NEW YORK ACADEMY OF SCIENCES
Issue: *Cooley's Anemia: Ninth Symposium*

Thalassemia as a global health problem: recent progress toward its control in the developing countries

D.J. Weatherall

Weatherall Institute of Molecular Medicine, University of Oxford, John Radcliffe Hospital, Headington, Oxford, United Kingdom.

Addresses for correspondence: D.J. Weatherall, Weatherall Institute of Molecular Medicine, University of Oxford, John Radcliffe Hospital, Headington, Oxford, OX3 9DS, UK. liz.rose@imm.ox.ac.uk

The thalassemias, together with sickle cell anemia and its variants, are by far the most common monogenic diseases. They occur at their highest frequency in countries of the developing world where their control and management is hampered by a lack of knowledge of their true prevalence, adequate services for their management and control, and support by their governments and international health agencies. However, there has been some progress recently in addressing these problems and there are several ways in which the lot of children with thalassemia in poor countries could be improved in the future. Over the last 20 years there has been considerable improvement in the control and management of the thalassemias in the richer countries of the world. Unfortunately, however, this is not the case for many of the developing countries, where there have been few improvements in the control of the numbers of births of babies with thalassemia or in the care of thalassemic children since the frequency of the problem started to become evident in the 1960s. Here, I will try to assess the current situation in these countries and examine some of the potential approaches for improving the current situation.

Keywords: thalassemia; population control; malaria; genetic modifiers; adaptation; prevention; management

Why are the hemoglobin disorders so common and why is their frequency likely to increase?

There is now extensive evidence that the unusually high frequency of the hemoglobin disorders compared with other monogenic diseases reflects natural selection due to the relative resistance of carriers against *P. falciparum* malaria.[1] It has also become apparent recently that the unequal distribution of these conditions both within and between different countries reflects complex epistatic interactions between the genes for carriers for different varieties of these diseases with respect to the relative resistance of carriers to malaria.[2,3] Other factors that help maintain the gene frequency for these conditions at a high level include the widespread practice of consanguineous marriage, which may be practiced by up to 25% of the world's population, increased maternal age and gene drift and founder effects.

Even if malaria transmission is significantly reduced it will take many generations to have a significant effect on the carrier rates for these diseases. Meanwhile, many of the poorer countries of the world are going through an epidemiological transition reflecting improvements in hygiene, nutrition, public health care, and other factors which are combining to reduce both neonatal and childhood mortality rates. It follows therefore that babies with severe forms of thalassemia who previously would have died undiagnosed early in life, are now surviving to present for diagnosis and treatment. Hence the global burden of disease caused by the thalassemias and related diseases is likely to increase, a phenomena that has already been observed in some countries.[4]

The extent of the problem

If any progress is to be made toward bringing the attention of governments and international health agencies to the increasing problem of thalassemia

doi: 10.1111/j.1749-6632.2010.05546.x

in the developing world it will be essential to be able to provide at least an approximate outline of the true extent of the problem. In a recent study it was estimated that over seven million babies are born with either a congenital abnormality or genetic disease every year, and that up to 90% of these births occur in low or middle income countries.[5] Of these conditions, approximately 25% are made up of five disorders, two of which, the inherited disorders of hemoglobin and glucose-6-phosphate dehydrogenase deficiency, are monogenic diseases. It is estimated that in excess of 300,000 children are born each year with either thalassemia or sickle cell anemia.

A breakdown of the raw data used to produce these figures for the births of hemoglobin disorders[6] is shown in Table 1. One of the most striking and possibly unexpected features of these data are the finding that the serious forms of β-thalassemia are almost equally divided between β-thalassemia major and HbE β-thalassemia. This reflects the extremely high frequency of the latter disorder in parts of India, Bangladesh, Burma, and throughout Southeast Asia. The symptomatic forms of α-thalassemia, HbH disease, and Hb Bart's hydrops fetalis are also mainly confined to Southeast Asia.

The results of these recent surveys must be reviewed with caution however. Unfortunately, because large scale population surveys of the hemoglobin variants were carried out mainly before the 1980s,[7] and often were only based on relatively small samples from limited numbers of centers in individual countries, they can only be taken as a rough approximation of the true global load of the thalassemias. More recent micro-mapping, that is studies which have achieved adequate sample-size estimates from many different parts of an individual country, have shown that there is a remarkable heterogeneity in the distribution of these conditions within populations separated by only short geographical distances.[8,9] To provide a better estimate of the global burden of the hemoglobin disorders it will be necessary to carry out micro-mapping of many of the high frequency regions in the future. Such data that are available suggest that, if anything, the current global frequency of the thalassemias may be an underestimate.

Table 1. **A breakdown of the annual number of births with the different hemoglobin disorders from available data[7]**

Annual births with major hemoglobin disorders	
β-thalassemia major	22,989
HbE β-thalassemia	19,128
HbH disease	9,568
Hb Bart's hydrops (α°/α°)	5,183
SS disease	217,331
S β-thalassemia	11,074
SC disease	54,736

Requirement for a better understanding of the mechanisms for the heterogeneity of common Asian forms of thalassemia

The findings in Table 1 are of considerable importance with respect to the future of global control of thalassemia. The fact that β-thalassemia major is much more common in Europe and the Middle East which, in World Health Organization (WHO) classifications also includes Pakistan, and that by far the commonest forms of thalassemia in Asia are those like HbE β-thalassemia with remarkably variable phenotypes, has important implications for future planning for the control and management of the thalassemias. Throughout the USA, Europe, and many parts of the Middle East effective prenatal screening and diagnosis programs have been established and conditions for treatment of children born with thalassemia major have improved enormously. On the other hand, this is not the case in many Asian countries. Given the considerable phenotypic differences between the severe forms of thalassemia in these countries and the forms of β-thalassemia major in the rest of the world, it cannot be assumed that the approaches to control and management that have been successful in the latter are necessarily those that are appropriate to the control of thalassemia in Asia.

The clinical diversity of HbE β-thalassemia and HbH disease

The clinical phenotype of HbE β-thalassemia varies from a condition indistinguishable from thalassemia major to a disorder that is compatible with survival into adult life with minimal treatment.[10] At least some progress has been made toward an understanding of the genetic, adaptive, and environmental factors that underlie this heterogeneity. Because most of the β-thalassemia alleles that are common in Asian countries are of the severe variety, phenotypic modification due to the co-inheritance of a mild β allele with HbE is relatively uncommon in Asia.[10] However, in most Asian countries there is a relatively high frequency of one or other of the deletion forms of α^+-thalassemia and there is now extensive evidence that their co-inheritance with HbE β-thalassemia has a marked effect on reducing the severity of the resulting phenotype.[11,12] Similarly, in countries where the α genes have been analyzed in detail it is clear that up to 2–3% of their populations carry increased numbers of α gene loci, with three, four, or even more α genes per haploid genome.[13] These α globin gene arrangements, when inherited with HbE β-thalassemia, are associated with severe genotypes. There is also good evidence that those patients with HbE β-thalassemia who produce unusually high levels of HbF also tend to have a milder disease.[13]

There is also growing evidence that the frequency of the complications of HbE β-thalassemia may be modified by genetic factors. For example, the very high frequency of gallstones and profound jaundice that is observed in countries like Sri Lanka and probably eastern parts of India and Bangladesh are related to the very high frequency of a polymorphism in the promoter region of UGTA1A, the variant that results in Gilbert's disease and which reaches an extremely high frequency in some of these populations.[14] It also seems very likely that the remarkable variability in the rate of iron absorption from the gastrointestinal tract, which in some cases causes severe iron loading in the absence of regular transfusion, has a genetic basis although so far a search for polymorphisms of the genes involved in the regulation of iron absorption have not provided a basis for the remarkable variability of iron accumulation in this disease.

A number of studies have been carried out recently regarding variability in adaptation to the severe anemia of HbE β-thalassemia. Because of the relatively low levels of HbF compared with other forms of β-thalassemia intermedia, patients with this condition are better able to right-shift their oxygen dissociation curves and therefore adapt better to anemia. And studies of erythropoietin responses have suggested that there is a decline in the rate of erythropoietin production for a given hemoglobin level with age, thus accounting at least in part for the remarkably unstable phenotypes of this condition in early life.[15]

Although environmental factors as modifiers of the course of thalassemia have been completely neglected, very recent work in Sri Lanka suggests that patients with HbE β-thalassemia may be more susceptible to malaria, particularly that due to *Plasmodium vivax*, and that those with particularly high antibodies to this condition tend to have significantly greater splenomegaly and hence a more severe phenotype.[16] Since *P. vivax* malaria is proving to be a much more serious condition than hitherto realized, and is affecting millions of children in parts of Asia,[17] this will have to be taken into account in future control programs for HbE β-thalassemia in this part of the world.

It is also clear that the clinical picture of HbH disease shows considerable heterogeneity and at least in some cases this condition requires chronic transfusion. Although there has been some progress toward an understanding of the reasons for this diverse phenotype much more work is required to assess both the genetic and potential environmental factors involved.[18]

Implications for the control and management of thalassemia in Asia

The remarkable clinical heterogeneity of the different forms of severe thalassemia in Asia raises important questions about the optimal approach to their control and management. The broad clinical diversity of these conditions also raises particularly important practical and ethical issues about the development of prenatal diagnosis programmes for their control; it is quite clear that a significant proportion of patients with HbE thalassemia can grow and develop normally without treatment. The instability of the phenotype in the first few years of life together with a proneness to infection, including malaria, leads to many young children presenting with this disorder with marked anemia. They are then started on a blood transfusion regimen which is continued without stopping it to assess the steady-state hemoglobin level and other clinical parameters. Undoubtedly this leads to many children commencing on life-long transfusion therapy which in many cases may be unnecessary, thus wasting rare resources. Because the erythropoietin response to anemia declines with age, and, in the

Table 2. Current services available for the control and management of thalassemia in Asian countries

Country	Transfusion	Iron chelation			BMT	PND	National programs
		DFO	L1	Exjade			
Bangladesh	(+)	(+)	−	−	−	−	−
Cambodia	(+)	(+)	−	−	−	−	−
China: Guangxi	+	(+)	(+)		(+)	+	−
China: Hong Kong	+	+	+	(+)	+	+	+
China: Taiwan	+	+	+	(+)	+	+	+
India	(+)	(+)	(+)	−	(+)	(+)	−
Indonesia	(+)	(+)	(+)	−	−	(+)	−
Laos	(+)	(+)	−	−	−	−	−
Malaysia	+	+	+	(+)	+	+	+
Maldives	+	+	+	−	(+)	−	+
Myanmar	(+)	(+)	−	−	−	−	−
Philippines	+	(+)	−	(+)	−	−	−
Singapore	+	+	+	(+)	+	+	+
Sri Lanka	+	+	+	−	−	−	+
Thailand	+	+	+	(+)	+	+	+
Vietnam	(+)	(+)	(+)	−	(+)	−	−

+ Denotes availability, (+) denotes services only available to those who can afford it, (−) denotes a complete lack of availability.
BMT = bone marrow transplantation; PND = prenatal diagnosis. Data collected and updated with the help of Dr. Suthat Fucharoen and the Asian Thalassaemia Network.

majority of cases the rate of splenic enlargement behaves in the same way, there may be a case for transfusion throughout the early period of phenotypic instability and then stopping transfusion followed by a period of assessment of the steady-state hemoglobin, patterns of growth and development, and other clinical parameters.

In short, a great deal more work needs to be done to try to define the reasons for the clinical heterogeneity of HbE β-thalassemia, whether this information can be used to predict the future course of the disease, and, in particular, whether it is appropriate to leave children with this condition untransfused at a relatively low hemoglobin level provided that their growth and development and quality of life is satisfactory. Currently there is very little information about the clinical status of adults treated in this way. Further work is also needed on the role of environmental factors and whether, as now seems likely, some form of malaria prophylaxis will be essential, particularly in countries with a high frequency of *P. vivax* malaria transmission.

Current services for the control and management of thalassemia in Asia

While over the last 20 years there has been slow progress toward the development of improved services for the control and management of thalassemia in the richer countries, the situation in many Asian countries, as shown in Table 2, is still bleak. There are many populations without any form of screening or prenatal diagnosis programs and in many cases blood transfusion services are limited and iron chelation therapy is only available to the relatively few who can afford it. Although national programs have been established recently in a few countries, in many their governments still do not recognize the importance of the thalassemias.

Except for a few recent studies, appropriate micro-mapping surveys for the frequency of the different forms of thalassemia in Asian countries have not been embarked on and hence it is still difficult to provide their governments with a true picture of the burden of thalassemia. In short, services for the avoidance and management of thalassemia in many

Table 3. The major objectives of the development of South/South partnerships

South/South partnerships for thalassemia control
Research
Micromapping
Heterogeneity
Pharmacogenetics
Capacity building
Training control management
National program development

Asian countries are grossly inadequate and the data that are available for providing their governments with a true indication of the total burden of the disease are still inadequate.

The concept of South/South partnerships

Over many years there have been a number of prolonged partnerships between centers with expertise in thalassemia in a few of the rich countries and those in the poorer countries where there is limited knowledge of the thalassemia. In at least some cases these so-called North/South partnerships have led to the development of considerable expertise in the control and management in the poorer countries involved. In the main, they have been supported by research agencies in the rich countries and, in addition to training appropriate staff, have involved a considerable amount of basic and clinical research. In short, they have been an extremely cost-effective way of improving the lot of patients with thalassemia in many countries.

As is clear from Table 2 there are a number of countries in Asia with genuine expertise in the control and management of thalassemia. The realization that this was the case led to the concept of the development of South/South partnerships between those countries in which there is expertise in this field with those where no such knowledge exists. The objectives of partnerships of this type are summarized in Table 3. They include several research developments including micro-mapping of the frequency of different forms of thalassemia in these countries, work directed at a better understanding of the phenotypic heterogeneity of these conditions, and studies of the pharmacogenetics of the oral chelating agents that are available or becoming available. It seems very likely that there will be individual variation in the response and side effects of these agents, particularly as both the oral agents that are currently available are metabolized through either UGTA1A or one of its isoforms. The promoter polymorphism of UGTA1A is known to be associated with variable response to a variety of drugs and it will be extremely important to determine whether there are significant numbers of patients at risk for unusually slow or rapid clearance of these drugs before determining their optimal dosage.

As well as these activities South/South partnerships must also be involved in capacity building through training clinicians, nurses, and counselors, and developing national programs through collaboration with the governments of countries where none exist. In short, the concept of the South/South partnership is simply an extension of the successful North/South partnerships that have evolved over many years and is a cost-effective approach to improving conditions for children with thalassemia in many countries where virtually no services exist.

Involving governments and international health agencies

In 2002 the WHO produced a report entitled *Genomics and World Health* in which recommendations for the further development of North/South and South/South partnerships between different countries were recommended as an approach to both the control of common diseases like the hemoglobin disorders and also as a way of introducing simple DNA diagnostics for communicable disease into the developing countries.[19] The recommendations of this report were later accepted by the WHO Executive Board. In 2006 at the 118th session of the WHO Executive Board and at the 59th World Health Assembly resolutions were passed to urge Member States to develop programs for the prevention and management of the inherited hemoglobin disorders. In 2007 a meeting was held under the auspices of the WHO and Thalassaemia International Federation (TIF) that made further recommendations for the development of international partnerships for the better control of the hemoglobin disorders[20] but since then there has been no further action in pursuing these developments. The major international funding agencies have also focused their attention almost entirely on communicable disease; non-communicable disease in general, and genetic disease in particular, continue to be ignored.

In 2007 plans were established for updating the *Global Burden of Disease, Injuries, and Risk Factors* (GBD) program, an initiative that had been developed much earlier by the WHO through the work of Murray and Lopez and which attempts to provide detailed information about the health burden of all the common diseases and to list them in order of the magnitude of burden to individual countries throughout the world.[21] For the first time it was decided to include the inherited disorders of hemoglobin in this program. Although the expert group that was elected to take on this task is making a valiant attempt to produce data of this kind it has been extremely difficult to obtain, even from the richer countries. There is a paucity of accurate frequency data, and very limited information about mortality rates from different hemoglobin disorders or the frequency of complications and their sequelae. In short, there is a severe paucity of good epidemiological or demographic data. However, this is the case for many diseases and at least a start has been made in trying to bring the attention of the international health community to the importance of thalassemia and the sickling disorders. The GBD program has, in the past, had considerable influence on both international and national priorities for healthcare. It is hoped that the inclusion of the hemoglobin disorders in the new version of the GBD league table of the relative importance of different diseases will focus the attention of the international health community on their current neglect.

Conclusions

As the poorer countries go through the epidemiological transition whereby the health of their populations improves due to better nutrition, sanitation, and public health services, many babies with thalassemia or sickle-cell disorders who would previously have died in the first year or two of life will survive long enough to come for diagnosis and treatment. It is likely therefore that the already large number of babies born with thalassemia and related disorders and the high rates of morbidity and mortality associated with them will pose an increasing global health problem unless measures are taken to develop control and management programs in many of the poorer countries of the world. Hence there is an important place for the development of sustained North/South partnerships and, in particular, for trying to persuade the international health community that support for South/South partnerships is a highly cost-effective approach to the control of the hemoglobin disorders. Their inclusion in the GBD program may be of some help in this respect. It is also vital that over the next few years micro-mapping studies are done in many parts of the world as a basis for providing more accurate information about the true burden of these diseases.

It is equally important that further research into the reasons for the clinical diversity of HbE β-thalassemia, which is the main form of severe thalassemia in many of the poorer countries, is pursued. There is already evidence that rare resources are being wasted through unnecessary treatment because of lack of knowledge about the natural history of this disease.

Even if, through developments in gene therapy or other novel approaches to their management, more definitive treatment becomes available for the thalassemias in the near future, the cost is likely to be such that it will be a long time before it becomes widely available in the parts of the world where it is most needed. In short, it is vital that the international hematology community becomes involved in the control and management of thalassemia in those parts of the world where it is being completely ignored. Unfortunately, based on their current track record we cannot rely on international health agencies to fulfill this role.

Conflicts of interest

The author declares no conflicts of interest.

References

1. Weatherall, D.J. 2008. Genetic variation and susceptibility to infection: the red cell and malaria. *Br. J. Haematol.* **141:** 276–286.
2. Williams, T.N., T.W. Mwangi, S. Wambua, *et al.* 2005. Negative epistasis between the malaria-protective effects of alpha+-thalassemia and the sickle cell trait. *Nat. Genet.* **37:** 1253–1257.
3. Penman, B.S., O.G. Pybus, D.J. Weatherall & S. Gupta. 2009. Why is the sickle cell gene uncommon in the Mediterranean? *Proc. Natl. Acad. Sci. USA* **106:** 21242–21246.
4. Weatherall, D.J. & J.B., Clegg. 2001. *The Thalassaemia Syndromes*, 4th edn. Blackwell Science. Oxford.
5. Christianson, A., C.P. Howson & B. Modell. 2006. *March of Dimes Global Report on Birth Defects.* March of Dimes Birth Defects Foundation. New York.

6. Modell, B. & M. Darlison. 2008. Global epidemiology of haemoglobin disorders and derived service indicators. *Bull. World Health Organ.* **86:** 480–487.
7. Livingstone, F.B. 1985. *Frequencies of Hemoglobin Variants.* Oxford University Press. New York, Oxford.
8. de Silva, S., C.A. Fisher, A. Premawardhena, *et al.* 2000. Thalassaemia in Sri Lanka: implications for the future health burden of Asian populations. Sri Lanka Thalassaemia Study Group. *Lancet* **355:** 786–791.
9. Colah, R., A. Gorakshakar, S. Phanasgaonkar, *et al.* 2009. Epidemiology of beta-thalassaemia in Western India: mapping the frequencies and mutations in different geographic regions. In press.
10. Olivieri, N.F., G.M. Muraca, A. O'Donnell, *et al.* 2008. Studies in haemoglobin E beta-thalassaemia. *Br. J. Haematol.* **141:** 388–397.
11. Premawardhena, A., C.A. Fisher, N.F. Olivieri, *et al.* 2005. Haemoglobin E β thalassaemia in Sri Lanka. *Lancet* **366:** 1467–1470.
12. Winichagoon, P., S. Fucharoen, D.J. Weatherall & P. Wasi. 1985. Concomitant inheritance of α-thalassemia in β-thalassemia/Hb E. *Am. J. Hematol.* **20:** 217–222.
13. Fisher, C.A., A. Premawardhena, S. de Silva, *et al.* 2003. The molecular basis for the thalassaemias in Sri Lanka. *Br. J. Haematol.* **121:** 662–671.
14. Premawardhena, A., C.A. Fisher, F. Fathiu, *et al.* 2001. The frequency of jaundice and gallstones in haemoglobin E β thalassaemia is genetically determined. *Lancet* **357:** 1945–1946.
15. O'Donnell, A., A. Premawardhena, M. Arambepola, *et al.* 2007. Age-related changes in adaptation to severe anemia in childhood in developing countries. *Proc. Natl. Acad. Sci. USA* **104:** 9440–9444.
16. O'Donnell, A., A. Premawardhena, M. Arambepola, *et al.* 2009. Interaction of malaria with a common form of severe thalassemia in an Asian population. *Proc. Natl. Acad. Sci. USA* **106:** 18716–18721.
17. Mendis, K., B.J. Sina, P. Marchesini & R. Carter. 2001. The neglected burden of *Plasmodium vivax* malaria. *Am. J. Trop. Med. Hyg.* **64**(Suppl 1–2): 97–106.
18. Higgs, D.R. & D.J. Weatherall. 2009. The alpha thalassaemias. *Cell. Mol. Life Sci.* **66:** 1154–1162.
19. WHO. 2002. *Genomics and World Health.* WHO. Geneva.
20. WHO-TIF Meeting. 2007. Management of haemoglobin disorders. *Report of a Joint WHO-TIF Meeting*. Nicosia, Cyprus.
21. Global Burden of Disease. 2008. Available at: http://www.globalburden.org.

Ann. N.Y. Acad. Sci. ISSN 0077-8923

ANNALS OF THE NEW YORK ACADEMY OF SCIENCES
Issue: *Cooley's Anemia: Ninth Symposium*

Iron metabolism and ineffective erythropoiesis in β-thalassemia mouse models

Pedro Ramos,[1,2] Luca Melchiori[1] Sara Gardenghi,[1] Nico Van-Roijen,[3] Robert W. Grady,[1] Yelena Ginzburg,[4] and Stefano Rivella[1]

[1]Division of Hematology-Oncology, Department of Pediatrics, Children's Blood Foundation Laboratories, Weill Medical College of Cornell University, New York, New York. [2]Instituto de Ciencias Biomedicas Abel Salazar, Porto, Portugal. [3]Department of Molecular Cell Biology, Vrije Universiteit Medical Center, Amsterdam, the Netherlands. [4]Erythropoiesis Laboratory, Lindsley F. Kimball Research Institute, New York Blood Center, New York, New York

Address for correspondence: Stefano Rivella, 515 E. 71 Street Room S-702, New York, NY 10021. str2010@med.cornell.edu

β-thalassemia is a disease associated with decreased β-globin production leading to anemia, ineffective erythropoiesis, and iron overload. New mechanisms associated with modulation of erythropoiesis and iron metabolism have recently been discovered in thalassemic mice, improving our understanding of the pathophysiology of this disease. These discoveries have the potential to be translated into clinically-relevant therapeutic options to reduce ineffective erythropoiesis and iron overload. A new generation of therapies based on limiting ineffective erythropoiesis, iron absorption, and the correction of iron maldistribution could be on the way, possibly complementing and improving the current standard of patient care.

Keywords: β-thalassemia; ineffective erythropoiesis; Jak2; iron overload; hepcidin; transferrin

Introduction

β-thalassemia is a disease characterized by reduced or absent production of β-globin chains. The phenotype is associated with development of anemia, production of abnormal red blood cells (RBC), ineffective erythropoiesis (IE), and iron overload. More than 200 mutations in the β-globin gene or its promoter have been associated with this disease, contributing to a diverse phenotypic manifestation and adding an additional degree of complexity to the understanding and management of this disease. The most severe form, β-thalassemia major or Cooley's anemia, is caused by mutations that completely abrogate synthesis of β-globin protein. Patients affected by this form of the disease develop a severe anemia requiring a regular blood transfusion regimen to sustain life. On the other hand, mutations that allow for production of some β-globin protein lead to milder forms of the disease, β-thalassemia intermedia. Although these patients are usually transfusion independent, iron overload develops due to increased iron uptake in the duodenum, leading to organ damage.[1] In this paper, we will focus on novel experimental models modulating IE and iron overload in β-thalassemic mice to showcase their potential utility as new therapies for patients affected by this devastating disease.

Ineffective erythropoiesis in β-thalassemia

IE is defined as the failure of erythroid progenitors to differentiate either as a consequence of cell death or an intrinsic differentiation defect, leading to abnormal production of mature RBCs. The premature death or hemolysis of circulating RBCs can also contribute to this process. Feedback from anemia triggers an increase in erythropoietic activity and results in erythroid expansion in the bone marrow as well as *de novo* proliferation in the spleen and liver, a process known as extra medullary hematopoiesis (EMH). As a consequence, patients often develop hepatosplenomegaly, a common finding in β-thalassemic patients. In normal individuals, the main function of the spleen is to clear senescent RBCs from circulation. For this reason it is believed that the splenomegaly observed in β-thalassemia increases RBC sequestration, worsening the anemia

doi: 10.1111/j.1749-6632.2010.05596.x

and leading to an escalation of transfusion requirements. Patients often undergo splenectomy to reduce their transfusion requirement and limit iron overload.

Ferrokinetic studies conducted 50 years ago have served as the basis of our understanding of IE in β-thalassemia.[2,3] In these studies it was observed that β-thalassemic patients had 10 times the plasma iron turnover of normal individuals, while their output of RBCs into the peripheral blood was markedly reduced. This suggested that the percentage of thalassemic erythroid precursors undergoing apoptosis was dramatically increased compared to that of normal individuals. Subsequent reports confirmed the increased apoptosis of erythroid progenitors in bone marrow and other sites of extramedullary erythropoiesis in β-thalassemic patients.[4,5] Taken together, these studies confirmed that the majority of erythroid progenitors from β-thalassemic subjects die during the maturation process. Apoptosis is associated with accumulation of α-globin chains resulting from the reduction in β-globin synthesis. In normal erythropoiesis, erythroid progenitors possess mechanism to control iron uptake and coordinate the production of all hemoglobin components. Iron was shown to modulate heme biosynthesis, and heme bioavailability to control globin production via the heme-regulated inhibitor kinase system.[6,7] Under the pathological conditions of β-thalassemia excesses of these elements leads to increased oxidative stress and accumulation of hemichromes. This is hypothesized to cause alterations in the cytoskeletal membrane proteins band-3 and spectrin, and to induce membrane lipid peroxidation,[8,9] leading to exposure of the anionic phospholipids phosphatidylethanolamine and phosphatidylserine.[10] All of these alterations in thalassemic erythroid cells undoubtedly contribute to the increased apoptosis observed. In agreement with the hypothesis that β-globin accumulation contributes to the development of IE, Kong and colleagues showed that lack of α-hemoglobin stabilizing protein (AHSP) impairs erythropoiesis and worsens the β-thalassemia phenotype, with increased apoptosis of erythroid precursors.[11] In summary, markedly increased apoptosis of erythroid precursors and the decreased life span of β-thalassemic RBC in the peripheral blood seem to be major factors contributing to anemia and driving IE.

Although there is unequivocal evidence of increased apoptosis in β-thalassemic erythroid precursors the data suggests that the percentage of apoptotic cells is much lower than originally suggested by the ferrokinetic studies.[2–5,12] The original studies predicted between 60% and 80% mortality of erythroid precursors but these researchers did not have the benefit of taking into consideration the role of hepcidin in increased iron absorption or the fact that a significant fraction of this iron would be stored in the liver.[13,14] We recently reported that erythroid marrow expansion and EMH are also associated with increased proliferation and decreased differentiation of erythroid progenitor cells, in addition to increased apoptosis.[12,15] Our data, obtained in mouse models of β-thalassemia intermedia (*th3*/+) and major (*th3*/*th3*), indicated that cell-cycle promoting genes were upregulated in β-thalassemic erythroid precursors limiting their differentiation, and likely worsening IE.[12] Interestingly, use of a Jak2 inhibitor, to block the erythropoietin (Epo) signaling pathway, was effective in reducing the relative and absolute number of undifferentiated erythroid cells and had a profound beneficial effect on splenomegaly (Fig. 1).[12] These observations corroborated our hypothesis that hyper proliferation of erythroid precursors with limited cell differentiation is an intrinsic feature of IE in β-thalassemia. In our original studies, use of the Jak2 inhibitor was associated with mild worsening of the anemia. Our new data in *th3*/+ mice indicate that a tailored dose of the Jak2 inhibitor leads to improvement of IE without worsening of anemia.[15] Moreover, in *th3*/*th3* animals, we determined that if the inhibitor was administered together with blood transfusions, the splenomegaly was ameliorated and the effectiveness of the transfusions was improved.[15] Higher levels of hemoglobin were maintained over time compared to the situation in untreated transfused *th3*/*th3* animals[15] (and Melchiori 2010, unpublished data). Overall, these preclinical results support the use of Jak2 inhibitors to prevent splenectomy, especially under conditions of increased thrombotic risk.

In conclusion, apoptosis driven by accumulation of α-globin aggregates plays a major role in IE. However, our data suggest that additional mechanisms may exacerbate IE. Epo signals erythroid cells to expand, promoting their proliferation and leading to erythroid expansion. On the other hand, it is

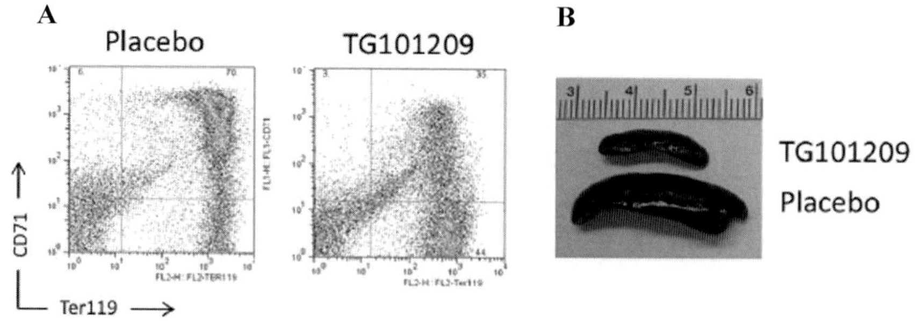

Figure 1. Effect of Jak2 on ineffective erythropoiesis in β-thalassemia. (A) Erythroid populations in splenic cell suspensions measured by classical CD71 and ter119 co-staining showing a decreased percentage of double positive cells in the animals treated with Jak2 inhibitor (right panel) compared to those of placebo treated mice (left panel). (B) Decrease in spleen size caused by treatment with the Jak2 inhibitor.

unlikely that the mechanisms leading to decreased cell differentiation depend on Epo production alone. We postulate that other factors contribute for this process including activation of unknown targets by iron, ROS, heme, and globin chain imbalance, possibly through heme-regulated inhibitor kinase.[16] This is an area of active research, especially because new tools have been identified to dissect erythropoiesis in normal and disease conditions.[17]

Preventing the need for splenectomy in β-thalassemia might also limit thrombosis in this disorder. It has been suggested that abnormal erythrocytes might predispose one to thrombotic events and that removal of the spleen might exacerbate this process.[18] Several observations suggest that a hypercoagulable state is present in β-thalassemia.[19,20] A number of abnormalities affecting coagulation have been seen in β-thalassemia, including activation of platelets, endothelium, and monocytes and altered levels of both coagulation factors and inhibitors.[19–21] Moreover, abnormal RBCs, through their increased cohesiveness, contribute to the higher risk from thrombotic complications. In addition, the asymmetry of thalassemic RBC membranes contributes to activation of important coagulation factors, such as thrombin enhancing the hypercoagulable state.[19–21]

Thus, use of Jak2 inhibitors may lead to new treatments for and better management of IE, EMH, splenomegaly and, potentially, thrombosis in this disease.

Hepcidin in β-thalassemia

Several studies, reviewed in,[16,22,23] dissected the role of hepcidin in β-thalassemia thereby adding to our understanding of the mechanisms affecting iron accumulation in this disorder. In particular, our study[14] revealed interesting differences that helped to further characterize the regulation of iron metabolism in β-thalassemia: (1) despite a greater degree of iron overload, animals affected by β-thalassemia major (*th3*/*th3*) had the lowest hepcidin expression, indicating that these animals are relatively insensitive to their iron burden under conditions of extreme IE; (2) mimicking the situation in human patients,[24] transfusion lead to increased hepcidin expression, hypothetically associated with decreased erythropoietic activity; (3) in mice affected by β-thalassemia intermedia (*th3*/+) hepcidin expression was disproportionally low compared to their iron load (Fig. 2).[14] However, hepcidin expression increased as the animals aged, with elevated iron intake from the duodenum seemingly associated with increased ferroportin expression in this organ. Low hepcidin expression has also been reported in patients affected by β-thalassemia.[13,25] These and other studies suggest that the expression of hepcidin is low due to the high erythropoietic activity.[26] A corollary of this scenario is that erythroid cells secrete a protein, called the erythroid factor, which suppresses hepcidin expression. Pak and colleagues corroborated this model showing that blockage of erythropoietic activity *in vivo* was sufficient to abolish the downregulation of hepcidin mediated by anemia, even in the presence of high levels of Epo.[26] Therefore, if an erythroid factor is secreted by erythroid progenitors, an increase in their number would augment the total amount of secreted erythroid factor, and result in a stronger downregulation of hepcidin. Sera from β-thalassemic patients suppressed hepcidin expression in a human hepatoma cell line, HepG2, further corroborating

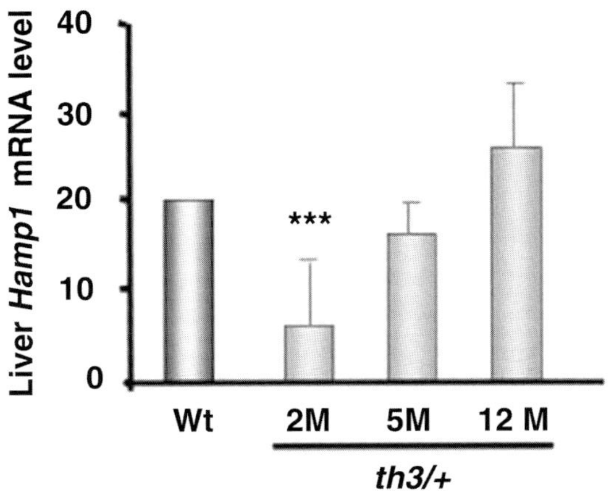

Figure 2. Hepcidin mRNA expression in liver samples from thalassemic mice. Hepcidin mRNA expression in the liver of *th3*/+ mice at different ages as measured by qPCR, showing very low levels of hepcidin expression in the early stages of the disease (2m) and an increase of hepcidin levels at later stages (1 year). The abbreviations 2m, 5m, and 12m indicate 2-month-old, 5-month-old, and 12-month-old mice.[14]

the existence of the erythroid factor. This effect was not observed using sera from normal individuals or from patients affected by hemochromatosis.[27] Based on all of these observations, and because we expect that β-thalassemia major is associated with a greater degree of IE, we hypothesized that the erythroid factor would be at its highest concentration exerting the greatest degree of hepcidin repression. We demonstrated that hepcidin expression in *th3/th3* mice is lower, despite a highest iron concentration in the liver, compared to *th3*/+ and normal mice.[14] However, under conditions of limited anemia and IE as in *th3*/+ animals, iron overload is able to exert an effect on increasing hepcidin expression. In fact, although the level of hepcidin was disproportionally low in these animals, hepcidin expression increased as the iron burden worsened.[14,16] This further supports the concept of independent pathways regulating hepcidin expression.

Recent studies introduced two members of the TGF-β superfamily, growth differentiation factor 15 (GDF15) and twisted gastrulation protein-1 (TWSG1), as potential candidates for the erythroid factor.[28,29] The corresponding genes were shown to be upregulated in undifferentiated erythroid cells and analysis of serum from β-thalassemic patients confirmed that their concentrations were elevated. Hepcidin expression in primary hepatocytes was shown to respond to both administration and blockage of these proteins in culture, suggesting that these erythroid derived factors are involved in the regulation of hepcidin in β-thalassemia. However, although they seem to contribute to hepcidin regulation in β-thalassemia, it is still not clear if they are involved in other conditions of anemia.

Modulation of iron metabolism and ineffective erythropoiesis in β-thalassemia

Iron overload is one of the major complications of β-thalassemia and new therapies to complement iron chelation are of great interest. This disease is characterized by an excess of iron over that needed to form hemoglobin, which accumulates progressively in the liver. Therefore, untransfused β-thalassemic patients and animals absorb more iron than they need to fulfill their requirements for erythropoiesis. Therapies that decrease iron uptake from the diet could prove efficient in reducing iron overload with minimal effect on anemia. This hypothesis was investigated by generating thalassemic animals overexpressing hepcidin. This resulted in decreased iron absorption and amelioration of anemia (Gardhengi 2010, unpublished data). Recently, using the *th1/th1* mouse model of β-thalassemia intermedia,[30] Dr. Ginzburg's group also suggested that iron maldistribution in β-thalassemia might contribute to IE.[31] In this study, iron delivery to erythroid cells in β-thalassemic mice was modulated by administration of apo-transferrin, showing a remarkable improvement of their phenotypic manifestations, including reduction of splenomegally and IE, improvement in hemoglobin concentration, increased hepcidin expression and reduced iron accumulation. Treatment with transferrin resulted in an increased number of RBCs, although the hemoglobin per cell (MCH) was decreased. These data suggest that decreasing iron availability, by decreasing either iron absorption or transferrin saturation, is beneficial to abnormal RBCs. Decreased iron availability likely results in more effective erythropoiesis as iron use within erythroid cells is limited to that needed for hemoglobin synthesis and less excess iron is available to generate free heme or α-globin precipitates, associated with shortened RBC survival.

Recently, a new line of investigation in our laboratory is also showing promising results. Although intrinsic properties of RBCs seem to drive IE and expansion of erythroid precursors increases iron absorption, we postulate that the microenvironment in the bone marrow affects erythroid maturation and differentiation under conditions of IE. Erythoid precursors mature in specialized structures called erythroblastic islands in which they associate with a central macrophage.[32] Moreover, macrophages within the reticuloendothelial system are also of crucial importance in the recycling of iron from senescent RBCs and play an important role in normal iron homeostasis. Finally, it has been proposed that macrophages participate in the regulation of hepcidin by a yet unknown mechanism.[33,34] Because of their multiple functions in erythropoiesis and iron homeostasis, we hypothesized that macrophages might modulate the thalassemic phenotype. A suicide technique to eliminate macrophages has been developed using liposome-mediated intracellular delivery of clodronate, a simple bisphosphonate (dichloromethylene diphosphonate, Cl2MDP).[35] Clodronate-containing liposomes are quickly ingested by macrophages via endocytosis, the liposome bilayers disrupted by lysosomal phospholipases, and the clodronate released into the cytoplasm. Subsequently, the clodronate can be metabolized to a nonhydrolysable analog of ATP, which causes collapse of the mitochondrial membrane potential, leading to apoptosis. Original studies have been performed to assess the effect of reducing or eliminating macrophages and macrophage-like cells in normal mice using clodronate. Splenic macrophages and hepatic Kupffer cells were targeted and eliminated by a single dose of intravenously injected clodronate. The effect is reversible because macrophage repopulation starts after about 1 week. Prolonged treatment with clodronate caused an almost complete depletion of macrophages from the spleen and a 58% reduction of those in the BM. These alterations were accompanied by an increase in both the life span and age-related changes of their RBCs, as well as a mild anemia associated with a reduced reticulocyte count.[36] Therefore, use of clodronate is an extremely efficient way to systematically reduce the number of macrophages.[35]

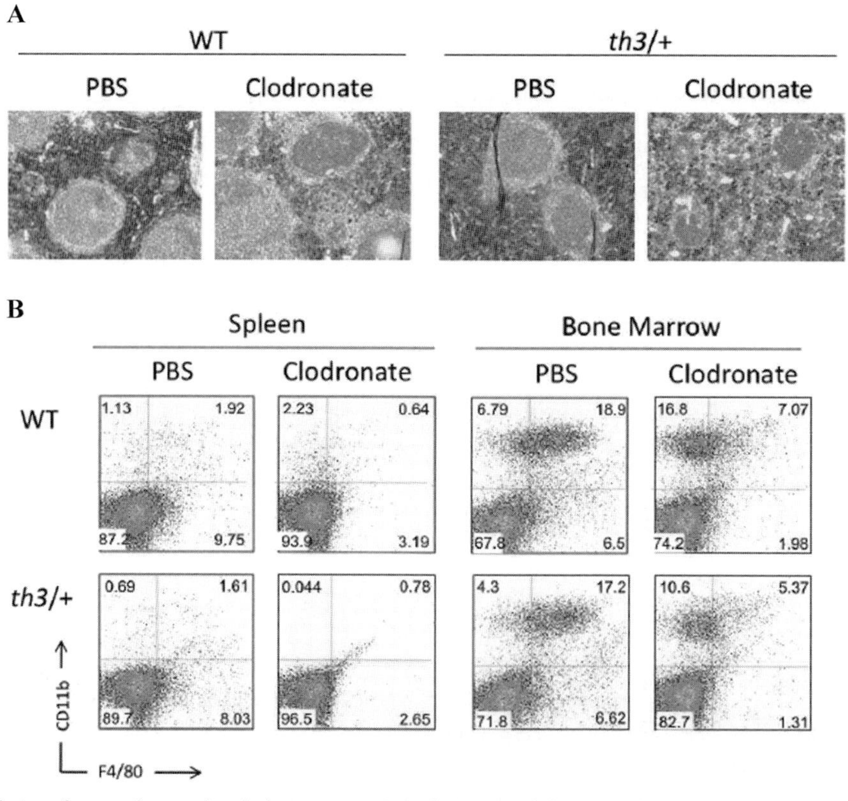

Figure 3. Depletion of macrophages using clodronate-containing liposomes. (A) Immunohistochemical staining of splenic sections from animals treated with PBS or clodronate-containing liposomes using the F4/80 antibody. (B) FACS analysis of cells from BM and spleen showing a reduction of F4/80 positive cells 48 hours after treatment with clodronate-containing liposomes.[37]

We performed some macrophage depletion studies using clodronate-containing liposomes. Using this approach, we confirmed by both flow cytometry and immunohistochemistry that macrophages in the spleen and bone marrow were markedly reduced (Fig. 3).[37] Preliminary studies indicate that while this treatment leads to reduced RBC synthesis in normal mice, elimination of macrophages positively affects iron metabolism and IE in mouse models of β-thalassemia. Further experiments are in progress to corroborate these observations and to more fully understand the role of macrophages in this disorder (Ramos 2010, unpublished data).

Future prospects

β-Thalassemia is a disease characterized by ineffective erythropoiesis, anemia, and iron overload. Recent studies shed light on the pathophysiology of β-thalassemia, including mechanisms driving ineffective erythropoiesis, with increased proliferation and decreased differentiation of erythroid progenitors in association with erythroid apoptosis, and increased iron absorption associated with inappropriately low hepcidin expression. In addition, studies in mice suggest that iron maldistribution may enhance IE and anemia in this disorder. Results obtained in mouse models of β-thalassemia suggest that use of Jak2 inhibitors, hepcidin, and transferrin might prove effective in limiting IE, iron absorption, or both. Additional studies related to the erythropoietic niche in the bone marrow, under conditions of chronic stress erythropoiesis and iron overload such as in β-thalassemia, will benefit our insight into the pathophysiology of this disorder and identify novel therapeutic targets to clinical practice. Human studies will be needed to corroborate these data and validate these approaches.

In conclusion, although the current treatments for β-thalassemia, blood transfusions and iron chelation, have proven to be effective in the management of this disease, recent observations suggest alternative strategies that may further improve the treatment of β-thalassemic patients.

Acknowledgments

This work was supported by the Cooley's Anemia Foundation-CAF, the Associazione Veneta Lotta alla Talassemia (AVLT) (S.G.), and by grants from the Carlo and Micol Schejola Foundation, the Children's Cancer and Blood Foundation and NIH-R21DK065169 (S.R.), R01DK55463 (R.W.G.), the American Portuguese Biomedical Fund (APBRF, USA)/Inova grant (P.R.). S.G. is a fellow of the Cooley's Anemia Foundation. P.R. is a fellow from Fundação para a Ciência e Tecnologia, Portugal (SFRH/BD/24813/2005).

Conflicts of interest

The authors declare no conflicts of interest.

References

1. Bannerman, R. M. *et al.* 1967. Thalassemia intermedia, with iron overload, cardiac failure, diabetes mellitus, hypopituitarism and porphyrinuria. *Am. J. Med.* **42:** 476–486.
2. Finch, C.A. & P. Sturgeon. 1957. Erythrokinetics in Cooley's anemia. *Blood* **12:** 64–73.
3. Finch, C.A. *et al.* 1970. Ferrokinetics in man. *Med. (Baltimore)* **49:** 17–53.
4. Yuan, J. *et al.* 1993. Accelerated programmed cell death (apoptosis) in erythroid precursors of patients with severe beta-thalassemia (Cooley's anemia). *Blood* **82:** 374–377.
5. Mathias, L.A. *et al.* 2000. Ineffective erythropoiesis in beta-thalassemia major is due to apoptosis at the polychromatophilic normoblast stage. *Exp. Hematol.* **28:** 1343–1353.
6. Ponka, P. 1997. Tissue-specific regulation of iron metabolism and heme synthesis: distinct control mechanisms in erythroid cells. *Blood* **89:** 1–25.
7. Chen, J.J. 2007. Regulation of protein synthesis by the heme-regulated eIF2alpha kinase: relevance to anemias. *Blood* **109:** 2693–2699.
8. Shinar, E. *et al.* 1987. Erythrocyte membrane skeleton abnormalities in severe beta-thalassemia. *Blood* **70:** 158–164.
9. Cappellini, M.D. *et al.* 1999. Metabolic indicators of oxidative stress correlate with haemichrome attachment to membrane, band 3 aggregation and erythrophagocytosis in beta-thalassaemia intermedia. *Br. J. Haematol.* **104:** 504–512.
10. Kuypers, F.A. *et al.* 1998. Membrane phospholipid asymmetry in human thalassemia. *Blood* **91:** 3044–3051.
11. Kong, Y. *et al.* 2004. Loss of alpha-hemoglobin-stabilizing protein impairs erythropoiesis and exacerbates beta-thalassemia. *J. Clin. Invest.* **114:** 1457–1466.
12. Libani, I.V. *et al.* 2008. Decreased differentiation of erythroid cells exacerbates ineffective erythropoiesis in beta-thalassemia. *Blood* **112:** 875–885.
13. Origa, R. *et al.* 2007. Liver iron concentrations and urinary hepcidin in beta-thalassemia. *Haematologica* **92:** 583–588.
14. Gardenghi, S. *et al.* 2007. Ineffective erythropoiesis in beta-thalassemia is characterized by increased iron absorption mediated by down-regulation of hepcidin and up-regulation of ferroportin. *Blood* **109:** 5027–5035.
15. Melchiori, L. *et al.* 2009. Use of Jak2 Inhibitors to limit ineffective erythropoiesis and iron absorption in Mice affected by β-thalassemia and other disorders of red cell production. *Blood* **114:** 2020.
16. Rivella, S. 2009. Ineffective erythropoiesis and thalassemias. *Curr. Opin. Hematol.* **16:** 187–194.

17. Chen, K. *et al.* 2009. Resolving the distinct stages in erythroid differentiation based on dynamic changes in membrane protein expression during erythropoiesis. *Proc. Natl. Acad. Sci. USA* **106:** 17413–17418.
18. Cappellini, M.D. *et al.* 2000. Venous thromboembolism and hypercoagulability in splenectomized patients with thalassaemia intermedia. *Br. J. Haematol.* **111:** 467–473.
19. Ataga, K.I., M.D. Cappellini & E.A. Rachmilewitz. 2007. Beta-thalassaemia and sickle cell anaemia as paradigms of hypercoagulability. *Br. J. Haematol.* **139:** 3–13.
20. Taher, A.T. *et al.* 2008. Thalassemia and hypercoagulability. *Blood Rev.* **22:** 283–292.
21. Eldor, A. & E.A. Rachmilewitz. 2002. The hypercoagulable state in thalassemia. *Blood* **99:** 36–43.
22. Rechavi, G. & S. Rivella. 2008. Regulation of iron absorption in hemoglobinopathies. *Curr. Mol. Med.* **8:** 646–662.
23. Rivella, S. & E. Rachmilewitz. 2009. Future alternative therapies for β-thalassemia. *Expert Rev. Hematol.* **2:** 685–697.
24. Jenkins, Z.A. *et al.* 2007. Iron homeostasis during transfusional iron overload in beta-thalassemia and sickle cell disease: changes in iron regulatory protein, hepcidin, and ferritin expression. *Pediatr. Hematol. Oncol.* **24:** 237–243.
25. Kattamis, A. *et al.* 2006. The effects of erythropoetic activity and iron burden on hepcidin expression in patients with thalassemia major. *Haematologica* **91:** 809–812.
26. Pak, M. *et al.* 2006. Suppression of hepcidin during anemia requires erythropoietic activity. *Blood* **108:** 3730–3735.
27. Weizer-Stern, O. *et al.* 2006. Downregulation of hepcidin and haemojuvelin expression in the hepatocyte cell-line HepG2 induced by thalassaemic sera. *Br. J. Haematol.* **135:** 129–138.
28. Tanno, T. *et al.* 2007. High levels of GDF15 in thalassemia suppress expression of the iron regulatory protein hepcidin. *Nat. Med.* **13:** 1096–1101.
29. Tanno, T. *et al.* 2009. Identification of TWSG1 as a second novel erythroid regulator of hepcidin expression in murine and human cells. *Blood* **114:** 181–186.
30. Skow, L.C. *et al.* 1983. A mouse model for beta-thalassemia. *Cell* **34:** 1043–1052.
31. Li, H. *et al.* 2010. Transferrin therapy ameliorates disease in beta-thalassemic mice. *Nat. Med.* **16:** 177–182.
32. Chasis, J.A. & N. Mohandas. 2008. Erythroblastic islands: niches for erythropoiesis. *Blood* **112:** 470–478.
33. Theurl, M. *et al.* 2008. Kupffer cells modulate iron homeostasis in mice via regulation of hepcidin expression. *J. Mol. Med.* **86:** 825–835.
34. Makui, H. *et al.* 2005. Contribution of Hfe expression in macrophages to the regulation of hepatic hepcidin levels and iron loading. *Blood* **106:** 2189–2195.
35. Van Rooijen, N. & A. Sanders. 1994. Liposome mediated depletion of macrophages: mechanism of action, preparation of liposomes and applications. *J. Immunol. Methods* **174:** 83–93.
36. Giuliani, A.L. *et al.* 2001. Changes in murine bone marrow macrophages and erythroid burst-forming cells following the intravenous injection of liposome-encapsulated dichloromethylene diphosphonate (Cl2MDP). *Eur. J. Haematol.* **66:** 221–229.
37. Ramos, P. *et al.* 2009. Macrophage depletion leads to modification of thalassemic phenotype. *Blood* **114:** 2023.

Ann. N.Y. Acad. Sci. ISSN 0077-8923

ANNALS OF THE NEW YORK ACADEMY OF SCIENCES
Issue: *Cooley's Anemia: Ninth Symposium*

Hepcidin in β-thalassemia

Elizabeta Nemeth
Department of Medicine, University of California at Los Angeles, Los Angeles, California

Address for correspondence: Elizabeta Nemeth, Ph.D., David Geffen School of Medicine at UCLA, CHS 37-131, 10833 LeConte Ave, Los Angeles, CA 90095. enemeth@mednet.ucla.edu

Iron overload is the principal cause of morbidity and mortality in β-thalassemia with or without transfusion dependence. Iron homeostasis is regulated by the hepatic peptide hormone hepcidin. Hepcidin controls dietary iron absorption, plasma iron concentrations, and tissue iron distribution. A deficiency in this hormone is the main or contributing factor of iron overload in iron-loading anemias such as β-thalassemia. Hepcidin deficiency results from a strong suppressive effect of the high erythropoietic activity on hepcidin expression. Although in thalassemia major patients iron absorption contributes less to the total iron load than transfusions, in non-transfused thalassemia, low hepcidin, and the consequent hyperabsorption of dietary iron is the major cause of systemic iron overload. Hepcidin diagnostics and future therapeutic agonists may help in management of patients with β-thalassemia.

Keywords: hepcidin; β-thalassemia; iron overload

Hepcidin regulates iron homeostasis

Hepcidin is a small peptide hormone secreted by hepatocytes, circulating in blood plasma and excreted in urine.[1] Hepcidin regulates iron concentration in the plasma and the distribution of iron among different tissues. Dysregulation of hepcidin production underlies many iron disorders. Chronic excess of hepcidin causes iron-restricted anemia[2] whereas hepcidin deficiency results in iron overload with iron deposition in the liver and other parenchyma.[3]

Hepcidin acts by regulating the cellular concentration of its receptor, ferroportin. Ferroportin is the sole known cellular iron exporter[4] and it exports iron into plasma from duodenal enterocytes which absorb dietary iron, macrophages of the spleen and liver which recycle iron from old erythrocytes, and hepatocytes which release stored iron according to body needs.[5–7] Hepcidin binding to ferroportin triggers internalization and degradation of the receptor.[8] Removal of ferroportin from the membrane stops cellular iron export leading to decreased supply of iron into plasma. Conversely, when hepcidin concentration is low, ferroportin remains on the cell surface, leading to increased iron absorption and export from macrophages. If uncontrolled, increased iron absorption eventually causes iron overload.

Regulation of hepcidin

Hepcidin is homeostatically regulated by iron and erythropoietic activity, but similar pathways are involved in hepcidin dysregulation in thalassemia.

Increased plasma and stored iron stimulates hepcidin production, which in turn blocks dietary iron absorption and further iron loading. Conversely, hepcidin is suppressed in iron deficiency,[9] allowing increased absorption of dietary iron and replenishment of iron stores. Hepcidin appears to be regulated by both plasma iron-transferrin and intracellular iron stores, and these signals likely use the bone morphogenetic protein (BMP) pathway to alter hepcidin expression. Although several BMPs can increase hepcidin production *in vitro* and *in vivo*,[10] BMP6 has recently emerged as the principal endogenous BMP that regulates hepcidin. BMP6 knockout mice develop severe iron overload but no other significant abnormalities.[11,12] BMP signaling to hepcidin is modulated by hemojuvelin (HJV), a co-receptor of the BMP pathway.[13] HJV mutations in humans or mice result in severe iron overload similar to that caused by hepcidin

doi: 10.1111/j.1749-6632.2010.05585.x

mutations.[14] It is possible that another HJV-interacting protein, neogenin, participates in hepcidin regulation by iron[15] because neogenin-deficient mice also displayed low hepcidin expression and developed liver iron overload.[16]

Hepcidin regulation by extracellular iron is thought to depend on sensing of iron-transferrin concentrations by transferrin receptor 2 (TfR2) and HFE. Mutations of TfR2 and HFE lead to hepcidin deficiency and the adult form of hereditary hemochromatosis.[17,18] Increase in iron-transferrin concentration appears to promote HFE/TfR2 interaction[19,20] and likely potentiates BMP pathway signaling. The mechanism by which intracellular iron regulates hepcidin expression is less understood. HFE and TfR2 do not appear to be required for hepcidin regulation by iron stores, as mice and humans with HFE and TfR2 mutations are still capable of decreasing hepcidin levels after iron depletion.[18] Expression of BMP6 mRNA was recently shown to increase with iron loading in mice, raising the possibility that BMP6 is a signal reflecting iron stores.[21]

As would be expected for the iron-regulatory hormone, hepcidin production is also regulated by the process that consumes the most iron, erythropoiesis.[22] Increased erythropoietic activity suppresses hepcidin production that allows the release of stored iron from macrophages and hepatocytes, and increased absorption of dietary iron, all resulting in greater supply of iron for hemoglobin synthesis. How erythropoiesis affects hepcidin production is not clear. Although injection of erythropoietin in humans and mice decreased hepcidin expression,[23,24] Epo by itself does not appear to be a direct regulator of hepcidin because pretreatment of mice with carboplatin, a cytotoxic inhibitor of erythropoiesis, completely abrogated the effect of Epo on hepcidin.[22] Similarly, mouse models of anemias caused by bleeding or hemolysis showed that hepcidin suppression depended on intact erythropoietic activity.[22,25] Erythropoietin administration in mice was found to reduce Smad signaling[24] suggesting that erythroid activity may affect hepcidin expression by modulating the BMP pathway.

The mediators of hepcidin suppression may include the production of soluble factors by the erythroid precursors in the bone marrow, decreased circulating or stored iron, and hypoxia. Two proteins produced by erythroid precursors, growth differentiation factor 15 (GDF15), and twisted gastrulation protein (TWSG1), have been proposed to mediate hepcidin suppression in anemias with ineffective erythropoiesis.[26,27] GDF15, a member of the TGF-β superfamily, and TWSG1, a BMP-binding protein, are both produced by developing erythroblasts and were shown to suppress hepcidin mRNA *in vitro*.[26,27] Very high levels of GDF15 were detected in β-thalassemia and congenital dyserythropoietic anemia type I, and elevated Twsg1 expression was found in a mouse model of thalassemia. However, whether these factors are the main suppressors of hepcidin in β-thalassemia remains to be determined. Furthermore, there is no evidence that these factors mediate physiologic hepcidin suppression in response to bleeding or to anemias with effective erythropoiesis.

HIF pathway was proposed as another regulator of hepcidin in anemias, and *in vivo* alterations of this pathway can affect hepcidin expression.[28] Hypoxia may exert its effect on hepcidin by increasing erythropoietin production in the kidney, and subsequent proliferation of erythroblasts in the bone marrow, but whether hypoxia can suppress hepcidin directly is still unresolved.[28,29]

Hepcidin production is also pathologically increased in inflammation and infection.[9,30–33] The resulting hypoferremia may represent a host defense strategy to limit iron availability to microorganisms, but can also lead to iron dysregulation and iron-restricted anemia in inflammatory diseases. Of inflammatory mediators regulating hepcidin, IL-6 was shown to be a prominent inducer *in vitro* and *in vivo*, but other cytokines such as IL-1 may also contribute.

The role of hepcidin in β-thalassemia

In iron-loading anemias not treated by frequent transfusions, such as β-thalassemia intermedia and congenital dyserythropoietic anemias, urinary and serum hepcidin are severely decreased.[34–36] Hepcidin deficiency in turn allows excessive iron absorption and development of systemic iron overload. The liver is most commonly affected by iron overload due to the avid uptake of non-transferrin bound iron by hepatocytes. Iron overload of other organs appears to correlate broadly with the rate of iron absorption. Rapid accumulation of iron, such as seen with severe hepcidin deficiency (juvenile hemochromatosis, thalassemia intermedia) is associated with prominent deposition of iron in the heart and some endocrine organs.

In β-thalassemia major, transfusions rather than dietary iron absorption are the predominant cause of iron overload. In chronically transfused patients, hepcidin concentrations are significantly higher than in nontransfused patients, presumably due to both increased iron load and the alleviation of ineffective erythropoiesis.[34,36] However, hepcidin concentrations decrease in the intervals between transfusions, as the effect of each transfusion wears off.[34–36] During those periods, decreased hepcidin and the resulting increase in intestinal iron absorption may be significant contributors to patients' iron load.

Different levels of hepcidin in thalassemia intermedia and major result in different cellular distribution of iron. Origa and colleagues[36] showed that nontransfused patients have liver iron concentrations similar to those of regularly transfused thalassemia patients. However, in nontransfused thalassemia, iron was deposited in hepatocytes, whereas higher hepcidin levels in transfused patients resulted in macrophage iron loading. As a consequence of this difference in cellular iron distribution, serum ferritin levels were much lower in nontransfused patients, and did not adequately reflect the patients' liver iron load. The specific pattern of cellular iron deposition may be important because different cell types exhibit differential tolerance to iron-mediated toxicity.[37]

Hepcidin diagnostics and therapeutics in β-thalassemia

Hepcidin measurements have only recently become possible with the development of assays for bioactive mature hepcidin in serum and urine. The methodologies include competitive ELISAs,[9,38] and mass spectrometry-based assays (MALDI-TOF MS, SELDI, and LC–MS/MS).[39–41] Determining hepcidin concentrations in patients with iron-loading anemias may be useful to identify the patients at higher risk of iron toxicity due to severely decreased hepcidin levels. However, the utility of hepcidin for the management of iron overload in β-thalassemia is not known and needs to be evaluated in larger clinical studies.

Continuous or nearly continuous chelation is the major therapeutic modality for β-thalassemia, either with parenteral agents and/or with oral chelators. However, compliance with chelation therapy is often inadequate and iron overload remains a major cause of morbidity and mortality. Hepcidin-targeted therapeutics may help improve treatment of iron overload in β-thalassemia. In thalassemia intermedia, hepcidin therapy would be expected to have beneficial effects by curbing hyperabsorption of dietary iron. It is possible that hepcidin agonists could be useful even in transfused thalassemia patients. Although intestinal iron absorption contributes less to the total iron load in these patients, hepcidin therapy may help in the intervals when endogenous hepcidin falls and intestinal iron uptake increases. Furthermore, considering that high hepcidin shifts iron distribution to macrophages where it is less toxic, pharmacologic doses of hepcidin may postpone the iron deposition and consequent damage in the parenchyma.

The first indication of the beneficial effect of hepcidin in β-thalassemia came from the group of Dr. Stefano Rivella (Weill Medical College of Cornell University, New York). They used the th3/+ mouse model of β-thalassemia, which exhibits features comparable to those of patients affected by β-thalassemia intermedia. Th3/+ hematopoietic stem cells were transplanted either into transgenic mice expressing hepcidin or into wild-type mice. After several months, mice with moderate overexpression of hepcidin had lower spleen and liver iron content, decreased inefficient erythropoiesis in the spleen, lower spleen weight and even improvement of hematological parameters (Gardenghi *et al.*, submitted). Thus transgenic hepcidin overexpression in β-thalassemia intermedia mice not only decreased iron overload but also ameliorated ineffective erythropoiesis and anemia.

Although these proof-of-principle studies show promise, no hepcidin therapies are yet available. Hepcidin has several characteristics that limit its potential use as a therapeutic. Because of its length and complex 4-disulfide structure it is very expensive to produce. Its relatively large size and susceptibility to inactivating proteolytic degradation at the N-terminus preclude efficient oral absorption. Rapid clearance of hepcidin through renal excretion may limit its efficacy *in vivo*. We have undertaken structure-function analysis of the hepcidin-ferroportin interaction and based on those findings developed small (7–9 amino acid) peptide agonists that mimic the activity of full-length hepcidin (E.

Nemeth, unpublished). In preliminary experiments using wild-type mice, we showed that minihepcidin acted as agonists *in vivo*. The small size should allow eventual development of orally available agonists.

Future preclinical and clinical studies will be necessary to assess the risks and relative benefits of hepcidin-targeted treatment approaches.

Acknowledgments

Supported by the grant from the National Institute of Health, R01 DK082717.

Conflicts of interest

Dr. Elizabeta Nemeth is a co-founder and the Chief Scientific Officer of Intrinsic LifeSciences, LLC, a biotech company developing iron-related diagnostics.

References

1. Park, C.H., E.V. Valore, A.J. Waring & T. Ganz. 2001. Hepcidin, a urinary antimicrobial peptide synthesized in the liver. *J. Biol. Chem.* **276:** 7806–7810.
2. Roy, C.N., H.H. Mak, I. Akpan, *et al.* 2007. Hepcidin antimicrobial peptide transgenic mice exhibit features of the anemia of inflammation. *Blood* **109:** 4038–4044.
3. Roetto, A., G. Papanikolaou, M. Politou, *et al.* 2003. Mutant antimicrobial peptide hepcidin is associated with severe juvenile hemochromatosis. *Nat. Genet.* **33:** 21–22.
4. Donovan, A., C.A. Lima, J.L. Pinkus, *et al.* 2005. The iron exporter ferroportin/Slc40a1 is essential for iron homeostasis. *Cell Metab.* **1:** 191–200.
5. Abboud, S. & D.J. Haile. 2000. A novel mammalian iron-regulated protein involved in intracellular iron metabolism. *J. Biol. Chem.* **275:** 19906–19912.
6. Donovan, A., A. Brownlie, Y. Zhou, *et al.* 2000. Positional cloning of zebrafish ferroportin1 identifies a conserved vertebrate iron exporter. *Nature* **403:** 776–781.
7. Mckie, A.T., P. Marciani, A. Rolfs, *et al.* 2000. A novel duodenal iron-regulated transporter, IREG1, implicated in the basolateral transfer of iron to the circulation. *Mol. Cell* **5:** 299–309.
8. Nemeth, E., M.S. Tuttle, J. Powelson, *et al.* 2004. Hepcidin regulates cellular iron efflux by binding to ferroportin and inducing its internalization. *Science* **306:** 2090–2093.
9. Ganz, T., G. Olbina, D. Girelli, *et al.* 2008. Immunoassay for human serum hepcidin. *Blood* **112:** 4292–4297.
10. Xia, Y., J.L. Babitt, Y. Sidis, *et al.* 2008. Hemojuvelin regulates hepcidin expression via a selective subset of BMP ligands and receptors independently of neogenin. *Blood* **111:** 5195–5204.
11. Andriopoulos, B., Jr., E. Corradini, Y. Xia, *et al.* 2009. BMP6 is a key endogenous regulator of hepcidin expression and iron metabolism. *Nat. Genet.* **41:** 482–487.
12. Meynard, D., L. Kautz, V. Darnaud, *et al.* 2009. Lack of the bone morphogenetic protein BMP6 induces massive iron overload. *Nat. Genet.* **41:** 478–481.
13. Babitt, J.L., F.W. Huang, D.M. Wrighting, *et al.* 2006. Bone morphogenetic protein signaling by hemojuvelin regulates hepcidin expression. *Nat. Genet.* **38:** 531–539.
14. Niederkofler, V., R. Salie & S. Arber. 2005. Hemojuvelin is essential for dietary iron sensing, and its mutation leads to severe iron overload. *J. Clin. Invest.* **115:** 2180–2186.
15. Zhang, A.S., F. Yang, K. Meyer, *et al.* 2008. Neogenin-mediated hemojuvelin shedding occurs after hemojuvelin traffics to the plasma membrane. *J. Biol. Chem.* **283:** 17494–17502.
16. Lee, D.H., L.J. Zhou, Z. Zhou, *et al.* 2010. Neogenin inhibits HJV secretion and regulates BMP induced hepcidin expression and iron homeostasis. *Blood* **115:** 3136–3145.
17. Nemeth, E., A. Roetto, G. Garozzo, *et al.* 2005. Hepcidin is decreased in TFR2 hemochromatosis. *Blood* **105:** 1803–1806.
18. Piperno, A., D. Girelli, E. Nemeth, *et al.* 2007. Blunted hepcidin response to oral iron challenge in HFE-related hemochromatosis. *Blood* **110:** 4096–4100.
19. Johnson, M.B., J. Chen, N. Murchison, *et al.* 2007. Transferrin receptor 2: evidence for ligand-induced stabilization and redirection to a recycling pathway. *Mol. Biol. Cell* **18:** 743–754.
20. Goswami, T. & N.C. Andrews. 2006. Hereditary hemochromatosis protein, HFE, interaction with transferrin receptor 2 suggests a molecular mechanism for mammalian iron sensing. *J. Biol. Chem.* **281:** 28494–28498.
21. Kautz, L., D. Meynard, A. Monnier, *et al.* 2008. Iron regulates phosphorylation of Smad1/5/8 and gene expression of Bmp6, Smad7, Id1, and Atoh8 in the mouse liver. *Blood* **112:** 1503–1509.
22. Pak, M., M.A. Lopez, V. Gabayan, *et al.* 2006. Suppression of hepcidin during anemia requires erythropoietic activity. *Blood* **108:** 3730–3735.
23. Ashby, D.R., D.P. Gale, M. Busbridge, *et al.* 2010. Erythropoietin administration in humans causes a marked and prolonged reduction in circulating hepcidin. *Haematologica* **95:** 505–508.
24. Huang, H., M. Constante, A. Layoun & M.M. Santos. 2009. Contribution of STAT3 and SMAD4 pathways to the regulation of hepcidin by opposing stimuli. *Blood* **113:** 3593–3599.
25. Vokurka, M., J. Krijt, K. Sulc & E. Necas. 2006. Hepcidin mRNA levels in mouse liver respond to inhibition of erythropoiesis. *Physiol. Res* **55:** 667–674.
26. Tanno, T., N.V. Bhanu, P.A. Oneal, *et al.* 2007. High levels of GDF15 in thalassemia suppress expression of the iron regulatory protein hepcidin. *Nat. Med.* **13:** 1096–1101.
27. Tanno, T., P. Porayette, O. Sripichai, *et al.* 2009. Identification of TWSG1 as a second novel erythroid regulator of hepcidin expression in murine and human cells. *Blood* **114:** 181–186.
28. Peyssonnaux, C., A.S. Zinkernagel, R.A. Schuepbach, *et al.* 2007. Regulation of iron homeostasis by the hypoxia-inducible transcription factors (HIFs). *J. Clin. Invest.* **117:** 1926–1932.
29. Choi, S.O., Y.S. Cho, H.L. Kim & J.W. Park. 2007. ROS mediate the hypoxic repression of the hepcidin gene by inhibiting C/EBPalpha and STAT-3. *Biochem. Biophys. Res. Commun.* **356:** 312–317.

30. Ganz, T. 2006. Molecular pathogenesis of anemia of chronic disease. *Pediatr. Blood Cancer* **46:** 554–557.
31. Semrin, G., D.S. Fishman, A. Bousvaros, *et al.* 2006. Impaired intestinal iron absorption in Crohn's disease correlates with disease activity and markers of inflammation. *Inflamm. Bowel Dis.* **12:** 1101–1106.
32. Sharma, S., E. Nemeth, Y.H. Chen, *et al.* 2008. Involvement of hepcidin in the anemia of multiple myeloma. *Clin. Cancer Res.* **14:** 3262–3267.
33. Nemeth, E., E.V. Valore, M. Territo, *et al.* 2003. Hepcidin, a putative mediator of anemia of inflammation, is a type II acute-phase protein. *Blood* **101:** 2461–2463.
34. Kearney, S.L., E. Nemeth, E.J. Neufeld, *et al.* 2007. Urinary hepcidin in congenital chronic anemias. *Pediatr. Blood Cancer* **48:** 57–63.
35. Nemeth, E. & T. Ganz. 2006. Hepcidin and iron-loading anemias. *Haematologica* **91:** 727–732.
36. Origa, R., R. Galanello, T. Ganz, *et al.* 2007. Liver iron concentrations and urinary hepcidin in beta-thalassemia *Haematologica* **92:** 583–588.
37. Britton, R.S., K.L. Leicester & B.R. Bacon. 2002. Iron toxicity and chelation therapy. *Int. J. Hematol.* **76:** 219–228.
38. Busbridge, M., C. Griffiths, D. Ashby, *et al.* 2009. Development of a novel immunoassay for the iron regulatory peptide hepcidin. *Br. J. Biomed. Sci.* **66:** 150–157.
39. Kemna, E.H., H. Tjalsma, V.N. Podust & D.W. Swinkels. 2007. Mass spectrometry-based hepcidin measurements in serum and urine: analytical aspects and clinical implications. *Clin. Chem.* **53:** 620–628.
40. Castagna, A., N. Campostrini, F. Zaninotto & D. Girelli. 2010. Hepcidin assay in serum by SELDI-TOF-MS and other approaches. *J. Proteomics* **73:** 527–536.
41. Bansal, S.S., J.M. Halket, J. Fusova, *et al.* 2009. Quantification of hepcidin using matrix-assisted laser desorption/ionization time-of-flight mass spectrometry. *Rapid Commun. Mass Spectrom.* **23:** 1531–1542.

Ann. N.Y. Acad. Sci. ISSN 0077-8923

ANNALS OF THE NEW YORK ACADEMY OF SCIENCES
Issue: *Cooley's Anemia: Ninth Symposium*

Therapy for β-globinopathies: a brief review and determinants for successful and safe correction

Ajay Perumbeti[1] and Punam Malik[1,2]

Divisions of [1]Hematology-Oncology, Cancer and Blood Institute, Cincinnati Children's Research Foundation, Cincinnati Children's Hospital Medical Center (CCHMC), Cincinnati, Ohio. [2]Experimental Hematology/Cancer Biology, Cancer and Blood Institute, Cincinnati Children's Research Foundation, Cincinnati Children's Hospital Medical Center (CCHMC), Cincinnati, Ohio

Address for correspondence: Punam Malik, M.D., Divisions of Experimental Hematology/Cancer Biology and Hematology Oncology, Cincinnati Children's Hospital Medical Center, ML 7013, 3333 Burnet Avenue, Cincinnati, OH 45229. Punam.Malik@cchmc.org

Gene therapy for β-globinopathies, particularly β-thalassemia and sickle cell anemia, hold much promise for the future, as a one time cure for these common and debilitating disorders. Correction of the β-globinopathies using lentivirus vectors (LV) carrying the β- or γ-globin genes and elements of the locus control region has been well established in murine models, and a good idea of "what it will take to cure these diseases" has been developed in the first decade of the twenty-first century. A clinical trial using one such vector has been initiated in France while other trials are in development. Vector improvements to enhance the safety and efficiency of LV are being explored, while newer strategies, like homologous recombination in induced pluripotent cells for correction of sickle cell anemia, has been shown as a proof-of-concept. Here we provide a review of current progress in genetic correction of β-globin disorders.

Keywords: thalassemia; sickle cell disease; lentivirus vectors; insulators; gene therapy

Introduction

Inherited β-globin disorders (β-globinopathies) such as thalassemia and sickle cell anemia are the most common monogenic disorders world-wide that cause significant morbidity, mortality, and health care expenditures.[1] A one-time genetic correction has long been conceived as the ultimate method of cure. Current gene therapy technology has resulted in a permanent correction of other monogenic disorders, such as X-linked severe combined immune deficiency (X-linked SCID), adenine deaminase deficient SCID (ADA-SCID), and chronic granulomatous disease (CGD).[2–6] In immunodeficiency diseases, relatively small proportions of gene modified hematopoietic stem cells (HSC) can give rise to sufficient long-lived T cells, and a relatively small amount of transgene protein expression in the differentiated T cell progeny is adequate to produce a phenotypic correction. In β-globinopathies, this is not the case. An enormous amount of gene expression in individual red blood cells (RBC), especially in RBC from patients with Cooley's anemia, is necessary; additionally, engraftment of a large proportion of gene corrected HSC that repopulate the bone marrow is necessary in order to affect cure. HIV-1 based lentivirus vectors (LV) hold the promise of delivering high expression and transducing a high proportion of HSC and have revolutionized genetic therapy approaches for β-globinopathies.

HIV-based lentivirus vectors

Efficient delivery of large locus control region (LCR) elements and β-globin gene has been a challenging task with the conventional retroviral (RV) vectors. Numerous investigators have worked on defining critical elements within the LCR that are necessary for high level of expression human β-globin. LV vectors (i) carry some unique cis elements that allow efficient packaging of the intron-containing β-globin

doi: 10.1111/j.1749-6632.2010.05584.x

expression cassette, and allow stable transmission of the β or γ globin genes and LCR. (ii) They can carry larger cargo, allowing large LCR elements, necessary for high-level globin gene expression, to be inserted. (iii) LV vectors can enter through intact nuclear membrane of nondividing cells and integrate into nondividing HSC at high efficiency. This eliminates the need for prolonged *ex vivo* cytokine prestimulation to force HSC division, a phenomenon shown to result in significant loss of "stemness." (iv) Self inactivating (SIN) LV vectors are safer as they carry no viral transcriptional elements and can be efficiently concentrated without significant loss in titers; a feature important for globin vectors that are typically produced at very low titers. (v) SIN LV vectors are relatively resistant to proviral silencing due to lack of viral transcriptional elements,[7–9] a phenomenon that has been observed commonly with conventional RV vectors in animal models[10] and in a recent clinical trial for CGD.[11]

Gene therapy for Cooley's anemia

Potential strategies for gene therapy of Cooley's anemia have employed "additive gene therapy," delivering the human β-globin gene (hβ), recombinant hβ genes, or human γ-globin (hγ) genes and the β-globin LCR enhancer into the HSC genome. Correction of thalassemia mice was first shown by May and colleagues, who delivered the hβ transgene via a LV vector. Mice that have heterozygous deletion of the mouse β^{major} and β^{minor} globin genes on one allele are commonly used as a model of thalassemia,[12] and have a phenotype that resembles thalassemia intermedia with moderate anemia (hemoglobin [Hb] 8–10 gm/dL), allowing survival to adulthood. Homozygous deletion of the murine β-globin genes is lethal at embryonic days 14.5–15 due to a switch from embryonic mouse globin expression to adult β^{major} and β^{minor} globin expression when hematopoiesis is confined to fetal liver. When the fetal liver cells from E14.5 embryos are transplanted into lethally irradiated normal mice, the mice engraft with fetal liver HSC and develop severe anemia [Hb of 2–3 g/dL], like humans with Cooley's anemia, and die within 6 weeks. Genetic correction of the fetal liver HSC, using the same hβ vector developed by the Sadelain group that corrected thalassemia intermedia phenotype, also rescued lethality in this model; an average 4 gm/dL increase in Hb. Notable in their experiments was the variable correction among the different mice, showing that position effects play a significant role in therapeutic correction of Cooley's anemia phenotype.[13]

Subsequently several groups have shown correction in the thalassemia intermedia mouse model: Imren and colleagues showed correction of thalassemia intermedia used a LV vector with a mutated hβ ($h\beta^{T87Q}$) that also has antisickling properties.[14] Emery and colleagues used a hγ and the smaller α-globin enhancer (HS-40) in a RV vector along with the chicken hypersensitivity site (cHS4) insulator element, and showed 5–45% hγ-expressing RBC in the thalassemia intermedia mouse model.[15] Persons and colleagues, showed that level of expression of a γ-globin transgene delivered by a LV vector corrected thalassemia intermedia phenotype in mice, but expression was dependent on the site of vector integration and copy number.[16] Taken together, these studies underscore the variable expression due to position effects, despite inclusion of the LCR.

We showed the first evidence of effective genetic correction of human Cooley's anemia using an *in vitro* and an *in vivo* xenograft model of human erythropoiesis with a cHS4 insulated β-globin LV vector, BG-I. The BG-I vector was used to transduce $CD34^+$ cells from four patients with thalassemia major, of which three of four patients had β° thalassemia major.[17] There was reversal of ineffective erythropoiesis and effective RBC production. Genetically modified thalassemia major $CD34^+$ cells were transplanted into splenectomized $\beta 2M^{null}$-NOD-SCID mice, and 3–4 months later, effective production of human glycophorin A expressing erythroid cells were observed in circulation.[17] Miccio and colleagues showed hβ gene with a minimal 2.7 Kb HS2 and HS-3 fragment could produce efficacious amounts of hβ protein. Importantly, they demonstrated a selective advantage to erythroid progenitors and their expansion in mice.[18]

In attempts to improve expression to correct Cooley's anemia, Lisowski and colleagues from the Sadelain lab showed that the addition of HS1 of the LCR in the LV vector did not improve hβ expression, but the addition of HS4 in addition to HS2 and HS3 improved the expression from 27% to 41% per vector copy.[19] Persons and colleagues showed that use of a larger LCR fragment could improve overall expression of hγ protein.[20]

Our group subsequently showed that the cHS4 insulator element flanking hβ/LCR contributes to

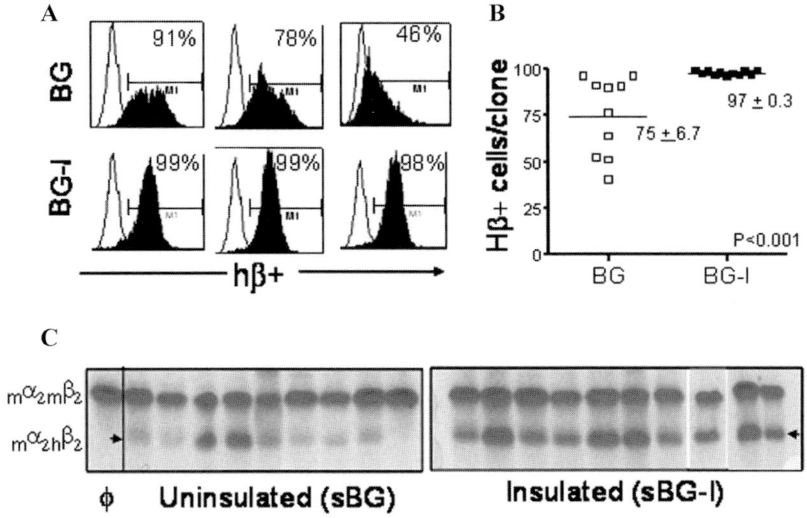

Figure 1. Insulated β-globin LV vectors express at a uniform level in MEL cell clones and in the thalassemia intermedia mouse model. (A) MEL cells were transduced with the insulated β-globin vector (BG-I) or the same vector without the insulator (BG). Single copy clones were screened by PCR and qPCR, differentiated and analyzed for human β-globin (hβ) expression by FACS. FACS histograms of three representative BG and BG-I MEL clones are shown. (B) Cumulative data on the proportion of hβ expressing MEL cells from in clones derived from BG (open square) or BG-I (filled squares) transduced cells. Each symbol represents one clone carrying one proviral integrant. (C) Thalassemia mice were transplanted with Lineage (−), Sca (+), Kit (+) primitive progenitor cells transduced with uninsulated or insulated β-globin vectors and expression of hβ (tetramers of murine α and human β-globin) were analyzed by electrophoresis. Consistent levels of hβ-expression were seen by flanking the β-globin gene with the cHS4 insulator element.

reduced the variability of transgene expression, thus protecting the provirus from chromosomal position effects, resulting in an overall two to fourfold higher expression.[8] The effect of insulated versus uninsulated β-globin LV vectors in mouse erythroleukemia (MEL) cell clones and in thalassemia intermedia mice is shown in Figure 1. The uniform, and therefore, overall higher expression from insulated vectors corrects the human Cooley's anemia phenotype.[17]

The β^{87} LV vector developed by Leboulch and colleagues is now in a clinical trial in France for the treatment of sickle cell anemia and thalassemia. One patient with hemoglobin E-β° thalassemia transplanted with $h\beta^{87}$-modified CD34^{+} hematopoietic cells has become transfusion independent (American Society of Gene Therapy Meeting, oral presentation, 2009). Of note, this transfusion dependence has occurred at the expense of a dominant integrant that is contributing approximately 85% of the β^{87} globin. The LV is integrated in the HMGA2 gene intron in this clone, resulting in dysregulation of HMGA2, although the expression of β^{87} globin is unaltered. So far, this "clonal dominance" seen at a molecular level has not caused any adverse event, and has been beneficial to the patient.[21]

Of the newer technologies in development, Ye and colleagues produced human iPS cells from skin fibroblasts of patients with thalassemia major, and concominantly showed that human iPS cells could be also be made from amniotic fluid cells and chorionic villus cells sampled for prenatal diagnostic for genetic and chromosomal disorders in the fetus.[2] This proof of principle study opens the door for possible prenatal production of iPS cells as a source for autologous HSC for gene therapy and transplantation in the early neonatal period.

Gene therapy for sickle cell disease

The strategy for gene therapy for sickle cell disease (SCD) is more complex, since it relies on production of an anti-polymerization globin in a cell producing a full complement of globin chains. The well known natural models for this antipolymerization effect are that patients with SCD are typically asymptomatic in the first 6 months of life when circulating sickle RBC have high amounts of fetal hemoglobin (Hb F), and patients with SCD and hereditary persistence of fetal hemoglobin have amelioration of disease. Both the naturally occurring Hb F and modified antisickling β-globins have been studied in the context of gene therapy for SCD.

Humanized murine models that result in murine RBC with human hemoglobin, that have been used for this purpose are the Berkeley sickle mice developed by Patszy and colleagues,[22] and the knockout transgenic (KO-TG) sickle mice developed by the Tim Townes group.[23–24] Gene transfer experiments are done by transplanting gene modified murine sickle stem/progenitor cells into lethally irradiated normal mice, since sickle mice do not tolerate myeloablative irradiation. Transplant of unmodified HSC (mock controls) would convert a normal mouse to a sickle mouse following engraftment while genetic correction would correct the SCD phenotype.

To circumvent the problem of low hγ expression in adult/postnatal RBC, synthetic antisickling β-globins (β^{T87Q}, β^{AS3}) were designed by the Leboulch and Townes groups, respectively, which prevent contacts between β-sickle (β^S) globin and α-globin, thus preventing polymer formation.[25–27] Pawliuk and colleagues showed correction of humanized Berkeley sickle mice with delivery of β^{T87Q} LV vector.[28] Levasseur and colleagues, showed correction of the KO-TG sickle mice using a highly HSC enriched population [Lineage(−) Sca(+), c-Kit(+) cells] and showed that expression of 20–25% $h\beta^{AS3}$ could completely correct SCD in primary and secondary mice.[23] The $h\beta^{AS3}$ globin carries three mutations and is functionally more potent than β^{T87Q} globin; and as potent as hγ in inhibiting sickle polymer formation. In an attempt to reduce $h\beta^S$ concomitantly, Samakoglu and colleagues expressed hγ with a small hairpin RNA targeting $h\beta^S$ mRNA via a LV. There was reduction in $h\beta^S$ mRNA along with increased expression of hγ mRNA in human CD34 cell erythroid progeny.[29] This approach was effective, although the findings need confirmation with protein expression and *in vivo* models, the latter necessary to assess the toxicity of shRNA vectors. Subsequently, our group[9] and that of Persons[30] showed genetic correction of SCD by expressing hγ globin, using the same approach.

Requirements for successful genetic correction

While the above approaches have yielded elegant proof-of-concept data, major concerns for current models have been (i) using a "disease prevention" model, attained by transplantation of genetically corrected or uncorrected progenitors into myeloablated "normal" mice, and (ii) lack of disease sequelae/organ pathology in recipient mice. (iii) complete donor chimerism with myeloablative regiments results in a high chimerism in gene corrected HSC in mice, findings that are not practically achieved in humans. Indeed, it has taken two decades of multiple clinical trials in ADA-SCID before critical determinants for successful correction were defined. Therefore, there is a strong need for assessing requirements for successful correction of the disease in humans using carefully designed animal models, after initial proof of concept studies.

To examine the minimal proportion of gene corrected long-term repopulating cells necessary to causer repopulation of genetically corrected RBC and ameliorate SCD phenotype, we transplanted varying doses of gene transduced Berkeley sickle HSC into Berkeley sickle recipients exposed to nonmyeloablative, conditioning. We have used a modified hβ LV vector, where the exons of hβ are replaced by hγ exons, but the introns, promoter, and 3′ and 5′ untranslated regions are those of hβ-globin gene. A careful quantification of the hematological correction, functional correction (degree of sickling, RBC half life, and deformability) and correction of organ pathology showed that if genetically modified HSC comprise 20% of more of the repopulated donor marrow, the total Hb F produced is greater than 10%, there are at least 60% Hb F containing RBC (F cells) and the Hb F per F cell is 30% of the total globin in the RBC, it results in effective and successful correction of SCD in the Berkeley mice[9] (illustrated in Fig. 2). More importantly, we could achieve this with nonmyeloablative conditioning in this model, suggesting the same could be tried in human trials initially.

Newer modalities that are upcoming are the gene correction approach with homologous recombination.[24] Hanna and colleagues generated iPS cells from the "knock-in" mouse tail fibroblasts, performed homologous recombination and selected corrected clones, and differentiated them into HSC *in vitro* via gene transfer of the HoxB4 transcription factor. HSC developed from murine iPS cells were transplanted into lethally irradiated normal mice and resulted in normal erythropoiesis and correction SCD.[31] The pluripotency and unlimited growth potential of iPS cells can potentially overcome inefficient gene delivery by homologous recombination, allowing the ability to screen specific

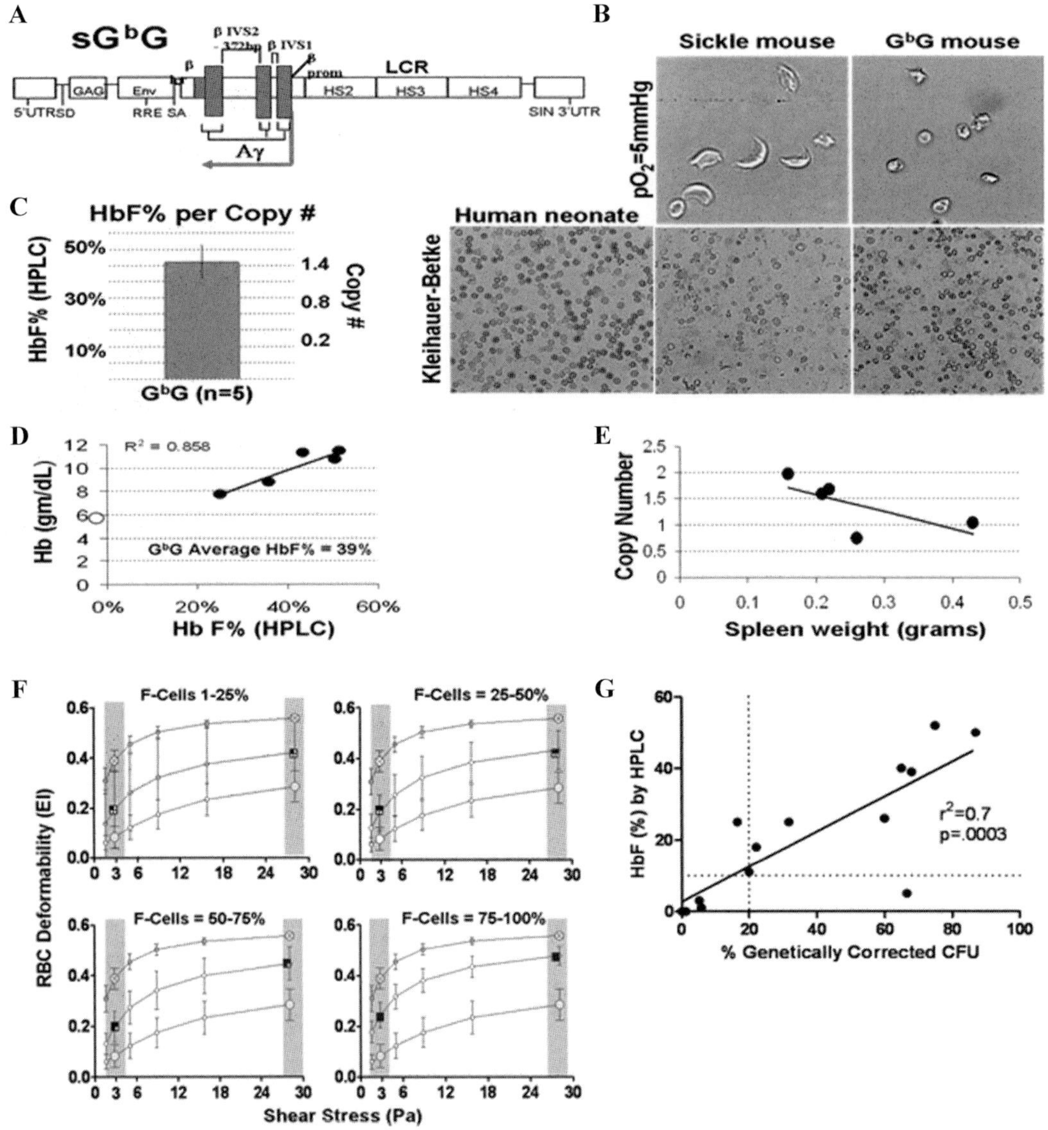

Figure 2. Critical determinants required for correction of SCD in Berkeley sickle mice. (A) sGbG vector encodes Aγ-globin exons, β-globin promoter and introns, and HS2, HS3, and HS4 elements of the LCR. (B) Top panels show that GbG mice (sickle mice transplanted with sG^bG genetically modified HSC) RBC are more resistant to hypoxia induced sickling than "mock" transplanted sickle mice, labeled sickle mouse. The bottom panel shows Hb F expression of GbG mice peripheral blood, as demonstrated by the Kleihauer–Betke assay. GbG mice show high Hb F expression with relatively low copies of transgene (C), increasing hemoglobin with increases in Hb F expression (D), and reduction of extramedullary hematopoiesis as demonstrated by reduced spleen size with increasing copies of transgene (E). (F) Peripheral blood from sickle mice was exposed to shear stress and RBC deformability was measured using laser assisted optical rotational cell analyzer (LORCA). GbG mice showed significant improvements in RBC deformability at low and high shear pressures as F-cells increased. Circle with "x" depicts wildtype mice, open circle depicts mock transplanted sickle mice, and dark box depicts GhG corrected sickle mice. Shaded areas depict low (3Pa) and high (27Pa) shear stress, representing flow through small angle vessels, respectively. (G) CFU-S assay was performed on GbG mice 6–11.5 months of following transplant, showing that when the proportion of GbG modified HSC were roughly 18–20%, the percentage of Hb F was greater than 10%. This level of chimerism and Hb F correlated with improved hematological and functional parameters of SCD and improved survival (data not shown).

clones with genetic correction. Moreover, iPS cells would be more readily available and be free of the ethical concerns associated with ES cells. Human ES cells, differentiated *in vitro* into hematopoietic cells, only give rise to erythroid cells producing embryonic and fetal globins.[32] Proof-of-concept studies on human iPSC and their differentiation into hematopoietic cells has been shown *in vitro*, but these cells are not transplantable.[33] Transplantable HSC that contribute to definitive erythropoiesis are needed, and this area is under active investigation. These approaches are novel and exciting, but are farther away from translation into the clinic. Much work needs to be done to show their safety and feasibility for human use.

Safety of LV vectors for β-globinopathies

Safety of gene therapy is of paramount importance for additive gene therapy with randomly integrating vectors. Of particular concern are gains of function in the form of (1) insertional activation of oncogenes, or (2) dysregulation of gene expression resulting in increased/unregulated target cell proliferation. Loss of function resulting from disruption of a cellular tumor suppressor gene that results in loss of heterozygosity could also potentially occur.

The potential for leukemogenesis with gene therapy has been shown to be more than a hypothetical risk by the development of T-cell leukemia in five of twenty patients in the French and British human gene therapy clinical trials for X-linked severe combined immunodeficiency (X-SCID), and myelodysplastic syndrome in two of two subjects in the clinical gene transfer trial for CGD,[6] using gamma-retroviral vectors. In both trials, there was insertional activation of surrounding cellular protooncogenes by the viral long terminal repeat (LTR) enhancer. Strangely, no such predilection was observed in the gene transfer trial for adenosine deaminase deficiency performed using a similar retroviral vector despite a similar duration of follow up.[2] The adverse events from the X-SCID and CGD trials has prompted deeper investigations into vector genotoxicity and shown that presence of ubiquitous enhancers in viral vectors are not be desirable. Experimentally, self-inactivating LV and RV vectors containing internal promoters/enhancers show reduced genotoxicity, although strong ubiquitously active enhancers can dysregulate genes independent of vector type/design.[34]

Genotoxicity of the locus control region in globin vectors

Imren and colleagues showed integration of LCR-containing hβ-globin LV vector near putative oncogenes in primary human cells,[35] although expression of the proto-oncogenes was not analyzed in their study. Recently, some global perturbation of gene expression in colony forming units-spleen (CFU-S) with the LCR driven LV was reported in microarray analysis.[36] It was also reported that the chicken β-globin hypersensitive site-4 (cHS4) insulator in RV results in reduced perturbation of gene expression in microarray analysis.[37]

The LCR is a strong long-range lineage-specific-enhancer, that has been shown to be in an active chromatin configuration prior to erythroid lineage commitment in multipotent HSC.[38] We therefore explored the genotoxicity of β-globin LCR, with/without insulator elements using primary murine hematopoietic progenitors to generate *in vitro* immortalization assay mutant clones.[39] LCR-containing LV vectors had approximately 200-fold lower transforming potential when compared to the conventional RV vectors with intact LTRs (Fig. 3). The LCR perturbed expression of a few genes in a 300Kb proviral vicinity, although no upregulation of genes associated with cancer, including an erythroid-specific transcription factor occurred. A further two- to three-fold reduction in transforming activity was observed with insulated LCR-containing LV vectors. It is to be noted these results from mock transduced lineage negative progenitors, and those transduced with vectors carrying the hβ promoter but no LCR did not transform any lineage negative progenitors clearly demonstrated that the low level of transforming potential was due to the LCR enhancer. It also showed the robustness and sensitivity of the *in vitro* immortalization assay. *In vivo* models for vector induced leukemias at best generate tumors in one in ten mice, when studied long-term in secondary transplants. Our data suggest that thousands of mice would be required to demonstrate genotoxicity *in vivo* with self-inactivating erythroid lineage specific vectors.[39]

Preliminary results from the first trial on gene therapy for thalassemia and SCD by Leboulch and colleagues were presented at the American Society

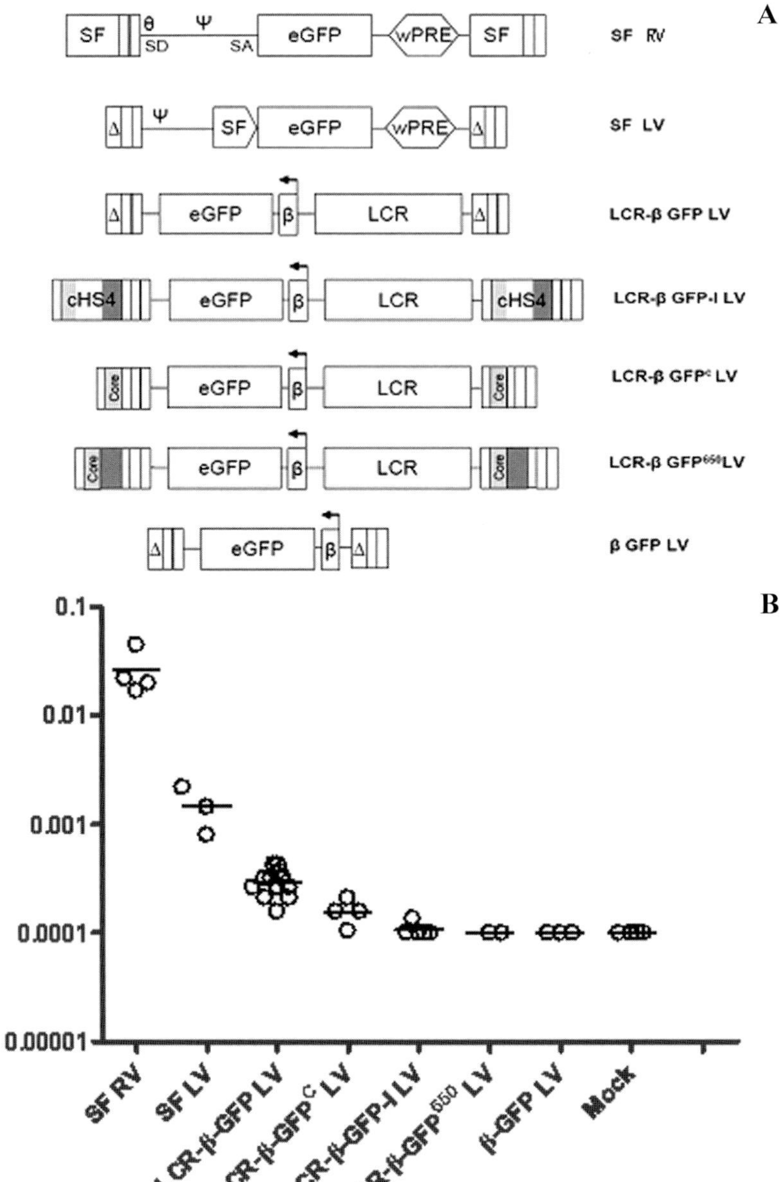

Figure 3. The relative transforming capability of LCR-containing LV vectors in the *in vitro* immortalization assay using primary murine lineage negative progenitor cells. (A) Vector maps. SFFV LTR (SF) driven retroviral vector (SF RV) was the positive control for a genotoxic vector. The SFFV promoter enhancer was also placed internally in a self inactivating lentivirus vector (SF LV) as a second positive control. The LCR enhancer and **β** globin-promoter containing LV encoded eGFP (LCR-**β**-GFP) was flanked by different lengths of the cHS4 insulator—the insulator core (LCR-**β**-GFP^{C}), full length insulator (LCR-**β**-GFP-I), or the core combined with the 3′ 400 bp region (LCR-**β**-GFP^{650}). A vector without the LCR enhancer (**β**-GFP) and mock were negative controls. (B) Frequency of generation of *in vitro* immortalized mutant (IVIM) clones from lineage-negative primary murine hematopoietic cells scored at 2 weeks (actual replating frequency)[39] per vector copy for each vector is shown. The replating frequency of the LCR-**β**-GFP vector was extremely low, and significantly lower than the SF RV ($P < 0.001$) and SF LV ($P < 0.01$). The replating frequency of the insulated vectors was lower than the uninsulated LCR-**β**-GFP vector ($P < 0.05$). No IVIM clones were derived in mock or enhancerless (**β**-GFP) vector.

of Gene Therapy annual meeting 2009. One patient with hemoglobin E-ß^0-thalassemia was given with genetically modified CD34$^+$ cells (using the hβ^{T87Q} LV vector) in June 2007 demonstrated long-term gene marked cells and the therapeutic benefit of becoming transfusion independent. Integration analysis revealed a dominant clone with integration within the HMGA2 gene detected in myeloid and erythroid cells, but not lymphoid cells (NIH Office of Biotechnology Activities, News and events, Recombinant DNA news, June 15, 2009 based on a press release by French Health Products Safety Agency (Agence Française de Sécurité Sanitaire des Produits de Santé; AFSSAPS). The HMGA2 gene expression is increased in the erythroid cells, but not the myeloid cells, showing dysregulation of this gene by the LCR in the erythroid lineage. This clone has resulted in a net increase in the patient's fetal hemoglobin and the vector-derived β^{87} globin, resulting in transfusion independence. Therefore, this insertional dysregulation has resulted in a clinical benefit and cure of the disease. However, this is also the first clinical evidence of the emergence of a dominant cell population in a human clinical trial with LV vectors, and whether this clinically beneficial effect of this clonal dominance is sustainable long-term remains to be seen. In the meanwhile, the AFSSAPS has allowed the trial to accrue more patients.[21]

Conclusion

Gene therapy for Cooley's anemia and SCD hold much promise for the future. Correction and cure has been well established in murine models and human models of the disease with HIV-1 based LV vectors. A good estimate of "what it will take to cure these diseases," has now been assessed in the first decade of the 21st century. The current limitations for genetic correction are vector production, efficient gene delivery into a high proportion of engraftable HSC, which would be curative in the human setting. Long-term safety needs to be established in clinical trials. Currently clinical trials are being developed by several laboratories that have performed correction in animal models and a clinical trial is underway in France by Leboulch and colleagues. As progress is made in these areas, gene therapy will live up to its promise of curing the most common monogenic diseases in the world.

Conflicts of interest

The authors declare no conflicts of interest.

References

1. Kauf, T.L., T.D. Coates, L. Huazhi, *et al.* 2009. The cost of health care for children and adults with sickle cell disease. *Am. J. Hematol.* **84:** 323–327.
2. Aiuti, A. *et al.* 2009. Gene therapy for immunodeficiency due to adenosine deaminase deficiency. *N. Engl. J. Med.* **360:** 447–458.
3. Hacein-Bey-Abina, S. *et al.* 2003. LMO2-associated clonal T cell proliferation in two patients after gene therapy for SCID-X1. *Science (New York, N.Y.)* **302:** 415–419.
4. Hacein-Bey-Abina, S. *et al.* 2008. Insertional oncogenesis in 4 patients after retrovirus-mediated gene therapy of SCID-X1. *J. Clin. Invest.* **118:** 3132–3142.
5. Gaspar, H.B. *et al.* 2004. Gene therapy of X-linked severe combined immunodeficiency by use of a pseudotyped gammaretroviral vector. *Lancet* **364:** 2181–2187.
6. Ott, M.G. *et al.* 2006. Correction of X-linked chronic granulomatous disease by gene therapy, augmented by insertional activation of MDS1-EVI1, PRDM16 or SETBP1. *Nat. Med.* **12:** 401–409.
7. Mohamedali, A. *et al.* 2004. Self-inactivating lentiviral vectors resist proviral methylation but do not confer position-independent expression in hematopoietic stem cells. *Mol. Ther.* **10:** 249–259.
8. Arumugam, P.I. *et al.* 2007. Improved human beta-globin expression from self-inactivating lentiviral vectors carrying the chicken hypersensitive site-4 (cHS4) insulator element. *Mol. Ther.* **15:** 1863–1871.
9. Perumbeti, A. *et al.* 2009. A novel human gamma-globin gene vector for genetic correction of sickle cell anemia in a humanized sickle mouse model: critical determinants for successful correction. *Blood* **114:** 1174–1185.
10. Challita, P.M. & D.B. Kohn. 1994. Lack of expression from a retroviral vector after transduction of murine hematopoietic stem cells is associated with methylation in vivo. *Proc. Natl. Acad. Sci. USA* **91:** 2567–2571.
11. Stein, S. *et al.* 2010. Genomic instability and myelodysplasia with monosomy 7 consequent to EVI1 activation after gene therapy for chronic granulomatous disease. *Nat. Med.* **16:** 198–204.
12. Ciavatta, D.J., T.M. Ryan, S.C. Farmer & T.M. Townes. 1995. Mouse model of human beta zero thalassemia: targeted deletion of the mouse beta maj- and beta min-globin genes in embryonic stem cells. *Proc. Natl. Acad. Sci. USA* **92:** 9259–9263.
13. Rivella, S., C. May, A. Chadburn, *et al.* 2003. A novel murine model of Cooley anemia and its rescue by lentiviral-mediated human beta-globin gene transfer. *Blood* **101:** 2932–2939.
14. Imren, S. *et al.* 2002. Permanent and panerythroid correction of murine beta thalassemia by multiple lentiviral integration in hematopoietic stem cells. *Proc. Natl. Acad. Sci. USA* **99:** 14380–14385.
15. Emery, D.W. *et al.* 2002. Development of virus vectors for gene therapy of beta chain hemoglobinopathies: flanking

with a chromatin insulator reduces gamma-globin gene silencing in vivo. *Blood* **100:** 2012–2019.
16. Persons, D.A., P.W. Hargrove, Allay, E.R., *et al.* 2003. The degree of phenotypic correction of murine beta-thalassemia intermedia following lentiviral-mediated transfer of a human gamma-globin gene is influenced by chromosomal position effects and vector copy number. *Blood* **101:** 2175–2183.
17. Puthenveetil, G. *et al.* 2004. Successful correction of the human beta-thalassemia major phenotype using a lentiviral vector. *Blood* **104:** 3445–3453.
18. Miccio, A. *et al.* 2008. In vivo selection of genetically modified erythroblastic progenitors leads to long-term correction of beta-thalassemia. *Proc. Natl. Acad. Sci. USA* **105:** 10547–10552.
19. Lisowski, L. & M. Sadelain. 2007. Locus control region elements HS1 and HS4 enhance the therapeutic efficacy of globin gene transfer in beta-thalassemic mice. *Blood* **110:** 4175–4178.
20. Hanawa, H. *et al.* 2004. Extended beta-globin locus control region elements promote consistent therapeutic expression of a gamma-globin lentiviral vector in murine beta-thalassemia. *Blood* **104:** 2281–2290.
21. Kaiser, J. 2009. Gene therapy. Beta-thalassemia treatment succeeds, with a caveat. *Science (New York, N.Y.)* **326:** 1468–1469.
22. Paszty, C. *et al.* 1997. Transgenic knockout mice with exclusively human sickle hemoglobin and sickle cell disease. *Science (New York, N.Y.)* **278:** 876–878.
23. Levasseur, D.N., T.M. Ryan, K.M. Pawlik & T.M. Townes. 2003. Correction of a mouse model of sickle cell disease: lentiviral/antisickling beta-globin gene transduction of unmobilized, purified hematopoietic stem cells. *Blood* **102:** 4312–4319.
24. Wu, L.C. *et al.* 2006. Correction of sickle cell disease by homologous recombination in embryonic stem cells. *Blood* **108:** 1183–1188.
25. McCune, S.L., M.P. Reilly, M.J. Chomo, *et al.* 1994. Recombinant human hemoglobins designed for gene therapy of sickle cell disease. *Proc. Natl. Acad. Sci. USA* **91:** 9852–9856.
26. Levasseur, D.N. *et al.* 2004. A recombinant human hemoglobin with anti-sickling properties greater than fetal hemoglobin. *J. Biol. Chem.* **279:** 27518–27524.
27. Oh, I.H., A. Lau & C.J. Eaves. 2000. During ontogeny primitive ($CD34^{(+)}CD38^{(-)}$) hematopoietic cells show altered expression of a subset of genes associated with early cytokine and differentiation responses of their adult counterparts. *Blood* **96:** 4160–4168.
28. Pawliuk, R. *et al.* 2001. Correction of sickle cell disease in transgenic mouse models by gene therapy. *Science (New York, N.Y.)* **294:** 2368–2371.
29. Samakoglu, S. *et al.* 2006. A genetic strategy to treat sickle cell anemia by coregulating globin transgene expression and RNA interference. *Nat. Biotechnol.* **24:** 89–94.
30. Pestina, T.I. *et al.* 2009. Correction of murine sickle cell disease using gamma-globin lentiviral vectors to mediate high-level expression of fetal hemoglobin. *Mol. Ther.* **17:** 245–252.
31. Hanna, J. *et al.* 2007. Treatment of sickle cell anemia mouse model with iPS cells generated from autologous skin. *Science (New York, N.Y.)* **318:** 1920–1923.
32. Qiu, C., E.N. Olivier, M. Velho & E.E. Bouhassira. 2008. Globin switches in yolk sac-like primitive and fetal-like definitive red blood cells produced from human embryonic stem cells. *Blood* **111:** 2400–2408.
33. Lengerke, C. *et al.* 2009. Hematopoietic development from human induced pluripotent stem cells. *Ann. N.Y. Acad. Sci.* **1176:** 219–227.
34. Maruggi, G. *et al.* 2009. Transcriptional enhancers induce insertional gene deregulation independently from the vector type and design. *Mol. Ther.* **17:** 851–856.
35. Imren, S. *et al.* 2004. High-level beta-globin expression and preferred intragenic integration after lentiviral transduction of human cord blood stem cells. *J. Clin. Invest.* **114:** 953–962.
36. Hargrove, P.W. *et al.* 2008. Globin lentiviral vector insertions can perturb the expression of endogenous genes in beta-thalassemic hematopoietic cells. *Mol. Ther.* **16:** 525–533.
37. Li, C.L., D. Xiong, G. Stamatoyannopoulos & D.W. Emery. 2009. Genomic and functional assays demonstrate reduced gammaretroviral vector genotoxicity associated with use of the cHS4 chromatin insulator. *Mol. Ther.* **17:** 716–724.
38. Jimenez, G., S.D. Griffiths, A.M. Ford, *et al.* 1992. Activation of the beta-globin locus control region precedes commitment to the erythroid lineage. *Proc. Natl. Acad. Sci. USA* **89:** 10618–10622.
39. Arumugam, P.I. *et al.* 2009. Genotoxic potential of lineage-specific lentivirus vectors carrying the beta-Globin locus control region. *Mol. Ther.* **17:** 1929–1937.

Ann. N.Y. Acad. Sci. ISSN 0077-8923

ANNALS OF THE NEW YORK ACADEMY OF SCIENCES
Issue: *Cooley's Anemia: Ninth Symposium*

Humanized mouse models of Cooley's anemia: correct fetal-to-adult hemoglobin switching, disease onset, and disease pathology

Yongliang Huo, Sean C. McConnell, Shanrun Liu, Tingting Zhang, Rui Yang, Jinxiang Ren, and Thomas M. Ryan
Department of Biochemistry and Molecular Genetics, University of Alabama at Birmingham, Birmingham, Alabama

Address for correspondence: Thomas M. Ryan, PhD, Department of Biochemistry and Molecular Genetics, University of Alabama at Birmingham, 1918 University Building, MCLM 566A, Birmingham, AL 35294. tryan@uab.edu

β thalassemia major or Cooley's Anemia (CA) has been difficult to model in mice due to their lack of a fetal hemoglobin gene equivalent. This summary describes novel preclinical humanized mouse models of CA that survive on human fetal hemoglobin at birth and are blood-transfusion dependent for life upon completion of their human fetal-to-adult hemoglobin switch after birth. These CA models are the first to recapitulate the temporal onset of the disease in human patients. These novel humanized CA disease models are useful for the study of the regulation of globin gene expression, synthesis, and switching; examining the onset of disease pathology; development of transfusion and iron chelation therapies; induction of fetal hemoglobin synthesis; and the testing of novel genetic and cell-based therapies for the correction of thalassemia.

Keywords: thalassemia; HPFH; transfusion; mouse model; hemoglobin switching

Introduction

Hemoglobin is a tetramer consisting of two α globin chains and two β globin chains. Thalassemia is caused by an imbalance in α and β globin chain production. The most severe form of β thalassemia, β-thalassemia major or Cooley's Anemia (CA), is caused by complete absence of the adult β globin chains. Newborn CA patients are initially healthy due to high levels of fetal hemoglobin but develop severe anemia upon completion of their fetal to adult hemoglobin switch at about 1 year of age.[1,2] In a futile response to correct their anemia, CA patients expand the production of short-lived thalassemic erythroid progenitors in their bone marrow in a process termed ineffective erythropoiesis.[3] For survival into adulthood, CA patients require lifelong regular blood transfusion.[4] A preclinical CA animal model that more closely mimics the developmental onset and disease pathology of thalassemia in humans will greatly facilitate the study of CA.

Modeling human hemoglobin disorders in mice is complicated by the fact that mice do not have a true fetal hemoglobin. Both humans and mice change the type of α and β globin chains produced in the blood during development.[2,5,6] This hemoglobin switching occurs in two distinct cell types. The first type, the primitive erythroid cell, arises early in development in the yolk sac blood islands. These primitive erythroid cells are large, nucleated, and synthesize embryonic globin chains. The second type termed definitive erythroid cell arises when erythropoiesis shifts to the fetal liver. Definitive erythroid cells are smaller, enucleated, and synthesize predominantly adult (mouse) or fetal (humans) globin chains. When definitive erythropoiesis shifts to the bone marrow after birth, mice continue to express the same adult globin genes synthesized during fetal development, but human definitive erythroid cells undergo a fetal to adult hemoglobin switch.

Murine models of β thalassemia have been made by deleting the adult mouse β goblin genes or replacing the adult mouse β globin genes with

doi: 10.1111/j.1749-6632.2010.05547.x

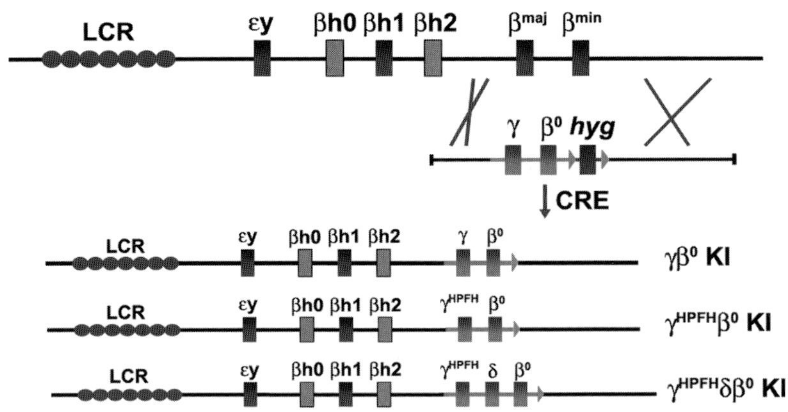

Figure 1. Gene-targeting strategy in ES cells used to replace the adult mouse β globin genes with human globin genes in the mouse β globin locus. Top line represents the wild-type mouse β globin locus. A single-targeting vector is drawn below the locus illustrating homologous recombination between 5′ and 3′ mouse homology regions. After removal of the hygromycin marker gene (hyg) by recombinase (CRE), the resulting human globin gene KI alleles are shown. Locus control region (LCR) represented by blue ovals, functional mouse embryonic genes (εy and βh1), and adult genes (β^{maj} and β^{min}) represented by blue boxes, mouse pseudogenes drawn as gray boxes, human genes are red boxes, hygromycin marker gene is brown box, loxP sites are green triangles.

nonfunctional human β globin transgenes.[7–12] Because murine fetal liver definitive erythropoiesis requires adult β globin gene expression, all of these mice die *in utero* when homozygous for the adult mouse β globin genes deletion. Mice have no fetal hemoglobin equivalent to sustain definitive erythropoiesis in the absence of their adult globin genes. Furthermore, attempts to produce mice that express high levels of human fetal hemoglobin in definitive erythroid cells by introducing human cosmid, BAC, or YAC transgenes that encompass the entire human β globin locus has been largely unsuccessful.[13–17] The human γ globin transgene expression in these models is predominantly confined to the primitive erythroid cells.[18–20] Modified human transgenes that contain the locus control region linked directly to human γ and β globin genes with much of the intergenic sequence deleted have been successful in producing human γ globin gene expression in definitive erythroid cells.[21,22] Indeed, such a delayed fetal to adult hemoglobin-switching transgene was important for the generation of a mouse model of sickle cell disease.[21] Recently, our group has used a delayed fetal to adult hemoglobin-switching cassette to generate murine models of CA that more faithfully recapitulate the hemoglobin switch that occurs in humans.[18,19]

The ideal mouse model of CA should have the following characteristics: express only human hemoglobin in their red blood cells (RBCs), complete the human γ to β globin gene switch after birth, synthesize no functional adult β globin chains in RBCs, require regular blood transfusions for life, and be genetically heritable. Recently, our group has made a series of humanized CA mouse models that have all of these qualities by targeted gene replacement of the adult mouse α and β globin genes with human α and $\gamma\beta^{\circ}$ globin genes in mouse embryonic stem (ES) cells.[18,19] Each model synthesizes high levels of human fetal hemoglobin at birth, but becomes severely anemic upon completion of their hemoglobin switch to a nonfunctional human β° globin allele after birth. Humanized CA mice exhibit increasing ineffective erythropoiesis and expire in the absence of life sustaining blood transfusions. These humanized CA mouse models will be useful for the study of the mechanism of human hemoglobin switching, examining the onset of disease pathology, developing novel methods for regulating iron toxicity, and for the testing of novel cellular and genetic therapies for the cure of CA.

Production of humanized mouse models of Cooley's Anemia

β thalassemia major in mouse models generated by deletion of the adult β globin genes results in early fetal death because the mouse does not have a fetal globin gene equivalent. We hypothesized that replacement of the mouse adult β globin genes with a human fetal to adult hemoglobin-switching cassette would produce animals with high levels of

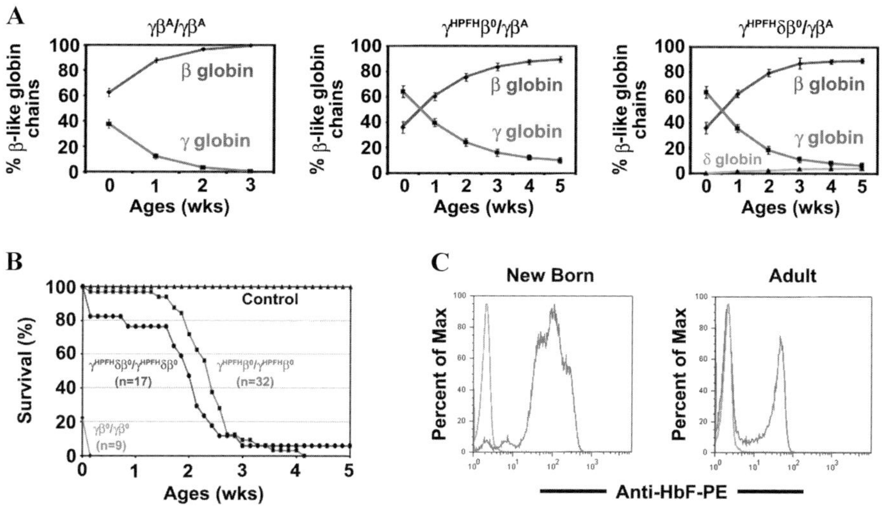

Figure 2. HPFH mutations modulate the human γ globin levels in CA mice. (A) Total β-like globin chains in peripheral blood hemolysates of humanized newborn to 5-week-old mice were separated by HPLC and quantified. High fetal γ globin levels at birth are replaced by adult β globin as the hemoglobin switch is completed after birth. Genotype of each humanized KI mouse shown at the top of each figure. Fetal γ globin chains shown in red, adult β globin in blue, and adult δ globin in orange. Values represent mean ± SEM. $n \geq 9$ at each time point. (B) Survival curves of humanized CA mice. The percentage of mice alive for each genotype is plotted with age. The few humanized γβ° KI CA mice that survive to birth die within the first 24 h. Incorporation of the HPFH mutation in the human γ globin gene promoter in CA mice results in 100% survival to birth and an average lifespan of 14 and 15 days for the $\gamma^{HPFH}\delta\beta^{\circ}$ and $\gamma^{HPFH}\beta^{\circ}$ CA mice, respectively. (C) F-cell distribution in newborn and adult heterozygous $\gamma^{HPFH}\beta^{\circ}/\gamma\beta^{A}$ KI mice. Peripheral mouse blood was fixed and stained with anti-human fetal hemoglobin monoclonal antibody and analyzed by flow cytometry. HbF is pancellularly distributed in newborn humanized mice, whereas adult mice have a heterocellular distribution. Green line is wild-type mouse control.

human fetal hemoglobin during fetal life. Using this strategy, we recently reported the production of two humanized mouse models of CA.[18,19] In this summary, we compare these models with an additional CA model. Each of these humanized models was produced by replacing the endogenous adult mouse α and β globin genes with human α and γβ or γδβ globin genes, respectively. Material and methods may be found online in the Supporting Information.

Figure 1 illustrates the gene-targeting strategy whereby human β-like globin genes were knocked into (KI) the murine β globin locus simultaneously deleting the adult murine β globin genes in ES cells. All three CA models have a nonfunctional human β° globin KI allele that contains a splice donor site mutation in the first base of intron 1 (IVS 1.1 G to A) that results in the production of no functional β globin chains.[19,23] The γβ° KI model contains a wild-type human γ globin promoter, whereas the $\gamma^{HPFH}\beta^{\circ}$ KI and $\gamma^{HPFH}\delta\beta^{\circ}$ KI models have the Greek-type hereditary persistence of fetal hemoglobin (HPFH) mutation in the γ globin gene promoter (−117 G to A).[24] The minor human adult δ globin gene is included in the $\gamma^{HPFH}\delta\beta^{\circ}$ KI model. Mice produced from each of these KI ES cells were bred to human α2α1 globin KI mice (T.M.R., unpublished data) generated by similar methodology to produce humanized CA mice that synthesize solely human hemoglobin in their RBCs.[18,19,25]

Completion of the fetal-to-adult hemoglobin switch after birth extends the postnatal lifespan of humanized CA mice

Humanized γβ KI mice synthesize high levels of fetal hemoglobin during fetal life that persists after birth. In Figure 2A, the human γ, δ, and β globin chain levels in hemolysates of humanized wild-type control ($\gamma\beta^{A}/\gamma\beta^{A}$) and compound heterozygous mice ($\gamma^{HPFH}\beta^{\circ}/\gamma\beta^{A}$ and $\gamma^{HPFH}\delta\beta^{\circ}/\gamma\beta^{A}$) are plotted over time. At birth, there are high levels of fetal hemoglobin in all three types of humanized mice illustrating the delayed hemoglobin switch inherent in the γβ KI cassette. In addition, the humanized mice all complete their fetal to adult hemoglobin switch after birth. Although the γ globin chains in humanized control mice ($\gamma\beta^A/\gamma\beta^A$) decrease to background levels by 3 weeks of age, the fetal chain levels in both the γ^{HPFH} KI mice persist into adulthood. Finally, there is also a fetal (HbF) to minor adult (HbA2) hemoglobin switch that occurs over time in humanized $\gamma^{HPFH}\delta\beta^{\circ}/\gamma\beta^A$ KI mice.[18]

The level of fetal globin chain production and the completion of the fetal to adult hemoglobin switch greatly influence the severity of anemia and the lifespan of humanized CA mice. Figure 2B is a plot of the survival curves for homozygous CA mice. Only 20% of humanized $\gamma\beta^{\circ}/\gamma\beta^{\circ}$ mice survive to birth. These CA mice are extremely pale and die within the first 24 h after birth.[19] In contrast, all humanized CA mice containing the HPFH mutation in the human γ globin gene promoter are alive at birth. As the high fetal hemoglobin levels in these CA mice declines over the first few weeks of life, the majority of the animals die around 2 weeks of age. At birth, virtually 100% of the RBCs in $\gamma\beta$ KI mice contain fetal hemoglobin. This pancellular distribution of HbF at birth is evident by flow cytometry in compound heterozygous $\gamma^{HPFH}\beta^{\circ}/\gamma\beta^A$ KI mice after staining with an anti-HbF antibody in Figure 2C. In adult mice, HbF is distributed heterocellularly being present in less than 50% of the circulating RBCs. All the above data suggest that $\gamma\beta$ globin KI mice synthesize high levels of fetal hemoglobin throughout fetal life and complete their fetal to adult hemoglobin switch after birth similar to humans.

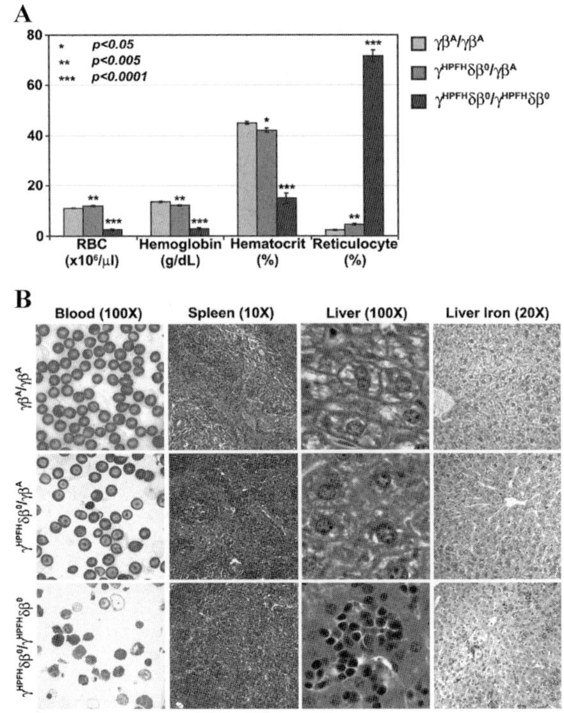

Figure 3. Hematological RBC indices and histopathology of humanized control, heterozygous, and homozygous CA mice. (A) RBC indices of peripheral blood from humanized mice showed a slight but significant anemia in heterozygous CA mice. Homozygous CA mice are severely anemic with marked reductions in RBC, hemoglobin, and hematocrit levels and an extreme reticulocytosis compared to control mice. Humanized control and heterozygous mice were analyzed eight weeks after birth. Moribund homozygous CA mice were analyzed prior to their euthanasia around two weeks of age. Values represent mean ± SEM. $n \geq 9$ for each mouse line. Statistical significances were determined compared to the $\gamma\beta^A/\gamma\beta^A$ control mice. *P* values were calculated by two-tailed unpaired Student's *t*-test. (B) Peripheral blood smear, spleen, and liver sections of humanized control ($\gamma\beta^A/\gamma\beta^A$), heterozygous ($\gamma^{HPFH}\delta\beta^{\circ}/\gamma\beta^A$), and homozygous ($\gamma^{HPFH}\delta\beta^{\circ}/\gamma^{HPFH}\delta\beta^{\circ}$) CA mice. Control mice have normocytic RBCs and typical splenic and hepatic structure. Heterozygous CA mice are slightly thalassemic with frequent RBC targeting, but little erythroid hyperplasia in the spleen or extramedullary hematopoiesis in the liver. Homozygous CA mice have numerous nucleated RBCs and erythroblasts in the peripheral blood, marked erythroid hyperplasia in the spleen and extramedullary hematopoiesis, and extensive iron overload in the liver.

Severe anemia, pathology, and death of humanized CA mice are prevented by serial blood transfusion

Humanized CA mice become severely anemic after birth. Compared to wild-type humanized controls, homozygous $\gamma^{HPFH}\delta\beta^{\circ}$ KI CA mice have marked reductions in their RBC, hemoglobin, and hematocrit levels (Fig. 3A). Homozygous CA mice have a massive reticulocytosis exceeding 70% of peripheral blood cells. Peripheral blood smears show numerous erythroblasts and nucleated RBCs, hypochromic RBCs, and anisopoikilocytosis (Fig. 3B). Heterozygous $\gamma^{HPFH}\delta\beta^{\circ}/\gamma\beta^A$ KI mice also show significant changes in their RBC indices, but are only mildly anemic. The persistent expression of fetal hemoglobin from the HPFH allele results in a much milder anemia compared to heterozygous β globin knockout or human $\gamma\beta^{\circ}$ globin KI mice.[8,18,19]

Histopathological sections of spleen and liver of humanized control ($\gamma\beta^A/\gamma\beta^A$), heterozygous ($\gamma^{HPFH}\delta\beta^{\circ}/\gamma\beta^A$), and homozygous ($\gamma^{HPFH}\delta\beta^{\circ}/\gamma^{HPFH}\delta\beta^{\circ}$) CA mice are shown in Figure 3B.

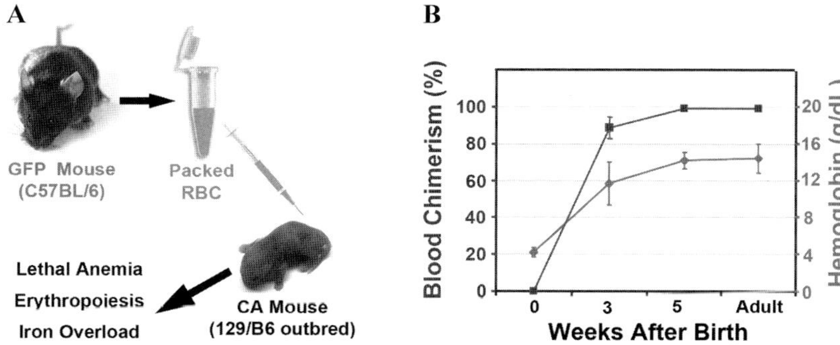

Figure 4. Humanized CA mice can be rescued from lethal anemia by blood transfusion. (A) Blood transfusion scheme for CA mice. Each week fresh peripheral RBCs were collected from GFP transgenic mice, pelleted through Ficoll, washed, resuspended to 70% hematocrit in saline, and transfused into CA mice. (B) Blood chimerism (blue line) and hemoglobin levels (red line) measured over time in transfused CA mice. The donor RBC chimerism was determined by measuring the percentage of GFP^+ RBCs in the peripheral blood by flow cytometry. Hemoglobin concentrations maintained at 14 g/dL efficiently suppressed endogenous erythropoiesis indicated by the virtual absence of GFP negative RBCs in the peripheral blood. Transfused CA mice live into adulthood free of anemia but develop severe iron overload.[18]

The severe anemia in CA mice causes a massive erythroid hyperplasia resulting in splenomegaly characterized by the loss of lymphoid white pulp regions and the expansion of the red pulp with erythroid progenitors. The livers of anemic CA mice have numerous foci of extramedullary erythropoiesis and increased iron deposition. In contrast, the heterozygous $\gamma^{HPFH}\delta\beta^{\circ}/\gamma\beta^{A}$ KI mice show little disease pathology consistent with their slight anemia.

The severe anemia and shortened lifespan of humanized CA mice are similar to human patients with β thalassemia major that do not receive treatment. The average age of death of CA mice is approximately equivalent to a 1- to 2-year-old human. To extend the life of CA mice, we transfused them with packed RBCs from GFP transgenic mice so that the donor RBCs could be tracked *in vivo* (Fig. 4). All the transfused CA mice were rescued from their lethal anemia and survived beyond weaning age. After five weekly transfusions, the endogenous erythropoiesis in the CA mice was effectively suppressed. Over 99% of the peripheral blood was from donor GFP transgenic mice and the hemoglobin level stabilized at 14 g/dL. After eight weeks of transfusion, the experiment was stopped and the CA mice were analyzed. All had marked reductions in spleen size and endogenous erythropoiesis was suppressed.[18] Importantly, the transfused CA mice had increased iron deposition in the liver similar to transfused CA patients.[18]

Summary of improvements in humanized CA mice over previous β thalassemia major mouse models

Successful generation of mice with true fetal hemoglobin during development was achieved by replacement of the adult mouse β globin genes with delayed switching human γβ globin KI cassettes. The definitive erythroid cells produced in these humanized KI mice switch from fetal to adult hemoglobin similar to humans rather than continuously express the endogenous mouse β^{maj} and β^{min} globins throughout both fetal and adult life in wild type mice. Presumably, the high-level expression of the human KI genes is enhanced through interactions with the murine β globin LCR sequences located far upstream (Fig. 1).

There are multiple improvements in these humanized KI mice over previous models of CA. For the first time, homozygous CA pups are alive at birth. Furthermore, similar to humans the high level of human α and γ globin chains synthesized during fetal life generates CA mice that survive upon human HbF at birth. Similarly, as the fetal to adult hemoglobin switch is completed after birth in humanized CA mice, the onset of anemia and disease pathology develops postnatally. Incorporation of an HPFH mutation in the human γ globin promoter and the minor adult δ globin gene in the KI allele extends the postnatal lifespan of the CA mice, making them more amenable for experimental manipulation. The disease in humanized CA mice is heritable in contrast to an adult transplant model of β thalassemia major produced by transplantation of early fetal liver cells from homozygous β globin knockout mice into irradiated wild-type mice.[26] Furthermore, disease in the transplant model occurs in adults only after senescence of the recipient's wild-type RBCs and is marked by abnormal erythroblast differentiation of the donor fetal erythroblasts in the absence of any hemolysis or reticulocytosis.[27] Anemia in humanized CA KI mice occurs postnatally as a consequence of hemoglobin switching and is marked by ineffective erythropoiesis, hemolysis, and reticulocytosis similar to human patients.[18]

Future studies

These novel preclinical humanized mouse models of CA are amenable to many diverse areas of study. Because they survive to birth and develop disease postnatally similar to humans, the pathophysiology of disease progression can be analyzed in parallel with transfusion and chelation therapy. Indeed, new transfusion regimens, iron chelators, or novel small molecules designed to make existing iron chelation therapy more efficient can be analyzed in these mice. Cellular and genetic therapies with stem or progenitor cells designed to cure or ameliorate CA are straightforwardly tested in this model. Because human fetal to adult hemoglobin switching is an integral component of this model, studies of the epigenetic changes during the silencing of the human γ globin KI allele or experiments designed to reactivate the γ globin KI allele in the adult could provide important insights into the mechanism of globin gene switching in humans. For example, the role that BCL11A, a modulator of γ globin levels identified in genome-wide association studies in humans,[28,29] may play in the regulation of fetal to adult globin gene switching in humanized CA KI mice could help identify important *cis*-regulatory sequences required for its action.[20,30]

Acknowledgments

This work was supported by National Institutes of Health grants R01 HL072351 (T.M.R.), R01 HL073440 (T.M.R.), and T32 GM008111 (S.C.M.). The authors thank the Cooley's Anemia Foundation RFA for Translational Research in Adult Thalassemia for support. S.C.M. and T.Z. were supported by Carmichael Scholarships. The authors thank UNICO Foundation, Mr. Joseph Ruisi, and the Thalassemia-Cooley's Anemia Group at UAB.

Conflicts of interest

The authors declare no conflicts of interest.

Supporting Information

Additional supporting information describing Materials and Methods may be found in the online version of this article:

Please note: Wiley-Blackwell are not responsible for the content or functionality of any supporting materials supplied by the authors. Any queries (other than missing material) should be directed to the corresponding author for the article.

References

1. Bunn, H. & B. Forget. 1986. *Hemoglobin: Molecular, Genetic, and Clinical Aspects*. W.B. Saunders. Philadelphia.
2. Nienhuis, A.W. & G. Stamatoyannopoulos. 1978. Hemoglobin switching. *Cell* **15:** 307–315.
3. Yuan, J., E. Angelucci, G. Lucarelli, *et al.* 1993. Accelerated programmed cell death (apoptosis) in erythroid precursors of patients with severe beta-thalassemia (Cooley's anemia). *Blood* **82:** 374–377.
4. Piomelli, S. & T. Loew. 1991. Management of thalassemia major (Cooley's anemia). *Hematol. Oncol. Clin. North Am.* **5:** 557–569.
5. Kingsley, P.D., J. Malik, R.L. Emerson, *et al.* 2006. "Maturational" globin switching in primary primitive erythroid cells. *Blood* **107:** 1665–1672.
6. Whitelaw, E., S.F. Tsai, P. Hogben & S.H. Orkin. 1990. Regulated expression of globin chains and the erythroid transcription factor GATA-1 during erythropoiesis in the developing mouse. *Mol. Cell Biol.* **10:** 6596–6606.
7. Shehee, W.R., P. Oliver & O. Smithies. 1993. Lethal thalassemia after insertional disruption of the mouse major adult beta-globin gene. *Proc. Natl. Acad. Sci. USA* **90:** 3177–3181.
8. Ciavatta, D.J., T.M. Ryan, S.C. Farmer & T.M. Townes. 1995. Mouse model of human beta zero thalassemia: targeted deletion of the mouse beta maj- and beta min-globin genes in embryonic stem cells. *Proc. Natl. Acad. Sci. USA* **92:** 9259–9263.
9. Yang, B., S. Kirby, J. Lewis, *et al.* 1995. A mouse model for beta-thalassemia. *Proc. Natl. Acad. Sci. USA* **92:** 11608–11612.
10. Jamsai, D., F. Zaibak, W. Khongnium, *et al.* 2005. A humanized mouse model for a common beta-thalassemia mutation. *Genomics* **85:** 453–461.
11. Lewis, J., B. Yang, R. Kim, *et al.* 1998. A common human beta globin splicing mutation modeled in mice. *Blood* **91:** 2152–2156.
12. Vadolas, J., M. Nefedov, H. Wardan, *et al.* 2006. Humanized beta-thalassemia mouse model containing the common

IVSI-110 splicing mutation. *J. Biol. Chem.* **281:** 7399–7405.
13. Behringer, R.R., T.M. Ryan, R.D. Palmiter, *et al.* 1990. Human gamma- to beta-globin gene switching in transgenic mice. *Genes Dev.* **4:** 380–389.
14. Gaensler, K.M., M. Kitamura & Y.W. Kan. 1993. Germ-line transmission and developmental regulation of a 150-kb yeast artificial chromosome containing the human beta-globin locus in transgenic mice. *Proc. Natl. Acad. Sci. USA* **90:** 11381–11385.
15. Kaufman, R.M., C.T. Pham & T.J. Ley. 1999. Transgenic analysis of a 100-kb human beta-globin cluster-containing DNA fragment propagated as a bacterial artificial chromosome. *Blood* **94:** 3178–3184.
16. Peterson, K.R., C.H. Clegg, C. Huxley, *et al.* 1993. Transgenic mice containing a 248-kb yeast artificial chromosome carrying the human beta-globin locus display proper developmental control of human globin genes. *Proc. Natl. Acad. Sci. USA* **90:** 7593–7597.
17. Strouboulis, J., N. Dillon & F. Grosveld. 1992. Developmental regulation of a complete 70-kb human beta-globin locus in transgenic mice. *Genes Dev.* **6:** 1857–1864.
18. Huo, Y., S.C McConnell & T.M. Ryan. 2009. Preclinical transfusion-dependent humanized mouse model of beta thalassemia major. *Blood* **113:** 4763–4770.
19. Huo, Y., S.M. McConnell, S.-R. Liu, *et al.* 2008. Humanized mouse model of Cooley's Anemia. *J. Biol. Chem.* **284:** 4889–4896.
20. Sankaran, V.G., J. Xu, T. Ragoczy, *et al.* 2009. Developmental and species-divergent globin switching are driven by BCL11A. *Nature* **460:** 1093–1097.
21. Ryan, T.M., D.J. Ciavatta & T.M. Townes. 1997. Knockout-transgenic mouse model of sickle cell disease. *Science* **278:** 873–876.
22. Ryan, T.M., C.W. Sun, J. Ren & T.M. Townes. 2000. Human gamma-globin gene promoter element regulates human beta-globin gene developmental specificity. *Nucleic Acids Res.* **28:** 2736–2740.
23. Treisman, R., S.H. Orkin & T. Maniatis. 1983. Specific transcription and RNA splicing defects in five cloned beta-thalassaemia genes. *Nature* **302:** 591–596.
24. Gelinas, R., B. Endlich, C. Pfeiffer, *et al.* 1985. G to A substitution in the distal CCAAT box of the A gamma-globin gene in Greek hereditary persistence of fetal haemoglobin. *Nature* **313:** 323–325.
25. Wu, L.C., C.W. Sun, T.M. Ryan, *et al.* 2006. Correction of sickle cell disease by homologous recombination in embryonic stem cells. *Blood* **108:** 1183–1188.
26. Rivella, S., C. May, A. Chadburn, *et al.* 2003. A novel murine model of Cooley anemia and its rescue by lentiviral-mediated human beta-globin gene transfer. *Blood* **101:** 2932–2939.
27. Libani, I.V., E.C. Guy, L. Melchiori, *et al.* 2008. Decreased differentiation of erythroid cells exacerbates ineffective erythropoiesis in beta-thalassemia. *Blood* **112:** 875–885.
28. Menzel, S., C. Garner, I. Gut, *et al.* 2007. A QTL influencing F cell production maps to a gene encoding a zinc-finger protein on chromosome 2p15. *Nat Genet.* **39:** 1197–1199.
29. Uda, M., R. Galanello, S. Sanna, *et al.* 2008. Genome-wide association study shows BCL11A associated with persistent fetal hemoglobin and amelioration of the phenotype of beta-thalassemia. *Proc. Natl. Acad. Sci. USA* **105:** 1620–1625.
30. Sankaran, V.G., T.F. Menne, J. Xu, *et al.* 2008. Human fetal hemoglobin expression is regulated by the developmental stage-specific repressor BCL11A. *Science* **322:** 1839–1842.

Ann. N.Y. Acad. Sci. ISSN 0077-8923

ANNALS OF THE NEW YORK ACADEMY OF SCIENCES
Issue: *Cooley's Anemia: Ninth Symposium*

Strategy for a multicenter phase I clinical trial to evaluate globin gene transfer in β-thalassemia

Michel Sadelain,[1] Isabelle Rivière,[1] Xiuyan Wang,[1] Farid Boulad,[2] Susan Prockop,[2] Patricia Giardina,[3] Aurelio Maggio,[4] Renzo Galanello,[5] Franco Locatelli,[6] and Evangelia Yannaki[7]

[1]Center for Cell Engineering, Memorial Sloan-Kettering Cancer Center, New York, New York. [2]Department of Pediatrics, Memorial Sloan-Kettering Cancer Center, New York, New York. [3]Department of Pediatrics, Weill-Cornell Medical College, New York, New York. [4]U.O.C. Ematologia II, Ospedali Riuniti Villa Sofia-Cervello, Palermo, Italy. [5]Dipartimento di scienze biomediche e biotechnologie, Ospedale Microcitemico, Cagliari, Italy. [6]Department of Pediatrics, Ospedale Bambino Gesu, Roma, Italy. [7]Gene and Cell Therapy Center, G. Papanicolaou Hospital, Thessaloniki, Greece

Address for correspondence: Michel Sadelain, M.D., Ph.D., Memorial Sloan-Kettering Cancer Center, 1275 York Avenue, New York, NY 10065. m-sadelain@ski.mskcc.org

Globin gene transfer in autologous hematopoietic stem cells offers a potentially curative treatment option for patients suffering from β-thalassemia major who lack an HLA-matched hematopoietic stem cell donor. Based on extensive preclinical investigation, we are initiating a phase I clinical trial using G-CSF mobilized, autologous CD34$^+$ cells transduced with a vector similar to the original TNS9 vector. Our first mobilizations in adult β-thalassemic subjects have been well tolerated and yielded the required CD34$^+$ cell dose. To minimize toxicity to enrolled subjects, and in the absence of a demonstrated requirement for myeloablative conditioning, our trial will use a reduced intensity conditioning regimen. Because low vector titers may adversely affect efficacy and safety, we have focused on vector manufacturing processes. We are now in a position to transfer our globin lentiviral vectors in a clinically relevant dosage (averaging 0.8 vector copy per cell in bulk CD34$^+$ cells) and to supply clinical grade vector to collaborating centers in the U.S.A. and in Europe. We anticipate that the first U.S. trial of globin gene transfer will start in 2010.

Keywords: cell therapy; globin gene regulation; lentiviral vector; non-myeloablative conditioning; stem cell engineering

Introduction

The β-thalassemias are genetic disorders caused by mutations in or near the β-globin gene, an erythroid-specific gene that is activated in late stages of adult erythropoiesis.[1–3] Over 120 different mutations that reduce or abolish β chain synthesis have been reported.[1–4] The only currently conceivable means to cure β-thalassemia major is to provide the affected subject with hematopoietic stem cells containing functional β-globin genes.[1–3] Presently, this can only be achieved by allogeneic bone marrow transplantation.[5,6] Successful transplantation corrects ineffective erythropoiesis and restores the generation of long-lived red blood cells, resulting in transfusion independence.[5,6] This option, however, is not available to the vast majority (70–80%) of thalassemic subjects, for whom a matched related donor cannot be found.[7] Because of the greater risks associated with matched-unrelated or mismatched transplants, most subjects have to settle for palliative therapy based on life-long red blood cell transfusion and daily treatment with an iron chelator to eliminate excess iron. While controlling the anemia, transfusion therapy does not correct ineffective erythropoiesis, and exacerbates iron accumulation in a variety of organs.

Over the past decade, retroviral-mediated gene transfer in hematopoietic stem cells (HSCs) has shown therapeutic benefit in other congenital blood disorders. Encouraging results have been obtained in subjects with adenosine deaminase (ADA)

doi: 10.1111/j.1749-6632.2010.05597.x

deficiency,[8] X-linked severe combined immune deficiency,[9,10] chronic granulomatous disease,[11] adrenoleukodystrophy,[12] and Wiskott–Aldrich syndrome.[13] These studies made use of nonspecific vectors that use ubiquitous promoters to express the deficient protein. Such a technology, however, is not adequate for globin gene transfer, which requires much higher-level expression of the transgene product but in restricted fashion, confining transgene expression to maturing erythroblasts.

The goal of globin gene transfer is to restore the capacity of the thalassemic subject's own HSCs to generate red blood cells containing normal hemoglobin which will reverse the ineffective erythropoiesis and correct the inherited anemia.[14–16] Autologous HSCs, which self-renew and generate all hematopoietic lineages including the erythroid lineage, are the cellular target of *ex vivo* globin gene transfer. The goal is to restore the subject's ability to produce red blood cells with an increased content of normal adult hemoglobin and achieve transfusion-independence.

Ten years ago, we demonstrated that the human β-globin gene could be expressed at therapeutic levels in hematopoietic chimeras and cure β-thalassemia in mice.[17] Several groups later confirmed these results in various models of thalassemia and sickle cell anemia (reviewed in Refs. 14–16). In 2007, we obtained approval from the Recombinant DNA Advisory Committee (RAC) to undertake a phase I study to assess the safety of this therapy in subjects with transfusion-dependent β-thalassemia major. The proposed treatment is based on the administration of autologous $CD34^+$ hematopoietic cells transduced with a lentiviral vector encoding the normal human β-globin gene, TNS9.3.55. We soon realized that the relatively low titers of globin vectors obtained with current lentiviral vector manufacturing processes did not meet standards for a safe and effective clinical study and would hinder clinical development. After spending nearly two years to improve vector titers, without compromising the therapeutic globin transcription unit, we are now ready to initiate the first U.S. trial testing this approach.

Globin gene transfer as curative treatment for β-thalassemia in mice

The goal of globin gene transfer for the treatment of β-thalassemia is to (1) achieve stable introduction of functional globin genes into the patient's own hematopoietic stem cells and (2) to correct the ineffective erythropoiesis and hemolytic anemia, thus obviating the need for lifelong transfusions and preventing further iron accumulation. Following extensive and systematic testing of different vector designs, we identified over 10 years ago a combination of genomic sequences that could be stably transferred by a lentiviral vector, termed TNS9, and correct the thalassemia syndrome in β-thalassemic mice.[17] In this and subsequent studies,[17–19] we demonstrated that mice harboring the TNS9 vector at an average vector copy number of 0.5–1.0 exhibit correction of anemia, regression of extra-medullary hematopoiesis, and absence of iron accumulation in peripheral tissues and organs.[18] In a lethal model of β-thalassemia major, we established, in which mice succumb to ineffective erythropoiesis within 60 days after developing severe anemia, massive splenomegaly, extramedullary hematopoiesis, and hepatic iron overload, we showed rescue following TNS9 transfer in the vast majority of treated mice.[19] In large cohorts of mice, we did not observe evidence of vector silencing over time, neither in primary, secondary, or even tertiary chimeras, nor any evidence of leukemia (unpublished observations). More recent studies showed that globin transgene expression could be further increased without increasing the vector copy number by including an additional segment of the human β-globin locus control region, known as HS1.[20] In view of the high performance of the TNS9 vector and the vast amount of data collected over years with this vector, we selected the TNS9 transcription unit for clinical investigation.

Clinical trial outline

Our phase I study will be conducted in subjects with transfusion-dependent β-thalassemia major. The proposed treatment is based on the administration of autologous $CD34^+$ hematopoietic cells transduced with the TNS9.3.55 vector, a lentiviral vector encoding the normal human β-globin gene. The cells are transduced *ex vivo*, frozen down, tested for transduction efficiency, sterility, and other release criteria, and returned to the donor after reduced intensity conditioning. The goal is to restore the subject's ability to produce red blood cells with an increased content of normal adult hemoglobin and achieve transfusion-independence.

Table 1. Summary of inclusion criteria

1. Subjects must have a confirmed diagnosis of β-thalassemia major and have been enrolled in a hypertransfusion program for at least 2 years.
2. Subjects must be 15 years or older.
3. Patients must NOT have an HLA-matched sibling.
4. Patients must be off hydroxyurea (HU) or erythropoietin (EPO) treatment for at least 3 months prior to entry onto the study.
5. Subjects must have a performance score of Karnofsky ≥70% at the time of entry into the study.
6. Subjects must have acceptable hepatic, cardiac, pulmonary, and renal function.
7. Each patient must be willing to participate as a research subject and must sign an informed consent form. Parent or legal guardians of patients who are minors will sign the informed consent form. Assents will be obtained as age appropriate.
8. Patients must be available for follow-up evaluations at days 30, 60, 180 after cell infusion, and yearly thereafter.

The primary objective of this study is to assess the safety and tolerability of autologous CD34$^+$ cells that have been transduced with TNS9.3.55. This will be evaluated by monitoring the effects of a low-dose, non-myeloablative conditioning regimen, the occurrence of insertional oncogenesis, and the generation of a replication-competent lentivirus (RCL).

The secondary objective of this study is to assess the level of engraftment of transduced CD34$^+$ cells and the biological activity of the TNS9.3.55 vector-encoded β-globin, that is, its expression level after normalization to vector copy number.

The key inclusion criteria for enrolling patients on this protocol are listed in Table 1.

Peripheral blood stem cell mobilization in subjects with β-thalassemia major

The TNS9.3.55 vector must be introduced in self-renewing hematopoietic cells to achieve long-term benefit. Such cells are a small fraction of the CD34$^+$ cells that can be collected from bone marrow or following mobilization. The latter approach yields more CD34$^+$ cells and is the preferred approach for collecting cells for genetic engineering.

A mobilization study base on the administration of G-CSF was previously performed by Li and colleagues in 20 patients with β-thalassemia aged 3–21 years (mean 11.9).[21] These investigators reported that CD34$^+$ cells were effectively mobilized by G-CSF (10–16 μg/day/kg) in the 20 thalassemia patients and 11 healthy donors. Although no significant difference was observed in levels of daily stem cell counts between the two groups of subjects, a 1-day delay in achieving peak levels of CD34$^+$ cells was observed in the majority of thalassemia patients. The peak increase of CD34$^+$ cells was 21.5- and 30.8 fold of the basal steady-state levels in thalassemia patients and healthy donors, respectively. Compositions of the apheresis products were reported to be similar in the two groups of subjects. G-CSF administration was well-tolerated and the authors concluded that collection of G-CSF-mobilized CD34$^+$ cells was feasible in patients with β-thalassemia.

Two studies evaluating CD34$^+$ cell mobilization in adult subjects with β-thalassemia major are currently in progress, one at the George Papanicolaou Hospital in Thessaloniki, Greece, led by Dr. E. Yannaki, and ours at MSKCC. Three subjects have been mobilized to date at MSKCC in New York. All were female subjects between the ages of 23 and 29. All three patients tolerated G-CSF with minimal side effects (fatigue and bone pain). No other adverse effects were observed (unpublished observations). The total CD34$^+$ cell counts collected were 8.0, 12.0, and 8.5 × 10^6 CD34$^+$ cells/kg. These values are within the range required for the therapeutic protocol.

Vector production and patient CD34$^+$ cell transduction

Lentiviral vectors that encode intron-containing therapeutic transgenes and large genomic fragments, such as segments derived from the locus control region (3.2 kb in the TNS9 vector), have lower titers than most other vectors, which typically only encode a promoter and a polyA-less cDNA in the sense orientation. Three years ago, we realized that the titer of typical globin vectors was too low to achieve adequate levels of gene transfer in human CD34$^+$ cells. Furthermore, low titers make vector production very onerous and are a dead-end for conducting multicenter trials or phase II trials. A central tenet of our strategy has thus been to augment the vector titer without compromising

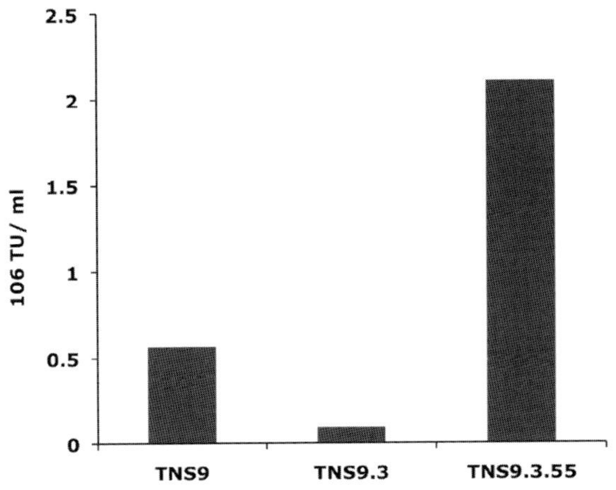

Figure 1. Comparative titer of TNS9, TNS9.3, and TNS9.3.55. Lentiviral vector titrations were performed in HeLa cells. Dilutions of the unconcentrated vector stocks were added to HeLa cells plated the previous day in six-well tissue culture plates. Hela cells were cultured for 15 days. Genomic DNA samples isolated from cell lysates were analyzed by quantitative Taqman PCR (Q-PCR) using HIV-gag specific probe and primers to determine the vectors titers (in 10^6 transduction units per mL). This data is representative of 3 independent experiments, showing a >10-fold improvement in vector titer when comparing TNS9.3 to TNS9.3.55.

or changing the β-globin transcription unit, that is, without modifying the globin gene, promoter, enhancers, and locus control region elements of the TNS9 vector. Through a series of modifications to the lentiviral components of TNS9 (unpublished observations), we were indeed able to substantially increase vector titers (Fig. 1), reaching levels that we deem to be sufficient to undertake a sound clinical study.

After collection and purification, the $CD34^+$ cells are transduced in the Gene Transfer and Somatic Cell Engineering Facility at MSKCC. The $CD34^+$ cells are prestimulated and transduced in the presence of Flt-3 ligand, Kit ligand, thrombopoietin, interleukin-3, and fibronectin. Transduction is performed on fresh cells whenever possible, or on frozen cells. An example of thalassemic $CD34^+$ cell transduction, obtained with clinical grade vector manufactured according to current good manufacturing practices (cGMP), is shown in Figure 2. Following transduction, the bulk of the $CD34^+$ cells are frozen down, while aliquots are tested for vector copy number and extensive biosafety, as per the U.S. Food and Drug Administration (FDA) guidelines.

Preparative regimen

Following extensive discussion with a number of transplant experts, we decided to initiate our clinical trial using a reduced intensity conditioning regimen to prepare the recipient before infusion of the transduced $CD34^+$ cells. The two reasons for that choice are that (1) this approach has previously been successful in the context of gene therapy for other blood disorders and (2) it is a safer first approach.

We decided to initially use busulfan at a total dose of 8 mg/kg, in consideration of the following points. (1) Studies in patients with immunodeficiency disorders[11,13] have shown successful engraftment of autologous-transduced cells. (2) Allogeneic stem cell transplantation for β-thalassemia using a higher dose of busulfan with fludarabine (instead of cyclophosphamide) was well tolerated.[22] (3) Allogeneic stem cell transplantation for disorders other than β-thalassemia using reduced intensity conditioning regimens has been successful.[23,24]

Risk/benefit considerations

The curative treatment of β-thalassemia major requires that the patient be provided hematopoietic stem cells that harbor functional β-globin genes. Currently, this can only be achieved by allogeneic bone marrow transplantation. Successful transplantation corrects ineffective erythropoiesis and restores the generation of long-lived red blood cells, resulting in transfusion independence. This option, however, is not available to the vast majority of subjects, for whom a matched related donor cannot be found. Because of the greater risks associated with matched-unrelated or mismatched transplants, most patients are given palliative therapy based on life-long red blood cell transfusion.[1–3,7]

For subjects lacking a matched donor, globin gene therapy offers the potential of curative stem cell transplantation without incurring the risk of graft-versus-host disease (GVHD) and without requiring immune suppression to prevent graft rejection. The risk/benefit analysis should be assessed in the light of the known risks associated with the alternative transplant modalities available to subjects lacking a matched, related donor.

Thalassemic subjects treated with allogeneic bone marrow grafts from unrelated donors are exposed

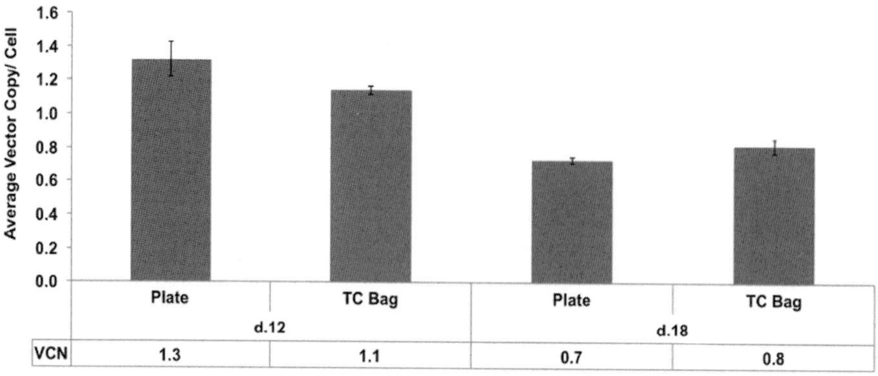

Figure 2. Vector copy number analysis in thalassemic CD34$^+$ cells transduced with the TNS9.3.55 lentiviral vector. Under MSKCC IRB protocol #08-030, a patient with ß-thalassemia major was treated with G-CSF to mobilize CD34$^+$ cells into peripheral blood and underwent an apheresis procedure. Purified CD34$^+$ were prestimulated for 24 h in serum-free XVIVO-10 with TPO, Flt-3L, SCF, and IL-3 in tissue culture plates or tissue culture (TC) bags, and subsequently transduced using TNS9.3.55 vector stocks. The cells were subsequently cultured in serum-free XVIVO-10 supplemented with cytokines. On day 4 of culture, cells were differentiated into erythroid lineage as per the MSKCC Gene Transfer and Somatic Cell Engineering Facility Standard Operating Procedure. Genomic DNA was extracted on days 12 and 18 of culture for determination of the average Vector Copy Number (VCN) in the bulk erythroid cultures by quantitative Taqman PCR (Q-PCR) using HIV-gag specific probe and primers.

to a risk of mortality of 20%, a disease-free survival of 66–69%, and a risk of chronic GvHD of 18% (reviewed in Ref. 7). Recent updates on the safety profile of retroviral-mediated gene transfer in autologous HSCs in 39 patients with immunodeficiencies (adenosine deaminase deficiency, X-linked severe combined immune deficiency (SCID) and chronic granulomatous disease)[8,11,25–27] show five cases of leukemia (all occurring in patients with X-linked SCID, including one fatal case), two cases of benign myeloid clonal expansion, and complete absence of GVHD. Assuming, as a worst case scenario, that the safety profile of globin lentiviral vectors is the same as that of gamma-retroviral vectors, and equating the risk of leukemia with the mortality risk, to date the risk of insertional oncogenesis (12%) is less than the mortality risk of 20% associated with unrelated bone marrow transplants. The significance of nontransformed myeloid clonal expansions is presently uncertain, although one may fear that they are preleukemic states. Our risk/benefit analysis was supported by the Recombinant DNA Advisory Committee, which reviewed in detail our trial proposal and unanimously voted in favor (http://oba.od.nih.gov/oba/rac/minutes/RAC_minutes_06-07.pdf; pages 14–18).

We propose to enroll patients aged 15 and above based on the following considerations. Patients 15–18 years old with evidence of early complications probably have higher risks of complications with allogeneic transplantation, especially if receiving grafts from unrelated donors. Therefore, we estimate that such patients would be appropriate candidates for our trial. We also believe that a 15-year-old child with β-thalassemia and evidence of significant hemochromatosis and possibly early hepatic fibrosis, should be as eligible to be enrolled on our protocol as a 20-year-old adult with the same findings. The age of 15 years was also chosen because, by that age, the probability of subsequently having an HLA-matched sibling born to the family is markedly decreased. The informed consent and assent procedures were extensively reviewed by our Institutional Review Board (IRB) and by the Recombinant DNA Advisory Committee.

Toward a multicenter evaluation of TNS9.3 vectors

Pending FDA approval, we are about to initiate a phase I clinical trial to evaluate the safety and tolerability of globin gene transfer in subjects with β-thalassemia major. The protocol will be offered to patients with transfusion-dependent β-thalassemia 15 years or older, who lack a matched, related donor, wherein the risk/benefit analysis provided above supports the investigation of a potentially curative treatment that does not require full myeloablation or immunosuppression. To minimize the risks to the patient, the genetically modified cells will be infused after extensive biosafety testing of the transduced cells and following the administration of a reduced intensity (non-myeloablative) conditioning regimen.

Complementing extensive studies in preclinical animal models of disease in mice and nonhuman primates, our strategy has been to conduct mobilization studies to assess the safety and efficacy of G-CSF mobilization in adult subject with β-thalassemia major while augmenting the vector titer without compromising or changing the TNS9 β-globin transcription unit.

Our own mobilization studies, still in progress, indicate that $CD34^+$ cells can be safely collected using G-CSF and that the cell yields in adult thalassemic subjects are within the required cell doses. Through a series of modifications to the lentiviral components of TNS9 (unpublished observations), we have now increased the vector titers to levels we deem to be sufficient to undertake a sound clinical study. This improved vector manufacturing places us in a position to provide vector to collaborating centers for multicenter clinical studies. We anticipate that the first U.S. trial of globin gene transfer will start in 2010.

Acknowledgments

The authors thank the Sloan-Kettering Institute, the Leonardo Giambrone Foundation, the National Heart, Lung, and Blood Institute, and the Cooley's Anemia Foundation for their financial support. The authors also thank Errant Gene Therapeutics, LLC for providing us with clinical grade lentiviral vector for our studies.

References

1. Weatherall, D.J. & J.B. Clegg. 1981. *The Thalassemia Syndrome*. Blackwell Scientific. Oxford, UK.
2. Stamatoyannopoulos, G., A.W. Nienhuis, P. Majers & H. Varmus. 1994. *The Molecular Basis of Blood Disorders*. W.B. Saunders. Philadelphia, PA.
3. Orkin, S.H. & D.G. Nathan. 1998. *Hematology of Infancy and Childhood*. W.B. Saunders. Philadelphia, PA.
4. Weatherall, D.J. 2001. Phenotype-genotype relationships in monogenic disease: lessons from the thalassaemias. *Nat. Rev. Genet.* **2:** 245–255.
5. Lucarelli, G., M. Andreani & E. Angelucci. 2002. The cure of thalassemia by bone marrow transplantation. *Blood Rev.* **16:** 81–85.
6. Boulad, F. 2006. Hematopoitic stem cell transplantation for the treatment of β-thalassemia. In *Pediatric Hematopoietic Stem Cell Transplantation*: 383–396. Informa Healthcare. New York.
7. Sadelain, M. *et al.* 2007. Therapeutic options for patients with severe beta-thalassemia: the need for globin gene therapy. *Hum. Gene. Ther.* **18:** 1–9.
8. Aiuti, A. *et al.* 2009. Gene therapy for immunodeficiency due to adenosine deaminase deficiency. *N. Engl. J. Med.* **360:** 447–458.
9. Cavazzana-Calvo, M. *et al.* 2000. Gene therapy of human severe combined immunodeficiency (SCID)-X1 disease. *Science* **288:** 669–672.
10. Hacein-Bey-Abina, S. *et al.* 2002. Sustained correction of X-linked severe combined immunodeficiency by ex vivo gene therapy. *N. Engl. J. Med.* **346:** 1185–1193.
11. Ott, M.G. *et al.* 2006. Correction of X-linked chronic granulomatous disease by gene therapy, augmented by insertional activation of MDS1-EVI1, PRDM16 or SETBP1. *Nat. Med.* **12:** 401–409.
12. Cartier, N. *et al.* 2009. Hematopoietic stem cell gene therapy with a lentiviral vector in X-linked adrenoleukodystrophy. *Science* **326:** 818–823.
13. Boztug, *et al.* 2010. Correction of Wiskott-Aldrich Syndrome by Hematopoietic Stem Cell Gene Therapy. *N. Engl. J. Med.* In press.
14. Sadelain, M. 2006. Recent advances in globin gene transfer for the treatment of beta-thalassemia and sickle cell anemia. *Curr. Opin. Hematol.* **13:** 142–148.
15. Persons, D.A. & J.F. Tisdale. 2004. Gene therapy for the hemoglobin disorders. *Semin. Hematol.* **41:** 279–286.
16. Sadelain, M. *et al.* 2008. Stem cell engineering for the treatment of severe hemoglobinopathies. *Curr. Mol. Med.* **8:** 690–697.
17. May, C. *et al.* 2000. Therapeutic haemoglobin synthesis in beta-thalassaemic mice expressing lentivirus-encoded human beta-globin. *Nature* **406:** 82–86.
18. May, C. *et al.* 2002. Successful treatment of murine beta-thalassemia intermedia by transfer of the human beta-globin gene. *Blood* **99:** 1902–1908.
19. Rivella, S. *et al.* 2003. A novel murine model of Cooley anemia and its rescue by lentiviral-mediated human beta-globin gene transfer. *Blood* **101:** 2932–2939.
20. Lisowski, L. & M. Sadelain. 2008. Current status of globin gene therapy for the treatment of beta-thalassaemia. *Br. J. Haematol.* **141:** 335–345.
21. Li, C.K. *et al.* 2002. Morbidity and mortality patterns of thalassaemia major patients in Hong Kong: retrospective study. *Hong Kong Med. J.* **8:** 255–260.
22. Boulad F. 2005. High dose busulfan and fludarabine with anti-thymocyte globulin (ATG) followed by unmodified marrow grafts from HLA-matched siblings for the treatment of high risk hemoglobinopathies (HGBpathies). *Blood* **106:** 575a.
23. Horn, B. *et al.* 2006. Reduced intensity conditioning using intravenous busulfan, fludarabine and rabbit ATG for children with nonmalignant disorders and CML. *Bone Marrow Transplant*. **37:** 263–269.
24. Giralt, S. 2005. Reduced-intensity conditioning regimens for hematologic malignancies: what have we learned over

the last 10 years? *Hematol. Am. Soc. Hematol. Educ. Program* 384–389.

25. Alexander, B.L. *et al.* 2007. Progress and prospects: gene therapy clinical trials (part 1). *Gene Ther.* **14:** 1439–1447.
26. Hacein-Bey-Abina, S., *et al.* 2008. Insertional oncogenesis in 4 patients after retrovirus-mediated gene therapy of SCID-X1. *J. Clin. Invest.* **118:** 3132–3142.
27. Howe, S.J. *et al.* 2008. Insertional mutagenesis combined with acquired somatic mutations causes leukemogenesis following gene therapy of SCID-X1 patients. *J. Clin. Invest.* **118:** 3143–3150.

Ann. N.Y. Acad. Sci. ISSN 0077-8923

ANNALS OF THE NEW YORK ACADEMY OF SCIENCES
Issue: *Cooley's Anemia: Ninth Symposium*

Hematopoietic stem cell mobilization strategies for gene therapy of beta thalassemia and sickle cell disease

Evangelia Yannaki[1] and George Stamatoyannopoulos[2]

[1]Gene and Cell Therapy Center, Hematology-BMT Unit, George Papanicolaou Hospital, Thessaloniki, Greece. [2]Medical Genetics, University of Washington, Seattle, Washington

Address for correspondence: Evangelia Yannaki, M.D., G.Papanicolaou Hospital, Gene and Cell Therapy Center, Hematology-BMT Unit, Thessaloniki 57010, Greece. eyannaki@u.washington.edu

Effective gene therapy for hemoglobinopathies will require high numbers of autologous gene-engineered hematopoetic stem cells to be reintroduced into the patients. Stem cell mobilization using G-CSF is the most convenient and effective approach to achieve this goal, but it can have severe side effects in sickle cell anemia and be potentially harmful in the case of severe thalassemia. Hence, the optimal way of collection of hematopoetic stem cells from patients with thalassemia and sickle cell disease needs to be determined. In this paper, we review the possible risks of G-CSF mobilization in hemoglobinopathies and we outline the approaches used in an on-going clinical trial in which pretreatment with hydroxyurea is used to reduce potential risks of G-CSF administration to patients with severe beta thalassemia.

Keywords: mobilization; thalassemia; G-CSF; sickle cell disease

Introduction

Gene therapy for hemoglobinopathies will require infusion to the patient of large numbers of gene-engineered stem cells for two reasons. First, because in these disorders, a reduced intensity conditioning should optimally be applied and this will only partially ablate the endogenous bone marrow; hence, high numbers of corrected cells will be required to physically compete for niche space against the large pool of unmodified stem cells. Second, the engrafted gene-corrected stem cells will not have any selective advantage compared with the endogenous stem cells. Thus, the application of gene therapy for hemoglobinopathies will first need to meet the challenge of obtaining the target stem cells in sufficient numbers.

Treatment with certain forms of chemotherapy or cytokines can induce the egress of hematopoietic stem and progenitor cells from the marrow into the peripheral blood through a process termed *mobilization.*[1] Currently, mobilized peripheral blood represents the most frequent source of HSCs for autologous or allogeneic bone marrow transplantation[2] due to the higher yields of $CD34^+$ stem/progenitor cells and the earlier hematopoietic recovery achieved after transplantation of mobilized blood compared to bone marrow harvested cells.[3] The cytokine granulocyte colony stimulating factor (G-CSF) is the most widely used and clinically accepted inducer of peripheral blood stem cell mobilization.[3–5] Compared to bone marrow harvesting, mobilization with G-CSF provides three- to fourfold higher yields of transplantable $CD34^+$ cells under a minimally invasive procedure.[3] In addition, the gene transfer rates of mobilized blood stem cells may be higher compared to steady-state bone marrow cells, although this is still an issue of debate.[6–8]

Mobilization with G-CSF, in normal donors and in patients with hematologic malignancies, is well tolerated with only mild side effects (low fever, bone pain, and fatigue), although not completely without toxicity. There is a documented, transient enlargement of the spleen during G-CSF-mobilization,[9,10] which very rarely can result in splenic rupture. Among the millions of normal donors and patients whose stem cells were mobilized using G-CSF, 17 cases of splenic rupture have been reported.[11–15]

doi: 10.1111/j.1749-6632.2010.05576.x

A transient procoagulant effect of G-CSF which can precipitate myocardial infarction or cerebral ischemia in high-risk individuals has also been described.[16,17] A large analysis of 1488 donors registered with the International or the European Bone Marrow Transplantation Registry showed only a low rate (1.1%) of serious complications after G-CSF mobilization and peripheral blood stem cell collection, which was comparable to the rate of serious complications following bone marrow harvesting.[18]

Autologous transplantation of hematopoietic stem cells for the treatment of thalassemia and SCD would have been justified only in a gene therapy setting and as consequence, the mobilization and collection of PBSCs in patients with hemoglobinopathies have been largely unexplored. Gene therapy experiments using murine models of thalassemia intermedia, thalassemia major, and sickle cell disease during the last 10 years,[19–24] have paved the way to the initiation of the first gene therapy clinical studies in patients with beta-thalassemia.[25] Due to the need of infusing to the patients large numbers of gene-corrected cells and the limited published information on the safety and efficacy of hematopoietic stem cell mobilization in patients with hemoglobinopathies, studies on the optimization of mobilization strategies in this target population are required.

Mobilization of hemopoietic stem cells in sickle cell disease

G-CSF, although generally safe when used in cancer patients and healthy donors for mobilization, has been reported to precipitate severe and sometimes fatal sickle cell crisis in patients with SCD.[26–30] Thus far, 11 adults (18–58 years old) with SCD (homozygous for HbSS or compound heterozygotes for HbS/HbC or HbS/β^+thalassemia) have been reported in the literature to have been submitted to stem cell mobilization with G-CSF.[31] Indications for G-CSF usage was back up collection for allogeneic transplantation, chemotherapy-induced neutropenia or autologous transplantation in SCD individuals suffering from a concomitant hematologic malignancy. Of the 11 subjects, 2 developed multiorgan failure which was fatal in 1, 4 developed complications that required hospitalization and 4 experienced no complications.[31] One subject received G-CSF twice; one was complicated with vasocclusive crisis whereas the other was well tolerated.[29]

The pathophysiology of SCD, including the propensity for vasoocclusion and the existence of a chronic inflammatory state associated with leukocytosis, increased serum levels of C-reactive protein and cell activation, as well as the G-CSF-induced leukocytosis with activation of WBCs and procoagulability, account for the severe side effects. Precautions taken before mobilization, namely red cell exchange and red cell transfusion to reduce the levels of HbS below 30%, have resulted in uneventful mobilization of SCD patients.[29] Unfortunately, there is no evidence for an apparent "threshold" leukocyte count, G-CSF dose and administration schedule or HbS percentage for which complications related to sickling could be anticipated. Indeed, multiorgan failure or vasoocclusive crisis have occurred in SCD individuals with peak leukocyte counts as low as $6.4 \times 10^9/L$[28] or high as $105 \times 10^9/L$[30] and with either low (2.5 mcg/kg)[26] or standard (10 mcg/kg)[30] daily G-CSF doses. In addition, no sequelae occurred in a patient who was mobilized without any preceding precaution and with starting HbS level of 75%.[30]

The risk-benefit assessment in subjects with SCD does not justify the routine usage of G-CSF. For stem cell mobilization, when autologous stem cells need to be collected, alternative strategies may be used for SCD patients. It has been reported that significant numbers of primitive progenitors such as myeloid-lymphoid-initiating cells and SCID-repopulating cells are spontaneously mobilized during pain crises, theoretically yielding sufficient numbers of $CD34^+$cells/kg.[32] However, severe acute pain was experienced by a nonmobilized SC patient who was scheduled to undergo cytarapheresis and subsequent exchange transfusion for pain management.[33] The pain started 1 h after the initiation of the leukapheresis procedure and culminated during the "rinse-back" phase when the remaining blood in the -hypoxic- separation chamber was returned to the patient. Due to the unpredictable response of SCD patients to G-CSF or leukapheresis, the conventional bone marrow harvest under local or general anesthesia with careful perioperative management is at present the safest method for obtaining hematopoietic stem cells for gene transfer.

Recently, a novel mobilizing agent (former AMD3100, plerixafor, mozobil) has been launched in the market. Mozobil rapidly peripheralizes stem cells and minimizes the days of exposure to the mobilizing agent as well as the days of leukaphereses.[34] It reversibly inhibits the CXCR4-SDF1 interaction within the bone marrow microenvironment and, in contrast to G-CSF, does not induce bone marrow hyperplasia and consequently bone pain or hyperleukocytosis.[35] Because Mozobil has a different mode of action and a better safety profile compared to G-CSF,[36] it is worth being explored as a mobilizing agent for sickle cell patients.

Mobilization of hemopoietic stem cells in thalassemia

Mobilization of hemopoietic stem cells in thalassemia is not expected to be associated with the side effects of mobilization observed in sickle cell patients. Li and colleagues[37] reported that G-CSF-mobilization in pediatric patients with beta-thalassemia had no serious adverse effects; yields of $CD34^+$ cells were comparable to the yields of normal donors both in numbers and content with one day delay in reaching the peak in peripheral blood. In adult thalassemic patients however, where there is considerable and age-dependent organ damage due to accumulated iron and probably an as yet unknown effect of the multiple transfusions and chronic chelation on the bone marrow stem cell reservoir, mobilization may be impaired or associated with increased risks compared to children.

Clinical features of thalassemia potentially affecting safety and efficacy of G-CSF-mobilization

To satisfy the increased erythropoietic demand, thalassemic patients have a several fold expansion of erythropoiesis, a greatly expanded bone marrow space and extramedullary hemopoiesis within liver and spleen. Splenic hemopoiesis could result in sequestration of stem and progenitor cells in the spleen during mobilization, effectively reducing the yield of $CD34^+$ cells. In a preclinical study of G-CSF-mobilization in a thalassemia intermedia mouse model (HBB^{th-3}), increased trapping of HSCs in the enlarged thalassemic spleen was responsible for the inefficient mobilization of Lin−Sca-1^+c-kit$^+$ cells and it was completely restored after splenectomy.[38]

Chronic splenomegaly could also increase the risk of splenic rupture because of further splenic enlargement during G-CSF administration. On the other hand, in conditions of chronic splenomegaly it is possible that the spleen becomes more flexible because splenic size fluctuates in response to the degree of extramedullary erythropoiesis or hypersplenism. In this case, compared to normal individuals, the spleen may not be subjected to abrupt size changes during G-CSF mobilization, and thus the risk of rupture may be even lower. In G-CSF-treated HBB^{th-3} mice no sequelae of splenic rupture was observed, however, hemorrhagic infarcts were detected in the spleen.[38]

G-SCF could also exacerbate the leukocytosis often associated with β-thalassemia patients that have undergone splenectomy, which in addition to secondary thrombocytosis of splenectomized subjects, may lead to an increased risk of thrombosis. Splenectomized thalassemic patients are theoretically at higher risk to develop a thrombotic event during G-CSF mobilization because of inherent hypercoagulability and high numbers of circulating damaged thalassemic red cells contributing to thrombin generation.[39] In terms of efficacy, splenectomized thalassemic patients could be a priori considered effective mobilizers because of the absence of a site trapping hematopoietic stem cells from the circulation.

In patients with severe organ impairment due to iron-overload, the G-CSF-induced substantial increases in the circulating activated neutrophils, may precipitate complications due to organ sequestration and vasoocclusion. Progressive organ damage by the accumulated iron may jeopardize the safety of mobilization in adult patients.

A stem cell mobilization study of adult patients with beta-thalassemia major

From the demographic data on patients with beta-thalassemia major in Greece, we expect that the majority of subjects seeking gene therapy in the future will be severely affected persons between 25 and 40 years of age. Hence, our study seeks to assess the safety and efficacy of G-CSF-mobilization with or without hydroxyurea (HU) pretreament, in adults with severe beta-thalassemia. The study is conducted in George Papanicolaou Hospital, Thessaloniki, Greece and is sponsored by NHI.

Rationale for the incorporation of hydroxyurea in the mobilization procedure

The incorporation of HU aims to potentially increase the safety and efficacy of G-CSF mobilization. In nonspenectomized patients, HU is used prior to G-CSF mobilization to reduce extramedullary hemopoiesis[40] and thereby the degree of splenomegaly, thus minimizing the potential risks of CD34$^+$cell sequestration and splenic rupture. In splenectomized subjects, HU is used to reduce the high platelet and white blood cell counts and the risk of an exuberant increase in white blood cells in response to G-CSF. In all patients, HU cessation is expected to result in a modest increase in circulating CD34$^+$ cells, as studies in sickle cell patients demonstrate.[33] HU-induced peripheralization of hemopoietic stem cells in combination with G-CSF mobilization could theoretically result in higher yields of CD34$^+$cells. We hope that our study will produce data that will determine whether HU confers an important safety advantage, without decreasing efficacy of mobilization or gene transfer.

Study design

Twenty-four adult patients with beta-thalassemia major, from whom 12 are splenectomized and 12 nonsplenectomized, will be included. Half of the subjects in both cohorts receive HU (20 mg/kg/day the nonsplenectomized, 25–30 mg/kg/day the splenectomized) for one month prior to mobilization and half do not. Due to their increased risk of thrombosis, splenectomized patients whose platelet counts exceed 500 × 10^3 per microliter are enrolled in the HU arm. HU is stopped 1–2 weeks prior to treatment with G-CSF. G-CSF at 5 mcg/kg twice daily, starts when CD34$^+$ cells rise to $\geq 1/\mu L$, and it is administered for 4–7 days. During the period of G-CSF administration and leukapheresis the subjects are hospitalized and monitored daily. Spleen volume is measured with abdominal ultrasound and physical examination at baseline and every other day after G-CSF initiation. For safety, when spleen volume increases more than 80% over baseline, mobilization is stopped. Two consecutive leukaphereses are performed, with a target cell yield of >2 × 10^6CD34$^+$/kg. Leukapheresis products are being processed by a CliniMacs device for CD34$^+$selection.

An aliquot of the selection product is kept to assess the ability of the thalassemic CD34$^+$ cells to be transduced with a β-globin lentiviral vector and engraft immunodeficient mice as well as the clonogenic capacity of mobilized cells. The bulk of the final product is cryopreserved and retained unmanipulated for a subsequent clinical gene transfer trial.

The study is not designed to provide any therapeutic benefit to the participating subjects at this stage, but it will provide important information that will help the design of stem cell mobilization strategies in patients with thalassemia major.

Acknowledgments

This work was supported by NIH Grant 2U01HL066947.

Conflicts of interest

The authors declare no conflicts of interest.

References

1. Papayannopoulou, T. & D. Scadden. 2008. Stem-cell ecology and stem cells in motion. *Blood* **111:** 3923–3930.
2. Gratwohl, A, H. Baldomero, K. Frauendorfer & A. Urbano-Ispizua. 2006. EBMT activity survey 2004 and changes in disease indication over the past 15 years: Joint Accreditation Committee, International Society for Cellular Therapy; European Group for Blood and Marrow Transplantation. *Bone Marrow Transplant*. **37:** 1069–1085.
3. To, L.B., D.N. Haylock, P.J. Simmons & C.A. Juttner. 1997. The biology and clinical uses of blood stem cells. *Blood* **89:** 2233–2258.
4. Welte, K., E. Platzer, L. Lu, *et al.* 1985. Purification and biochemical characterization of human pluripotent hematopoietic colony-stimulating factor. *Proc. Natl. Acad. Sci. USA* **82:** 1526–1530.
5. Horowitz, M.M. & D.L. Confer. 2005. Evaluation of hematopoietic stem cell donors. *Hematol. Am. Soc. Hematol. Educ. Program.* 469–475.
6. Dunbar, C.E., N.E. Seidel, S. Doren, *et al.* 1996. Improved retroviral gene transfer into murine and rhesus peripheral blood or bone marrow repopulating cells primed in vivo with stem cell factor and granulocyte colony-stimulating factor. *Proc. Natl. Acad. Sci. USA* **93:** 11871–1176.
7. Horn, P.A., K.A. Keyser, L.J. Peterson, *et al.* 2004. Efficient lentiviral gene transfer to canine repopulating cells using an overnight transduction protocol. *Blood* **103:** 37103716.
8. Thomasson, B., L. Peterson, J. Thompson, *et al.* 2003. Direct comparison of steady-state marrow, primed marrow, and mobilized peripheral blood for transduction of hematopoietic stem cells in dogs. *Hum. Gene Ther.* **14:** 1683–1686.
9. Platzbecker, U., G. Prange-Krex, M. Bornhäuser, *et al.* 2001. Spleen enlargement in healthy donors during G-CSF mobilization of PBPCs. *Transfusion* **41:** 184–189.
10. Stiff, P.J., W. Bensinger, M.H. Abidi, *et al.* 2009. Clinical and ultrasonic evaluation of spleen size during peripheral blood progenitor cell mobilization by filgrastim: results of an open-label trial in normal donors. *Biol. Blood Marrow Transplant*. **15:** 827–834.

11. Falzetti, F., F. Aversa, O. Minelli & A. Tabilio. 1999. Spontaneous rupture of spleen during peripheral blood stem cell mobilisation in a healthy donor. *Lancet* **353:** 555.
12. Becker, P.S., M. Wagle, S. Matous, *et al.* 1997. Spontaneous splenic rupture following administration of granulocyte colony-stimulating factor (G-CSF) occurrence in allogeneic donor of peripheral blood stem cells. *Biol. Blood Marrow Transplant*. **3:** 45–49.
13. Brown, S.L. & D.C. Dale. 1997. Spontaneous rupture following administration of of granulocyte colony-stimulating factor (G-CSF): occurrence in an allogeneic donor of peripheral blood stem cells. *Biol. Blood Marrow Transplant*. **3:** 45–49.
14. Balaguer, H., A. Galmes, G. Ventayol, *et al.* 2004. Splenic rupture after granulocyte-colony-stimulating factor mobilization in a peripheral blood progenitor cell donor. *Transfusion* **44:** 1260–1261.
15. Dincer, A.P., J. Gottschall & D.A. Margolis. 2004. Splenic rupture in a prarental donor undergoing peripheral blood progenitor cell mobilization. *J. Pediatr. Hematol. Oncol.* **26:** 761–763.
16. Fukumoto, Y., T. Miyamoto, T. Okamura, *et al.* 1997. Angina pectoris occurring during granulocyte colony-stimulating factor-combined preparatory regimen for autologous peripheral blood stem cell transplantation in a patient with acute myelogenous leukaemia. *Br. J. Haematol.* **97:** 666–668.
17. Lindemann, A. & B. Rumberger. 1993. Vascular complications in patients treated with granulocyte colony-stimulating factor (G-CSF). *Eur. J. Cancer.* **29A:** 2338–2339.
18. Anderlini, P., J.D. Rizzo, M.L. Nugent, *et al.*; IBMTR Statistical Center of the International Bone Marrow Transplant Registry, Medical College of Wisconcin, Milwaukee, WI, USA; EBMT, Kiel, Germany. 2001. Peripheral blood stem cell donation: an analysis from the International Bone Marrow Transplant Registry (IBMTR) and European Group for Blood and Marrow Transplant (EBMT) databases. *Bone Marrow Transplant*. **27:** 689–692.
19. Pawliuk, R., K.A. Westerman, M.E. Fabry, *et al.* 2001. Correction of sickle cell disease in transgenic mouse models by gene therapy. *Science* **294:** 2368–2371.
20. May, C., S. Rivella, J. Callegari, *et al.* 2000. Therapeutic haemoglobin synthesis in beta-thalassaemic mice expressing lentivirus-encoded human beta-globin. *Nature* **406:** 82–86.
21. Imren, S., E. Payen, K.A. Westerman, *et al.* 2002. Permanent and panerythroid correction of murine beta thalassemia by multiple lentiviral integration in hematopoietic stem cells. *Proc. Natl. Acad. Sci. USA* **99:** 14380–14385.
22. Rivella, S., C. May, A. Chadburn, *et al.* 2003. A novel murine model of Cooley anemia and its rescue by lentiviral-mediated human beta-globin gene transfer. *Blood* **101:** 2932–2939.
23. Puthenveetil, G., J. Scholes, D. Carbonell, *et al.* 2004. Successful correction of the human beta-thalassemia Major phenotype using a lentiviral vector. *Blood* **104:** 3445–3453.
24. Miccio, A., R. Cesari, F. Lotti, *et al.* 2008. In vivo selection of genetically modified erythroblastic progenitors leads to long-term correction of beta-thalassemia. *Proc. Natl. Acad. Sci. USA* **105:** 10547–10552.
25. Bank, A., R. Dorazio & P. Leboulch. 2005. A phase I/II clinical trial of beta-globin gene therapy for beta-thalassemia. *Ann. N.Y. Acad. Sci.* **1054:** 308–316.
26. Abboud, M., J. Laver & C.A. Blau. 1998. Granulocytosis causing sickle-cell crisis. *Lancet* **351:** 959.
27. Adler, B.K., D.E. Salzman, M.H. Carabasi, *et al.* 2001. Fatal sickle cell crisis after granulocyte colony-stimulating factor administration. *Blood* **97:** 3313–3314.
28. Grigg, A.P. 2001. Granulocyte colony-stimulating factor-induced sickle cell crisis and multiorgan dysfunction in a patient with compound heterozygous sickle cell/beta$^+$ thalassemia. *Blood* **97:** 3998–3999.
29. Kamble, R.T., C.K. Tin-U & G. Carrum. 2006. Successful mobilization and transplantation of filgrastim mobilized hematopoietic stem cells in sickle cell-hemoglobin C disease. *Bone Marrow Transplant*. **37:** 1065–1066.
30. Rosenbaum, C., D. Peace, E. Rich & K. Van Besien. 2008. Granulocyte colony-stimulating factor-based stem cell mobilization in patients with sickle cell disease. *Biol. Blood Marrow Transplant*. **14:** 719–723.
31. Fitzhugh, C.D., M.M. Hsieh, C.D. Bolan, *et al.* 2009. Granulocyte colony-stimulating factor (G-CSF) administration in individuals with sickle cell disease: time for a moratorium? *Cytotherapy* **11:** 464–471.
32. Lamming, C.E., L. Augustin, M. Blackstad, *et al.* 2003. Spontaneous circulation of myeloid-lymphoid-initiating cells and SCID-repopulating cells in sickle cell crisis. *J. Clin. Invest.* **111:** 811–819.
33. Richard, R.E., N. Siritanaratkul, E. Jonlin, *et al.* 2005. Collection of blood stem cells from patients with sickle cell anemia. *Blood Cells Mol. Dis.* **35:** 384–388.
34. Hal, E. Broxmeyer, Christie M. Orschell, D. Wade Clapp, *et al.* 2005. Rapid mobilization of murine and human hematopoietic stem and progenitor cells with AMD3100, a CXCR4 antagonist. *J. Exp. Med.* **201:** 1307–1318.
35. Liles, W.C., H.E. Broxmeyer, E. Rodger, *et al.* 2003. Mobilization of hematopoietic progenitor cells in healthy volunteers by AMD3100, a CXCR4 antagonist. *Blood* **102:** 2728–2730.
36. Devine, S.M., R. Vij, M. Rettig, *et al.* 2008. Rapid mobilization of functional donor hematopoietic cells without G-CSF using AMD3100, an antagonist of the CXCR4/SDF-1 interaction. *Blood* **112:** 990–998.
37. Li, K., A. Wong, C.K. Li, *et al.* 1999. Granulocyte colony-stimulating factor-mobilized peripheral blood stem cells in β-thalassemia patients: kinetics of mobilization and composition of apheresis product. *Exp. Hematol.* **27:** 526–532.
38. Yannaki, E., N. Psatha, E. Athanasiou, *et al.* 2009. Mobilization of hematopoietic stem cells in a thalassemic mouse model: implications for human gene therapy of thalassemia. *Hum Gene Ther.* **21:** 299–310.
39. Cappellini, M.D., L. Robbiolo, B.M. Bottasso, *et al.* 2000. Venous thromboembolism and hypercoagulability in splenectomized patients with thalassaemia intermedia. *Br. J. Haematol.* **111:** 467–473.
40. Saxon, B.R., D. Rees & N.F. Olivieri. 1998. Regression of extramedullary hemopoiesis and augmentation of fetal hemoglobin concentration during hydroxyurea therapy in β-thalassemia. *Br. J. Haematol.* **101:** 416–419.

Ann. N.Y. Acad. Sci. ISSN 0077-8923

ANNALS OF THE NEW YORK ACADEMY OF SCIENCES
Issue: *Cooley's Anemia: Ninth Symposium*

Transcriptional silencing of fetal hemoglobin by BCL11A

Vijay G. Sankaran,[1,2] Jian Xu,[1,2,3] and Stuart H. Orkin[1,2,3,4]

[1]Division of Hematology/Oncology, Children's Hospital Boston, Harvard Medical School, Boston, Massachusetts. [2]Department of Pediatric Oncology, Dana-Farber Cancer Institute, Harvard Stem Cell Institute, Harvard Medical School, Boston, Massachusetts. [3]Howard Hughes Medical Institute, Boston, Massachusetts

Address for correspondence: Stuart H. Orkin, M.D., Dana-Farber Cancer Institute, 44 Binney Street, Dana 1642, Boston, MA 02115. stuart_orkin@dfci.harvard.edu

The β-thalassemia syndromes are a major global health problem. Increased levels of fetal hemoglobin (HbF) ameliorate the clinical symptoms seen in this disease. By taking advantage of the natural variation in the level of HbF in various populations, we and others identified several common genetic variants in three major loci that regulate HbF levels. One of these variants resides in the gene *BCL11A*. We have studied the role of this gene product and established that BCL11A maintains silencing of γ-*globin* expression in adult erythroid cells and functions as a direct transcriptional regulator of the fetal to adult hemoglobin switch in humans. Moreover, we found that BCL11A plays a central role in the evolutionarily divergent globin gene switches of mammals. As a factor critical for γ-*globin* gene silencing, BCL11A should be considered as a therapeutic target to increase HbF in a directed manner in β-thalassemia patients.

Keywords: thalassemia; fetal hemoglobin; globin switching; BCL11A; transcription

The thalassemia syndromes remain major sources of morbidity and mortality worldwide, particularly in the developing world.[1] It is estimated that nearly two percent of death and disability adjusted life years among children in Asia are attributable to the thalassemia syndromes. However, despite their simple Mendelian inheritance, these disorders, exhibit considerable heterogeneity in their clinical manifestations.[2] The basis for this is not entirely clear, although in the case of the β-thalassemias it can be attributed in part to the ameliorating effect of increased levels of fetal hemoglobin (HbF) in patients.[2,3]

The production of hemoglobin is carefully regulated to achieve balanced synthesis of the α- and β-globin chains. These chains then combine as a tetramer of two α- and two β-globin polypeptides along with a heme moiety to form the adult hemoglobin molecule.[4] In β-thalassemia, the production of the β-globin polypeptide is reduced as a result of mutations in this gene, which results in excess unstable α-globin chains precipitating in red blood cell precursors, causing toxicity and death of these cells.[4,5] Anemia results due to ineffective production of mature red blood cells, leading to the numerous clinical manifestations that are frequently observed in β-thalassemia.

Over the course of human gestation and in early infancy, a different β-like globin polypeptide is produced from duplicated γ-*globin* genes within the β-globin cluster. This fetal globin polypeptide, γ-globin, combines with α-globin chains and a heme moiety to form HbF. Nonanemic adults typically express low levels of γ-*globin*, resulting in less than 1% of total hemoglobin being HbF. The clinical symptoms of patients with β-thalassemia and other disorders of the β-globin molecule are less severe among those who have higher levels of HbF. In the context of β-thalassemia, this less severe clinical phenotype is attributable to the fact that γ-globin chains can help compensate for the imbalance present from reduced β-globin production.

Because of the important contribution of HbF expression to the clinical severity of β-hemoglobin disorders, there has been a great interest in understanding how the γ-*globin* genes are regulated at the

doi: 10.1111/j.1749-6632.2010.05574.x

transcriptional level within the β-globin locus and how the fetal to adult (γ- to β-) globin switch occurs in the course of human ontogeny.[6,7] However, until recently, only limited insight has been gained into how this process is controlled in humans.

It has long been appreciated that in both nonanemic populations and cohorts of patients with sickle cell disease or β-thalassemia, HbF levels vary considerably and appear to at least partially be genetically determined. Building on such observations, recent genetic association studies have used this natural variation to delineate common genetic polymorphisms that contribute to this variation.[8] The first study, involving a nonanemic Caucasian population, was performed to identify variants associated with HbF-containing cell (F-cell) levels in a chromosomal region previously identified through more traditional linkage approaches.[9,10] In this instance, polymorphisms associated with F-cell levels in an intergenic region between the genes *HBS1L* and *MYB* were identified.[9] Soon thereafter, genome-wide association studies (GWAS) for HbF levels were performed on the same population and with an independent cohort of Sardinian individuals.[11,12] Both studies confirmed the strong association with the *HBS1L-MYB* region on chromosome 6, found an association with variants in the β-*globin* locus, and identified a new HbF-associated locus on chromosome 2, within the gene *BCL11A*. These associations were subsequently confirmed in populations with sickle cell disease,[13–15] as well as other populations.[16] Furthermore, we demonstrated that these genetic variants ameliorate the severity of sickle cell disease,[13] consistent with the effect of higher levels of HbF in lessening symptoms in this disease.[17–19] In addition and of great interest, two well-designed studies in cohorts of patients with β-thalassemia have demonstrated that these variants contribute significantly to the clinical course of the disease and may explain up to 75% of the variation in clinical severity.[12,20,21]

Given the strong association of genetic variants in the *BCL11A* gene with HbF levels in numerous populations, we explored how these variants may affect *BCL11A* expression and whether this gene product might have a direct role in regulation of the HbF (γ-*globin*) genes (Fig. 1).[22] BCL11A acts as a transcriptional repressor in B lymphocytes,[23] but its role in red blood cell production was previously unexplored. We initially showed that the variants characteristic of higher levels of HbF are associated with lower levels of *BCL11A* mRNA expression. We

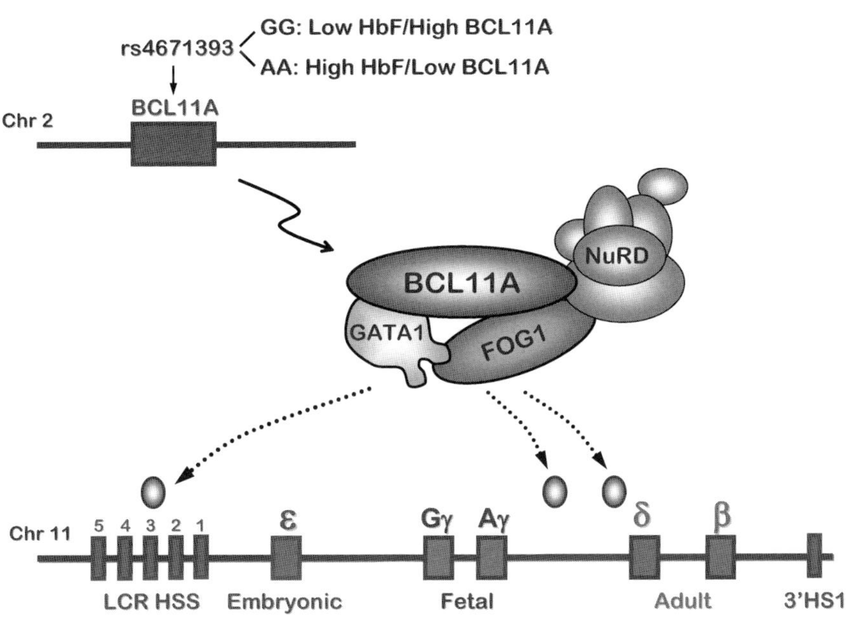

Figure 1. This diagram illustrates how a genetic variant within the *BCL11A* gene in humans that is associated with different levels of HbF is in turn associated with variation in expression of *BCL11A* (top of diagram). This variation in expression appears to have an effect on the function of BCL11A at the human β-globin locus, where it is thought to act with the erythroid transcription factors GATA-1 and FOG-1, as well as the NuRD remodeling and repressor complex to silence the γ-*globin* genes (bottom of diagram).

also found that BCL11A protein levels vary in red blood cell (erythroid) progenitors over the course of human ontogeny. BCL11A is expressed as short variant proteins in cells that robustly express γ-*globin* (primitive and fetal liver erythroid progenitors) and as full-length forms at the adult stage when the γ-*globin* genes are silenced. These findings suggested that BCL11A may function as a repressor of the human γ-*globin* genes.

Using a proteomic approach, we demonstrated that BCL11A interacts with the NuRD chromatin remodeling and repressor complex, the erythroid transcription factors GATA-1 and FOG-1, and the nuclear matrix component Matrin-3 in erythroid progenitors (Fig. 1). These findings suggest that full-length forms of BCL11A may act through interaction with these molecules to silence the γ-*globin* genes in erythroid progenitors. Of note, the NuRD repressor complex contains two histone deacetylases (HDAC), HDAC1 and HDAC2. It has been suggested that short-chain fatty acids and other therapeutic inducers of HbF may act as inhibitors of HDACs, possibly providing a connection between this mode of HbF induction and the role of this complex in repression of the γ-*globin* gene.[24,25] It is also interesting to note that the β-globin locus interacts with the nuclear periphery where the nuclear matrix is located at the early stages of erythropoiesis, before high-level transcription by RNA polymerase II begins.[26] One of the components isolated with BCL11A is the nuclear matrix component Matrin-3, suggesting a possible mechanism for recruitment to this nuclear region. Furthermore, we demonstrated that the interactions of BCL11A with GATA-1 are mediated through the zinc fingers of the GATA-1 transcription factor. In light of this finding, it is interesting to note that a patient with a mutation in the N-terminal zinc-finger of GATA-1 was found to have a phenotype of greatly elevated HbF levels with erythropoietic porphyria and β-thalassemia.[27] The exact cause of this phenotype is currently unclear.

To assess whether BCL11A has a direct role in regulating the γ-*globin* genes in humans, we used siRNA and shRNA knockdown approaches in human primary adult CD34-derived erythroid progenitors. Knockdown of BCL11A leads to robust elevations in the level of γ-*globin*, and furthermore in the production of mature HbF. We also showed that upon knockdown of BCL11A few global transcriptional expression differences with control cells are detected, while robust elevation of HbF expression occurs. Thus, BCL11A appears to act rather specifically to regulate the γ-*globin* genes. This hypothesis was strongly supported by the finding that BCL11A binds to chromatin located in the β-globin locus. Specifically, we found that BCL11A interacts with the third hypersensitive site of the locus control region (LCR) and distinct regions between the *A*γ- and δ-*globin* genes (Fig. 1). Notably, BCL11A fails to bind within the proximal promoters of the γ-*globin* genes. Collectively, these findings established BCL11A as a direct regulator of the HbF genes. Importantly, the discovery of BCL11A through genetic association studies constitutes strong, independent support for the *in vivo* role of BCL11A in humans.

The studies reviewed above address the role of BCL11A in silencing the γ-*globin* genes in adult erythroid cells. We then extended these findings to its role in developmental switching using mouse models.[28] Transgenic mice containing the entire human β-globin locus (with all regulatory elements in their normal configuration) failed to recapitulate the normal developmental regulation of the globin genes as seen in humans. Specifically, the γ-*globin* gene is treated largely as a mouse embryonic globin gene in the context of the mouse erythroid trans-acting environment. The γ-*globin* gene is predominantly expressed in the transient primitive erythroid lineage, but little expression is seen in definitive erythroid cells in these mice. This reveals an important limitation of this commonly used transgenic model. In addition, given that the *cis*-elements of the β-globin locus appear to be insufficient to ensure proper developmental regulation of the human β-like globin genes, these findings suggest that the evolutionary divergence in mammalian globin gene switching is likely mediated through modification of the expression of certain trans-acting factors. Given our prior findings on the role of BCL11A in regulating the human γ-*globin* genes, we assessed its expression pattern in stage-matched human and mouse erythroid progenitors at different times of development. Surprisingly, we found that BCL11A is not expressed in mouse primitive erythroid cells, but is expressed at similar levels in mouse fetal liver and bone marrow erythroid progenitors. In contrast, in humans, BCL11A is expressed as short variant proteins in the primitive and fetal liver erythroid cells, while only minor expression of the full-length forms are seen in the fetal liver cells. In the bone marrow, expression of full-length forms predominates. Thus, the divergent globin switching patterns of mouse and human may result from altered expression of BCL11A. To directly test this hypothesis, we examined globin gene expression in *Bcl11a* knockout mice. Remarkably, the mouse embryonic globin genes are dramatically upregulated in fetal liver definitive erythroid cells of *Bcl11a* knockout mice, where these genes are normally silent. However, erythropoiesis in the context of this knockout appears ostensibly normal. In the fetal liver of *Bcl11a* knockout mice harboring a human β-globin locus transgene, γ*-globin* expression is derepressed, identifying a failure of developmental switching in the absence of BCL11A.

Together these findings demonstrate that BCL11A is an important regulator of the fetal to adult hemoglobin switch in humans[22] and plays a critical role as a regulator of the divergence of mammalian globin switches that has occurred in the course of evolution.[28] Moreover, these findings suggest that loss of BCL11A is rather well tolerated in red blood cell differentiation *in vivo.* The above studies establish BCL11A as a central regulator of the fetal to adult hemoglobin switch, as well as a silencer of γ*-globin* gene expression in adult erythroid cells. As such, BCL11A is the first genetically and biochemically validated switching factor. Downregulation of BCL11A expression or function by siRNA or small molecules may offer a new therapeutic approach to directed activation of HbF in adult erythroid cells of patients with β-thalassemia and other disorders of β-hemoglobin.

Conflicts of interest

The authors declare no conflicts of interest.

References

1. Weatherall, D., O. Akinyanju, S. Fucharoen, *et al.* 2006. Inherited disorders of hemoglobin. *Disease Control Priorities in Developing Countries*, 2nd ed.: 663–680. Oxford University Press. New York.
2. Weatherall, D.J. 2001. Phenotype-genotype relationships in monogenic disease: lessons from the thalassaemias. *Nat. Rev. Genet.* **2:** 245–255.
3. Premawardhena, A., C.A. Fisher, N.F. Olivieri, *et al.* 2005. Haemoglobin E beta thalassaemia in Sri Lanka. *Lancet* **366:** 1467–1470.
4. Rund, D. & E. Rachmilewitz. 2005. Beta-thalassemia. *N. Engl. J. Med.* **353:** 1135–1146.
5. Olivieri, N.F. 1999. The beta-thalassemias. *N. Engl. J. Med.* **341:** 99–109.
6. Stamatoyannopoulos, G. 2005. Control of globin gene expression during development and erythroid differentiation. *Exp. Hematol.* **33:** 259–271.
7. Bank, A. 2006. Regulation of human fetal hemoglobin: new players, new complexities. *Blood* **107:** 435–443.
8. Thein, S.L. & S. Menzel. 2009. Discovering the genetics underlying foetal haemoglobin production in adults. *Br. J. Haematol.* **145:** 455–467.
9. Thein, S.L., S. Menzel, X. Peng, *et al.* 2007. Intergenic variants of HBS1L-MYB are responsible for a major quantitative trait locus on chromosome 6q23 influencing fetal hemoglobin levels in adults. *Proc. Natl Acad. Sci. USA* **104:** 11346–11351.
10. Craig, J.E., J. Rochette, C.A. Fisher, *et al.* 1996. Dissecting the loci controlling fetal haemoglobin production on chromosomes 11p and 6q by the regressive approach. *Nat. Genet.* **12:** 58–64.
11. Menzel, S., C. Garner, I. Gut, *et al.* 2007. A QTL influencing F cell production maps to a gene encoding a zinc-finger protein on chromosome 2p15. *Nat. Genet.* **39:** 1197–1199.
12. Uda, M., R. Galanello, S. Sanna, *et al.* 2008. Genome-wide association study shows BCL11A associated with persistent fetal hemoglobin and amelioration of the phenotype of beta-thalassemia. *Proc. Natl Acad. Sci. USA* **105:** 1620–1625.
13. Lettre, G., V.G. Sankaran, M.A. Bezerra, *et al.* 2008. DNA polymorphisms at the BCL11A, HBS1L-MYB, and beta-globin loci associate with fetal hemoglobin levels and pain crises in sickle cell disease. *Proc. Natl Acad. Sci. USA* **105:** 11869–11874.
14. Creary, L.E., P. Ulug, S. Menzel, *et al.* 2009. Genetic variation on chromosome 6 influences F cell levels in healthy individuals of African descent and HbF levels in sickle cell patients. *PLoS One* **4:** e4218.
15. Solovieff, N., J.N. Milton, S.W. Hartley, *et al.* 2010. Fetal hemoglobin in sickle cell anemia: genome-wide association studies suggest a regulatory region in the 5′ olfactory receptor gene cluster. *Blood* **115:** 1815–1822.
16. Sedgewick, A.E., N. Timofeev, P. Sebastiani, *et al.* 2008. BCL11A is a major HbF quantitative trait locus in three different populations with beta-hemoglobinopathies. *Blood Cells Mol. Dis.* **41:** 255–258.
17. Platt, O.S., D.J. Brambilla, W.F. Rosse, *et al.* 1994. Mortality in sickle cell disease. Life expectancy and risk factors for early death. *N. Engl. J. Med.* **330:** 1639–1644.
18. Platt, O.S., B.D. Thorington, D.J. Brambilla, *et al.* 1991. Pain in sickle cell disease. Rates and risk factors. *N. Engl. J. Med.* **325:** 11–16.
19. Castro, O., D.J. Brambilla, B. Thorington, *et al.* 1994. The acute chest syndrome in sickle cell disease: incidence and risk factors. The Cooperative Study of Sickle Cell Disease. *Blood* **84:** 643–649.
20. Galanello, R., S. Sanna, L. Perseu, *et al.* 2009. Amelioration of Sardinian beta0 thalassemia by genetic modifiers. *Blood* **114:** 3935–3937.
21. Nuinoon, M., W. Makarasara, T. Mushiroda, *et al.* 2010. A genome-wide association identified the common genetic variants influence disease severity in beta(0)-thalassemia/hemoglobin E. *Hum. Genet.* **127:** 303–314.
22. Sankaran, V.G., T.F. Menne, J. Xu, *et al.* 2008. Human fetal hemoglobin expression is regulated by the developmental stage-specific repressor BCL11A. *Science* **322:** 1839–1842.

23. Liu, P., J.R. Keller, M. Ortiz, *et al.* 2003. Bcl11a is essential for normal lymphoid development. *Nat. Immunol.* **4:** 525–532.
24. Fathallah, H., R.S. Weinberg, Y. Galperin, *et al.* 2007. Role of epigenetic modifications in normal globin gene regulation and butyrate-mediated induction of fetal hemoglobin. *Blood* **110:** 3391–3397.
25. Cao, H., G. Stamatoyannopoulos & M. Jung. 2004. Induction of human gamma globin gene expression by histone deacetylase inhibitors. *Blood* **103:** 701–709.
26. Ragoczy, T., M.A. Bender, A. Telling, *et al.* 2006. The locus control region is required for association of the murine beta-globin locus with engaged transcription factories during erythroid maturation. *Genes Dev.* **20:** 1447–1457.
27. Phillips, J.D., D.P. Steensma, M.A. Pulsipher, *et al.* 2007. Congenital erythropoietic porphyria due to a mutation in GATA1: the first trans-acting mutation causative for a human porphyria. *Blood* **109:** 2618–2621.
28. Sankaran, V.G., J. Xu, T. Ragoczy, *et al.* 2009. Developmental and species-divergent globin switching are driven by BCL11A. *Nature* **460:** 1093–1097.

Ann. N.Y. Acad. Sci. ISSN 0077-8923

ANNALS OF THE NEW YORK ACADEMY OF SCIENCES
Issue: *Cooley's Anemia: Ninth Symposium*

The challenge of obtaining therapeutic levels of genetically modified hematopoietic stem cells in β-thalassemia patients

Derek A. Persons
Division of Experimental Hematology, Department of Hematology, St. Jude Children's Research Hospital, Memphis, Tennessee

Address for correspondence: Derek Persons, M.D., Ph.D., Department of Hematology, 262 Danny Thomas Place, St. Jude Children's Research Hospital, Memphis, TN 38105. derek.persons@stjude.org

Hematopoietic stem cells (HSCs) function to provide the individual with a continuing supply of blood cells over many decades. To this end, HSCs have evolved unique mechanisms for self-preservation, including resistance to viral infection. Unfortunately, this characteristic may impede the ability to achieve high levels of gene transfer mediated by HIV-based lentiviral vectors. This is an important consideration for gene therapy efforts being undertaken for β-thalassemia. In particular, the study of β-thalassemia patients that underwent allogeneic stem cell transplantation and developed stable, long-term mixed chimerism suggests that HSC gene transfer levels of greater than 25% will be needed for a robust therapeutic effect in such patients. Available pre-clinical and clinical trial lentiviral gene transfer studies suggest that improvements are needed to achieve this goal. Here, we review what level of gene transfer is needed in the context of varying degrees of β-globin deficiency, what level is currently achievable, and the areas of research which may be fruitful in improving the likelihood of success for patients with the severest forms of β-thalassemia.

Keywords: β-thalassemia; gene therapy; lentiviral vector; hematopoietic stem cells

Introduction

Substantial progress has been made over the past decade in developing hematopoietic stem cell (HSC)-targeted gene transfer as a potentially curative treatment for β-thalassemia. Beginning in 2000 with the report of correction of a murine model of β-thalassemia using globin lentiviral vector gene transfer, several groups of investigators have made steady progress in this area.[1–6] Several potentially clinically useful globin lentiviral vector designs have been developed and studied in preclinical models. Using one of these designs, the first human clinical trial has begun in Paris and some success has been obtained in one patient with HbE/β-thalassemia as reported at the Cooley's Anemia 9th Symposium in October 2009 and at a meeting in December 2009 of the U.S. Recombinant DNA Advisory Committee.[7] However, available data and the results from this patient suggest that challenges remain before effective gene therapy can be realized for the most severe forms of β-thalassemia major. Herein, we review one of the major challenges, namely that of achieving therapeutic levels of engraftment with autologous HSCs genetically modified with a globin lentiviral vector. Several areas of research that seem relevant to this problem are discussed.

What is the therapeutic threshold level of engrafted, genetically modified HSCs for β-thalassemia?

Using murine transplantation models, we and others have shown that the majority of engrafting mouse HSCs can be genetically modified with lentiviral vectors.[2,4,8] However, nonhuman primate and human HSCs are much more resistant to lentiviral gene transfer. In studies using the rhesus macaque autologous transplantation model in the context of full myeloablation of the recipient

doi: 10.1111/j.1749-6632.2010.05581.x

animals, we achieved an average of 7% (range 3–12%) lentiviral vector-bearing peripheral blood cells 4 years after transplantation.[9] Recent work by the Kiem lab has also demonstrated levels of lentiviral gene transfer in pigtail macaques in the first year post-transplant comparable to those we observed at that time point.[10,11] Consistent with these preclinical results, HSC lentiviral gene marking levels of 10–15% in the context of myeloablation have recently been reported in two children in a clinical trial for adrenoleukodystrophy.[12] Similarly, and as mentioned above, a patient with HbE/β-thalassemia treated with myeloablation and transduced bone marrow CD34$^+$ cells also has about 10–15% genetically modified peripheral blood cells in a gene transfer clinical trial using a globin lentiviral vector. Thus, these various data are in agreement that it is currently possible to obtain engraftment with 10–15% genetically modified (transduced) repopulating cells.

Is this level of transduced cell engraftment adequate for a therapeutic response for patients with β-thalassemia? The outcome may depend on the underlying degree of β-globin deficiency and β-globin genotype of the patient. For patients with no production of β-globin (β°), the degree of HSC chimerism with gene-modified cells necessary for a therapeutic effect, as defined by transfusion independence, might be estimated from the clinical data of Andreani and colleagues.[13] They reported a series of β° patients that received allogeneic transplantation and maintained long-term mixed donor chimerism. Figure 1 shows the transfusion-independent hemoglobin (Hb) level as a function of peripheral blood (PB) leukocyte donor chimerism. Informative are two patients with 25% donor cells that had Hb levels of 8.3 and 9.3 g/dL, respectively. Donor cell chimerism levels of greater than 40% were needed to obtain Hb levels above 10 g/dL. Hb levels that equal or exceed the latter are likely preferable for overall long-term efficacy in order to suppress the erythroid drive, and the attendant complications, which remains at lower Hb levels. Thus, it might be concluded, based on available data, that improvements in HSC gene transfer and engraftment are needed to achieve the levels of genetically-modified HSC chimerism that appear to be required for a robust therapeutic effect in β° patients.

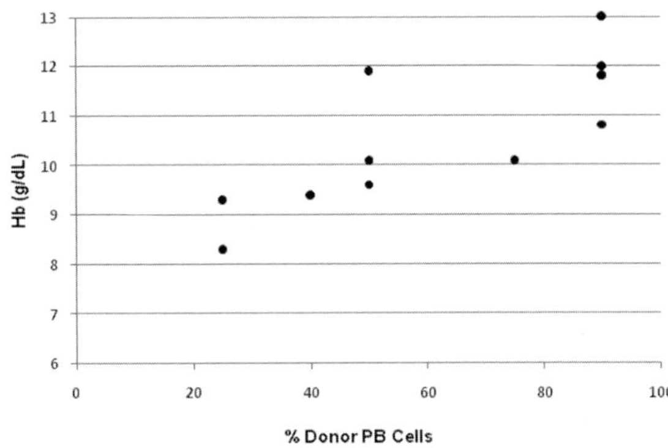

Figure 1. Transfusion-independent Hb level as a function of peripheral blood donor cell chimerism in β-thalassemic patients that received an allogeneic bone marrow transplant and developed stable mixed chimerism. Plotted data is from Andreani *et al.*[13]

In contrast, the presence of some intrinsic β-globin production may lower the required therapeutic threshold of engrafted, genetically modified cells. This could be due to: (1) the "baseline" level of endogenous Hb production from unmodified erythroid cells, intrinsically selected for the highest Hb content, and (2) the enhanced viability and contribution to the erythron and Hb concentration of genetically modified erythroid progeny that bear vector integrations producing marginally therapeutic levels of globin transgene expression. Indeed, it appears that modest levels of gene transfer can yield some benefit for transfusion-dependent patients with perhaps less severe forms of β-globin deficiency, such as the HbE/β-thalassemia patient in the Paris trial. Similarly, other patients with variable degrees of β-globin deficiency who nonetheless require transfusion to maintain quality of life might also derive some benefit with levels of genetically modified cells in the 10–20% range. Indeed, we previously showed that significant amelioration of murine β-thalassemia intermedia could be achieved with normal HSC chimerism levels of 10–20%.[14]

Factors limiting the gene transfer efficiency into primate and human HSCs

Cellular factors involved in lentiviral gene transfer into human HSCs

The resistance of primitive hematopoietic cells to infection by HIV-1, despite having the required membrane receptors, has been recognized for over a decade.[15,16] Therefore, it perhaps should not be surprising that HSCs possess intrinsic barriers to gene transfer mediated by HIV-based lentiviral vectors. Both previous studies and more recent genome wide screening approaches have identified a large number of host cell proteins that seem to be required for effective HIV replication in human T cells.[17–19] As a corollary, there may also be numerous host cell proteins that play a role in the restriction of HIV replication. Together, both sets of proteins likely influence the ability to transduce human HSCs with HIV-based lentiviral vectors. Several innate cellular mechanisms that restrict retroviral infection have been well-studied in cell line systems and in human T cells.[20,21] Cellular proteins in the TRIM5α and APOBEC3 families are examples of proteins that have been implicated in limiting HIV infection at viral post-entry steps by their interactions with uncoated viral cores, thereby impeding the necessary subsequent steps that ultimately result in proviral integration into the host cell DNA.[22,23] Little is known regarding the presence and activity of the various "promoting" or "restricting" factors in primitive hematopoietic cell populations.

However, recent studies by two groups have begun to uncover some of the mechanisms of resistance to lentiviral gene transfer that may be operative in HSCs. Naldini and colleagues have shown that lentiviral gene transfer into human $CD34^+$ cells may be limited by the proteasome through regulation of one or more of the cellular post-entry steps of the vector particle.[24] Experiments in which the proteasome inhibitor MG132 was included in the culture during lentiviral vector transduction demonstrated a nearly a fourfold increase in gene transfer into human $CD34^+$ cells. Interestingly, depletion of the cellular factor cyclophilin A, which is known to interact with the uncoated viral capsid, caused a reduction in gene transfer. It was speculated that the levels of endogenous cellular proteins important in facilitating the gene transfer process may be favorably altered by proteasomal inhibition. In a different study by Scadden and colleagues, the cell cycle protein p21, present at high levels in HSCs, was identified as a unique molecular barrier to HIV infection through its interactions with the viral integrase to inhibit chromosomal integration.[25] Continued investigation into the cellular factors that participate in the intracellular lentiviral gene transfer process seems critical in order to develop new approaches to increase the gene transfer rate into HSCs.

Low levels of HSC cycling during ex vivo *lentiviral transduction*

Observational studies using both quiescent human T cells and the quiescent subpopulation of human $CD34^+$ progenitor cells have shown that cells in the G_0 phase of the cell cycle are resistant to efficient gene transfer using HIV-1 based lentiviral vectors.[26–28] G_0 T cells have to traverse to the G_1b stage of the cell cycle before completion of reverse transcription can occur. This reverse transcription block cannot be overcome simply by supplying exogenous dNTPs.[29] Currently, the precise cellular proteins and molecular mechanisms that underlie the specific resistance of G_0 cells remain undefined but perhaps may involve some of those discussed above. These and other studies reinforce the observation that lentiviral gene transfer is much more efficient if cells, including human G_0 $CD34^+$ cells, are either activated and/or dividing. In fact, the efficiency of transduction of quiescent cells has been measured to be at least 10-fold less that of cells that are dividing.[30–32] It has been estimated that primate and human HSCs undergo cell division *in vivo* on average once every 30 and 45 weeks, respectively, compared to once every 2.5 weeks for mouse HSCs.[33,34] This intrinsic cycling difference and the likely inability using current culture conditions to induce proliferation of a large proportion of HSCs, without causing loss of pluripotency, may limit the gene transfer efficiency in primate and human HSCs.

Although approaches to induce proliferation and expand HSCs have been explored for many years, no significant breakthroughs have occurred. More recent data seems promising in that novel cytokine combinations, which include the use of newly identified angiopoietin-like proteins, can result in the *ex vivo* expansion of human cells that repopulate immunodeficient mice.[35,36] Studies to evaluate whether HSC gene transfer efficiencies can be improved using these novel culture conditions seem worthwhile. Similarly, other studies raise the possibility that cell-permeable transcription factors might also be used to increase HSC cycling.[37,38] Cell permeable HOXB4 can modestly increase the number of human repopulating cells during *ex vivo* culture. Recent work using a different HOX protein is also promising as a factor to induce HSC proliferation and expansion.[39] Overall, new strategies are needed to identify conditions that support the *ex vivo* proliferation of human HSCs, while maintaining their pluripotency.

Selection of genetically modified cells prior to transplantation

One approach to compensate for inefficient transduction of HSCs is the use of drug selection strategies to amplify and enrich a minor component of transduced HSCs. By including an appropriate drug resistance gene in the lentiviral vector and then treating the transplant recipient with the selective agent, it is possible to increase the proportion of genetically modified HSCs in a variety of preclinical models.[40] We have devoted significant efforts to evaluate whether the methylguanine methyltransferase (MGMT) drug resistance gene, which confers resistance to several potent hematopoietic toxins such as BCNU and temozolomide, could be used in this regard.[41,42] Cells expressing MGMT have the ability to repair the DNA lesions caused by these drugs prior to the induction of apoptosis. Normal HSCs express relatively low levels of endogenous MGMT and are therefore generally sensitive to these drugs.

Using this approach, we recently demonstrated that γ-globin/MGMT dual gene lentiviral vectors could be used effectively for *in vivo* selection of HSCs following cytotoxic drug administration, resulting in large increases in γ-globin expressing cells and resolution of anemia in a mouse model of β-thalassemia.[42] Perhaps more importantly, we also found that in the mouse system, MGMT-mediated *in vitro* selection could be used to enrich the number of globin vector-transduced β-thalassemic HSCs prior *to* transplantation. Mice receiving transplants of cells briefly cultured with the drug showed significant levels of HbF protein, compared to lower amounts in animals that received untreated cells. Mice given drug-selected HSCs had greater than 60% F cells on average, while mice receiving untreated HSCs averaged 18% F cells. Importantly, the former group showed a significantly high Hb level relative to the control group (Hb of 11.0 vs. 9.9). We observed no graft failures in the group receiving drug-treated cells. These data suggest that transduced HSCs can be selected in culture prior to transplantation using the MGMT system, at least in a model where starting numbers of HSC are not limiting and significant numbers remain after selection. One advantage of this approach is that it would eliminate the toxicity of drug administration to the patient. Future studies in large animals will be needed to evaluate the clinical feasibility of this strategy.

Conclusions

Results from several patients in recent gene therapy trials in which lentiviral vectors were used to transduce HSCs indicate that although clinical success can be achieved, the overall levels of engraftment with genetically modified HSCs that are currently possible are likely in the 10–15% range. While these levels may be sufficient to procure clinical improvement and transfusion independence in patients with β^{+}-thalassemias, higher levels of gene transfer will be needed to cure patients with β°-thalassemia. Therefore, patient selection will be an important factor in the current planning of upcoming clinical trials. Future studies to understand the molecular events in the lentiviral vector transduction process are needed to foster the development of approaches to improve HSC gene transfer efficiency. This will likely require a better understanding of cellular proteins that facilitate and or impede the gene transfer process.

Conflicts of interest

The author declares no conflicts of interest.

References

1. May, C., S. Rivella, J. Callegari, *et al.* 2000. Therapeutic haemoglobin synthesis in beta-thalassaemic mice expressing lentivirus-encoded human beta-globin. *Nature* **406:** 82–86.
2. Imren, S., E. Payen, K.A. Westerman, *et al.* 2002. Permanent and panerythroid correction of murine beta thalassemia by multiple lentiviral integration in hematopoietic stem cells. *Proc. Natl. Acad. Sci. USA* **99:** 14380–14385.
3. Persons, D.A., P.W. Hargrove, E.R. Allay, *et al.* 2003. The degree of phenotypic correction of murine beta -thalassemia intermedia following lentiviral-mediated transfer of a human gamma-globin gene is influenced by chromosomal position effects and vector copy number. *Blood* **101:** 2175–2183.
4. Hanawa, H., P.W. Hargrove, S. Kepes, *et al.* 2004. Extended beta-globin locus control region elements promote consistent therapeutic expression of a gamma-globin lentiviral vector in murine beta-thalassemia. *Blood* **104:** 2281–2290.
5. Puthenveetil, G., J. Scholes, D. Carbonell, *et al.* 2004. Successful correction of the human beta-thalassemia major phenotype using a lentiviral vector. *Blood* **104:** 3445–3453.

6. Miccio, A., R. Cesari, F. Lotti, *et al.* 2008. In vivo selection of genetically modified erythroblastic progenitors leads to long-term correction of beta-thalassemia. *Proc. Natl. Acad. Sci. USA* **105:** 10547–10552.
7. Kaiser, J. 2009. {beta}-Thalassemia Treatment Succeeds, With a Caveat. *Science* **326:** 1468–1469.
8. Levasseur, D.N., T. M. Ryan, K.M. Pawlik & T. M. Townes, *et al.* 2003. Correction of a mouse model of sickle cell disease: lentiviral/antisickling beta-globin gene transduction of unmobilized, purified hematopoietic stem cells. *Blood* **102:** 4312–4319.
9. Kim, Y.J., Y.S. Kim, A. Larochelle, *et al.* 2009. Sustained high level polyclonal hematopoietic marking and transgene expression four years following autologous transplantation of rhesus macaques with SIV lentiviral vector transduced CD34$^+$ cells. *Blood* **113:** 5747–5756.
10. Trobridge, G.D., B.C. Beard, C. Gooch, *et al.* 2008. Efficient transduction of pigtailed macaque hematopoietic repopulating cells with HIV-based lentiviral vectors. *Blood* **111:** 5537–5543.
11. Hanawa, H., P. Hematti, K. Keyvanfar, *et al.* 2004. Efficient gene transfer into rhesus repopulating hematopoietic stem cells using a simian immunodeficiency virus-based lentiviral vector system. *Blood* **103:** 4062–4069.
12. Cartier, N., S. Hacein-Bey-Abina, C.C. Bartholomae, *et al.* 2009. Hematopoietic stem cell gene therapy with a lentiviral vector in X-linked adrenoleukodystrophy. *Science* **326:** 818–823.
13. Andreani, M., S. Nesci, G. Lucarelli, *et al.* 2000. Long-term survival of ex-thalassemic patients with persistent mixed chimerism after bone marrow transplantation. *Bone Marrow Transplant.* **25:** 401–404.
14. Persons, D.A., E.R. Allay, D.E. Sabatino, *et al.* 2001. Functional requirements for phenotypic correction of murine beta-thalassemia: implications for human gene therapy. *Blood* **97:** 3275–3282.
15. Von, L.D., F.T. Hufert, T.E. Fenner, *et al.* 1990. CD34$^+$ hematopoietic progenitor cells are not a major reservoir of the human immunodeficiency virus. *Blood* **76:** 1281–1286.
16. Shen, H., T. Cheng, F.I. Preffer, *et al.* 1999. Intrinsic human immunodeficiency virus type 1 resistance of hematopoietic stem cells despite coreceptor expression. *J. Virol.* **73:** 728–737.
17. Goff, S.P. 2007. Host factors exploited by retroviruses. *Nat. Rev. Microbiol.* **5:** 253–263.
18. Brass, A.L., D.M. Dykxhoorn, Y. Benita, *et al.* 2008. Identification of host proteins required for HIV infection through a functional genomic screen. *Science* **319:** 921–926.
19. Konig, R., Y. Zhou, D. Elleder, *et al.* 2008. Global analysis of host-pathogen interactions that regulate early-stage HIV-1 replication. *Cell* **135:** 49–60.
20. Goff, S.P. 2004. HIV: replication trimmed back. *Nature* **427:** 791–793.
21. Strebel, K., J. Luban & K.T. Jeang. 2009. Human cellular restriction factors that target HIV-1 replication. *BMC Med.* **7:** 48.
22. Luban, J. 2007. Cyclophilin A, TRIM5, and resistance to human immunodeficiency virus type 1 infection. *J. Virol.* **81:** 1054–1061.
23. Chiu, Y.L., V.B. Soros, J.F. Kreisberg, *et al.* 2005. Cellular APOBEC3G restricts HIV-1 infection in resting CD4$^+$ T cells. *Nature* **435:** 108–114.
24. Santoni De Sio, F.R., A. Gritti, *et al.* 2008. Lentiviral vector gene transfer is limited by the proteasome at postentry steps in various types of stem cells. *Stem Cells* **26:** 2142–2152.
25. Zhang, J., D.T. Scadden & C.S. Crumpacker. 2007. Primitive hematopoietic cells resist HIV-1 infection via p21. *J. Clin. Invest.* **117:** 473–481.
26. Zack, J.A., A.M. Haislip, P. Krogstad & I.S. Chen. 1992. Incompletely reverse-transcribed human immunodeficiency virus type 1 genomes in quiescent cells can function as intermediates in the retroviral life cycle. *J. Virol.* **66:** 1717–1725.
27. Korin, Y.D. & J.A. Zack. 1998. Progression to the G1b phase of the cell cycle is required for completion of human immunodeficiency virus type 1 reverse transcription in T cells. *J. Virol.* **72:** 3161–3168.
28. Sutton, R.E., M.J. Reitsma, N. Uchida & P.O. Brown. 1999. Transduction of human progenitor hematopoietic stem cells by human immunodeficiency virus type 1-based vectors is cell cycle dependent. *J. Virol.* **73:** 3649–3660.
29. Korin, Y.D. & J.A. Zack. 1999. Nonproductive human immunodeficiency virus type 1 infection in nucleoside-treated G0 lymphocytes. *J. Virol.* **73:** 6526–6532.
30. O'Brien, W.A., A. Namazi, H. Kalhor, *et al.* 1994. Kinetics of human immunodeficiency virus type 1 reverse transcription in blood mononuclear phagocytes are slowed by limitations of nucleotide precursors. *J. Virol.* **68:** 1258–1263.
31. Trobridge, G. & D.W. Russell. 2004. Cell cycle requirements for transduction by foamy virus vectors compared to those of oncovirus and lentivirus vectors. *J. Virol.* **78:** 2327–2335.
32. Sutton, R.E., M.J. Reitsma, N. Uchida & P.O. Brown. 1999. Transduction of human progenitor hematopoietic stem cells by human immunodeficiency virus type 1-based vectors is cell cycle dependent. *J. Virol.* **73:** 3649–3660.
33. Shepherd, B.E., H.P. Kiem, P.M. Lansdorp, *et al.* 2007. Hematopoietic stem-cell behavior in nonhuman primates. *Blood* **110:** 1806–1813.
34. Shepherd, B.E., P. Guttorp, P.M. Lansdorp & J.L. Abkowitz. 2004. Estimating human hematopoietic stem cell kinetics using granulocyte telomere lengths. *Exp. Hematol.* **32:** 1040–1050.
35. Zhang, C.C., M. Kaba, G. Ge, *et al.* 2006. Angiopoietin-like proteins stimulate ex vivo expansion of hematopoietic stem cells. *Nat. Med.* **12:** 240–245.
36. Zhang, C.C., M. Kaba, S. Iizuka, *et al.* 2008. Angiopoietin-like 5 and IGFBP2 stimulate ex vivo expansion of human cord blood hematopoietic stem cells as assayed by NOD/SCID transplantation. *Blood* **111:** 3415–3423.
37. Krosl, J., P. Austin, N. Beslu, *et al.* 2003. In vitro expansion of hematopoietic stem cells by recombinant TAT-HOXB4 protein. *Nat. Med.* **9:** 1428–1432.
38. Amsellem, S., F. Pflumio, D. Bardinet, *et al.* 2003. Ex vivo expansion of human hematopoietic stem cells by direct delivery of the HOXB4 homeoprotein. *Nat. Med.* **9:** 1423–1427.

39. Ohta, H., S. Sekulovic, S. Bakovic, *et al.* 2007. Near-maximal expansions of hematopoietic stem cells in culture using NUP98-HOX fusions. *Exp. Hematol.* **35:** 817–830.
40. Persons, D.A. & A.W. Nienhuis. 2002. In vivo selection to improve gene therapy of hematopoietic disorders. *Curr. Opin. Mol. Ther.* **4:** 491–498.
41. Persons, D.A., E.R. Allay, N. Sawai, *et al.* 2003. Successful treatment of murine beta-thalassemia using in vivo selection of genetically modified, drug-resistant hematopoietic stem cells. *Blood* **102:** 506–513.
42. Zhao, H., T.I. Pestina, M. Nasimuzzaman, *et al.* 2009. Amelioration of murine beta-thalassemia through drug selection of hematopoietic stem cells transduced with a lentiviral vector encoding both gamma-globin and the MGMT drug-resistance gene. *Blood* **113:** 5747–5756.

Ann. N.Y. Acad. Sci. ISSN 0077-8923

ANNALS OF THE NEW YORK ACADEMY OF SCIENCES
Issue: *Cooley's Anemia: Ninth Symposium*

Deferiprone

Antonio Piga, Simona Roggero, Ilaria Salussolia, Davide Massano, Melania Serra, and Filomena Longo
Thalassemia Center, University of Turin, Orbassano, Italy

Address for correspondence: Prof. Antonio Piga, Centro Microcitemie-Pediatria, Dipartimento di Scienze Cliniche e Biologiche, Ospedale S. Luigi Gonzaga-Regione Gonzole, 10-10043 Orbassano (TO), Italy. antonio.piga@unito.it

Deferiprone (DFP) has been evaluated in a wide range of disorders, but most data come from transfusion-dependent thalassemia. The safety and tolerability profile includes gastrointestinal complaints, liver enzymes elevation, weight gain, arthropathy, neutropenia, and agranulocytosis. The last requires close monitoring of blood count and precludes the use of DFP in conditions with bone marrow abnormalities. The efficacy profile is similar among the three available chelators. For DFP, the choice of dosage is crucial to optimize the effect on liver iron concentration, according to the iron load degree and transfusional iron input. Growing evidence indicates that DFP, alone or in combination with deferoxamine, is effective in removing cardiac iron and preventing cardiac iron load. The available data consolidate an important role of DFP in the management of iron overload. There is a need to compare directly the relative value of the available chelators in the long-term prevention of iron toxicity by well-designed randomized controlled trials.

Keywords: thalassemia; iron; chelation; deferiprone

Introduction

Deferiprone (1,2-dimethyl-3-hydroxypyridin-4-one, or L1, DMHP, Kelfer, CP20, Ferriprox®) is an oral iron chelator from the bidentate hydroxypyridones family. It was synthesized in the eighties and early applied to humans, with a long but not systematic development as a drug.[1] Results of large and controlled studies in humans became available in the 1990s, allowing the approval of DFP in Europe and in a number of countries outside United States and Canada often as a second-line treatment for iron overload when DFO therapy is contraindicated or inadequate. Up to now deferiprone (DFP) has been extensively evaluated in thalassemia and tested in a wide range of disorders and it is approved in most countries for the treatment of transfusional iron overload. In these recent years DFP is increasingly studied for conditions where iron overload is not systemic but a dislocation of iron is present at the cellular level. An example is Friedreich ataxia, where mitochondrial iron load is a key component of the disease. Preliminary data suggest that, differently from DFO, DFP may be effective in many conditions of this type.[2,3]

Basic properties

DFP has a molecular weight of 139. After oral ingestion it is quickly absorbed, with peak plasma levels at 45–60 min. Ingestion at meals delays but does not reduce the absorption. DFP forms a stable 1:3 iron–chelator complex. The complex and free drug are excreted in urine almost totally. DFP is metabolized by glucuronidation.[4]

Side effects

Side effects of DFP therapy include agranulocytosis, which demand close monitoring, arthropathy, gastrointestinal symptoms, increase of transaminases levels, and weight gain.

Liver fibrosis

Data with concerns about the possibility of hepatic fibrosis induced by DFP[5] were not confirmed by independent review.[6] A further large study on liver biopsy before and after DFP treatment gave definitive evidence that DFP does not cause a progression of fibrosis in patients on long-term treatment.[7]

doi: 10.1111/j.1749-6632.2010.05586.x

Agranulocytosis

The most serious side effect of chelation therapy with DFP is agranulocytosis; different studies reported incidences varying from 0.5% to 3.6%.[8–10] In a large four-year prospective study, the rates of agranulocytosis (absolute neutrophil count (ANC) $<500 \times 10^9$/L) and milder forms of neutropenia (ANC, 500 to 1,500 × 109/L) were 0.2 and 2.8 per 100 patient-years, respectively.[11] Neutropenia occurs more commonly in patients with intact spleens and during infection or drug assumption. The time of onset of agranulocytosis and neutropenia may vary significantly (0–19 and 0–70 months, respectively) (Tricta, unpublished data). Both conditions are reversible upon discontinuation of the drug; some patients required temporary treatment with stimulating factors. For patients who develop agranulocytosis the drug should not be reintroduced.

The cause of agranulocytosis during therapy with DFP is uncertain. Studies in animals suggest a dose-dependent and time-dependent myelosuppression while clinical findings in patients with thalassemia seem to be more characteristic of an idiosyncratic response. Even if regular monitoring of blood count remains a critical component of DFP treatment, this does not preclude effective long-term therapy in the vast majority of patients. The use of DFP in pediatric age has been focused by Naithany on 44 children between 2 and 6 years of age. Mild side effects were frequent: gastrointestinal symptoms occurred in 27.2%, arthropathy in 9.1%, neutropenia in 4.5%, and thrombocytopenia in 45.5%. No episode of platelet count less than 50,000/μL or agranulocytosis was recorded.[12]

Arthropathy

The frequency of arthropathy varies from 2% to 30% among studies. It involves large joints, especially the knees. Differently from other side effects, the onset may be late, even after three years from the start of treatment. Symptoms may be mild and resolve in a few days after temporary discontinuation of the drug or reduction of the dose, or treatment with nonsteroid anti-inflammatory drugs.[13] Nevertheless, cartilage and subchondral bone alterations may persist even in asymptomatic patients and be detected by MRI.[14] Iron deposition, synovial hypertrophy, and proliferation with no inflammatory reaction, were observed on synovial exploration and biopsy; the cause of DFP-related arthropathy remains unknown; it has been hypothesized that an incomplete binding of iron to DFP, with formation of 1:1 and 2:1 complexes, may happen at synovial level, likely at low concentrations of DFP relative to iron.[15] These complexes are instable and generate free-radicals with tissue damage.[16]

Gastrointestinal symptoms

Nausea, vomiting, and abdominal pain are among the most frequent side effects, occur early, and in most of the cases do not require treatment discontinuation.

A mild and temporary increase of liver enzymes is frequent, while toxic hepatitis is rare. DFP is glucuronized almost totally by UGT1A6; genetic variations and differences in the expression of splice variants may account for individual variability in the metabolism that may account for these types of side effects and the individual efficacy profile.[17]

The recent availability of a liquid formulation of DFP appears to be an alternative for patients who are unable to tolerate or comply with the use of tablets.

Efficacy

On short terms, the efficacy of DFP may be assessed by quantifying the urinary iron excretion, whereas in longer term studies it is possible to quantify changes in body iron burden, assessed by trends in serum ferritin levels, liver iron concentration (LIC), and cardiac iron load.

Most of the available data have been obtained using the "standard" DFO dose of 75 mg/kg, whereas recent experience indicates the usefulness of a wider dose range in optimizing efficacy and safety profiles in the individual patient. For example, doses of DFP of 75 mg/kg of body weight/day give urinary iron excretion levels comparable to DFO treatment, even if the individual variability is large.[18,19]

A Cochrane systematic review did not find significant differences on reduction of iron overload between DFP and DFO in thalassemia.[20]

Growing data from the literature indicate a positive role of DFP in cardio protection. The first publications came from retrospective or nonrandomized clinical trials. Anderson and colleagues developed the MRI T2* technique as surrogate marker of cardiac iron status,[21] and found significantly better status in patients on long term DFP in comparison with DFO.[22]

The first study on primary outcomes as survival and heart disease was a retrospective analysis from our Centre reviewing a six-year follow-up period of regular iron chelation in a large series of consecutive thalassemic patients for survival and heart disease found significant differences in survival and in cardiac dysfunction between DFO-treated and DFP-treated patients.[23] In the setting of a natural history study on a larger Italian series of thalassemia major patients, DFP therapy was associated with significantly greater cardiac protection than DFO.[24]

In a small RCT, Peng found in DFP-treated patients significantly better MR changes than in DFO ones.[25] In a large RCT on β-thalassemia major patients with asymptomatic myocardial siderosis, DFP given for 1 year at 92 mg/kg was more effective than DFO at 43 mg/kg in changing myocardial iron and LVEF.[26]

In a prospective study with a 5-year follow-up, DFO treatment increased mortality, due mainly to heart disease, in comparison with DFP alone or the combined DFP–DFO chelation treatments.[27]

Combination therapy with DFP and DFO is not discussed in this chapter, as described in details elsewhere in this volume. Otherwise to focus on the relative contribution of DFP within combination treatments is improper, with the few exceptions of studies with a robust RCT and blind design as the paper from Tanner and colleagues.[28]

Conclusions

As a whole, these findings indicate that DFP may provide greater protection than DFO against the cardiotoxicity of iron,[29] it is likely that this advantage resides in the ability of DFP to cross the cell membrane, remove intracellular iron pools and shuttle iron to the circulation.

Conflicts of interest

The authors declare no conflicts of interest.

References

1. Kontoghiorghes, G.J. *et al.* 1987. 1,2-Dimethyl-3-hydroxypyrid-4-one, an orally active chelator for treatment of iron overload. *Lancet* **1:** 1294–1295.
2. Boddaert, N. *et al.* 2007. Selective iron chelation in Friedreich ataxia: biologic and clinical implications. *Blood* **110:** 401–408.
3. Sohn, Y.S. *et al.* 2008. Redistribution of accumulated cell iron: a modality of chelation with therapeutic implications. *Blood* **111:** 1690–1699.
4. Matsui, D. *et al.* 1991. Relationship between the pharmacokinetics and iron excretion pharmacodynamics of the new oral iron chelator 1,2-dimethyl-3-hydroxypyrid-4-one in patients with thalassemia. *Clin. Pharmacol. Ther.* **50:** 294–298.
5. Olivieri, N.F. *et al.* 1998. Long-term safety and effectiveness of iron-chelation therapy with deferiprone for thalassemia major. *N. Engl. J. Med.* **339:** 417–423.
6. Callea, F. 1998. Iron chelation with oral deferiprone in patients with thalassemia. *N. Engl. J. Med.* **339:** 1710–1711.
7. Wanless, I.R. *et al.* 2002. Lack of progressive hepatic fibrosis during long-term therapy with deferiprone in subjects with transfusion-dependent beta-thalassemia. *Blood* **100:** 1566–1569.
8. Ceci, A. *et al.* 2002. The safety and effectiveness of deferiprone in a large-scale, 3-year study in Italian patients. *Br. J. Haematol.* **118:** 330–336.
9. Al-Refaie, F.N., B. Wonke & A.V. Hoffbrand. 1994. Deferiprone-associated myelotoxicity. *Eur. J. Haematol.* **53:** 298–301.
10. Al-Refaie, F.N. *et al.* 1995. Results of long-term deferiprone (L1) therapy: a report by the International Study Group on Oral Iron Chelators. *Br. J. Haematol.* **91:** 224–229.
11. Cohen, A.R. *et al.* 2003. Safety and effectiveness of long-term therapy with the oral iron chelator deferiprone. *Blood* **102:** 1583–1587.
12. Naithani, R., J. Chandra & S. Sharma. 2005. Safety of oral iron chelator deferiprone in young thalassaemics. *Eur. J. Haematol.* **74:** 217–220.
13. Vlachaki, E. *et al.* 2008. Deferiprone-related arthropathy of the knee in a thalassemic patient: report of a case and review of the literature. *Clin. Rheumatol.* **27:** 1459–1461.
14. Kellenberger, C.J. *et al.* 2004. Radiographic and MRI features of deferiprone-related arthropathy of the knees in patients with beta-thalassemia. *Am. J. Roentgenol.* **183:** 989–994.
15. Hershko, C.M. *et al.* 2005. Iron chelation therapy. *Curr. Hematol. Rep.* **4:** 110–116.
16. Berkovitch M. *et al.* 1994. Arthropathy in thalassaemia patients receiving deferiprone. *Lancet* **343:** 1471–1472.
17. Benoit-Biancamano, M.O. *et al.* 2009. Deferiprone glucuronidation by human tissues and recombinant UDP glucuronosyltransferase 1A6: an in vitro investigation of genetic and splice variants. *Drug. Metab. Dispos.* **37:** 322–329.
18. Piga, A. *et al.* 2005. Deferiprone: new insight. *Ann. N.Y. Acad. Sci.* **1054:** 169–174.
19. Fischer R. *et al.* 2003. Monitoring long-term efficacy of iron chelation therapy by deferiprone and desferrioxamine in patients with beta-thalassaemia major: application of SQUID biomagnetic liver susceptometry. *Br. J. Haematol.* **121:** 938–948.
20. Roberts, D.J. *et al.* 2007. Oral deferiprone for iron chelation in people with thalassaemia. *Cochrane Database Syst. Rev.* **3:** CD004839.
21. Anderson, L.J. *et al.* 2001. Cardiovascular T2-star (T2*) magnetic resonance for the early diagnosis of myocardial iron overload. *Eur. Heart J.* **22:** 2171–2179.

22. Anderson, L.J. *et al.* 2002. Comparison of effects of oral deferiprone and subcutaneous desferrioxamine on myocardial iron concentrations and ventricular function in beta-thalassaemia. *Lancet* **360:** 516–520.
23. Piga, A. *et al.* 2003. Comparative effects of deferiprone and deferoxamine on survival and cardiac disease in patients with thalassemia major: a retrospective analysis. *Haematologica* **88:** 489–496.
24. Borgna-Pignatti C. *et al.* 2006. Cardiac morbidity and mortality in deferoxamine- or deferiprone-treated patients with thalassemia major. *Blood* **107:** 3733–3737.
25. Peng, C.T. *et al.* 2006. Deferiprone or deferoxamine vs. combination therapy in patients with beta-thalassemia major: a case study in Taiwan. *Hemoglobin* **30:** 125–130.
26. Pennell, D.J. *et al.* 2006. Randomized controlled trial of deferiprone or deferoxamine in beta-thalassemia major patients with asymptomatic myocardial siderosis. *Blood* **107:** 3738–3744.
27. Maggio, A. *et al.* 2009. Improving survival with deferiprone treatment in patients with thalassemia major: a prospective multicenter randomised clinical trial under the auspices of the Italian Society for Thalassemia and Hemoglobinopathies. *Blood Cells Mol. Dis.* **42:** 247–251.
28. Tanner, M.A. *et al.* 2007. A randomized, placebo-controlled, double-blind trial of the effect of combined therapy with deferoxamine and deferiprone on myocardial iron in thalassemia major using cardiovascular magnetic resonance. *Circulation* **115:** 1876–1884.
29. Hershko, C. *et al.* 2004. Purging iron from the heart. *Br. J. Haematol.* **125:** 545–551.

Ann. N.Y. Acad. Sci. ISSN 0077-8923

ANNALS OF THE NEW YORK ACADEMY OF SCIENCES
Issue: *Cooley's Anemia: Ninth Symposium*

Combined iron chelation therapy

Renzo Galanello,[1] Annalisa Agus,[1] Simona Campus,[1] Fabrice Danjou,[1] Patricia J. Giardina,[2] and Robert W. Grady[2]

[1]Pediatric Clinic 2, University of Cagliari, Italy and Thalassemia Unit Asl 8. [2]Weill Cornell Medical Center, New York, New York

Address for correspondence: Renzo Galanello, Professor of Pediatrics, Pediatric Clinic 2 and Thalassemia Unit Asl 8 - University of Cagliari, Via Jenner, 09121 Cagliari, Italy. renzo.galanello@mcweb.unica.it

Patients with thalassemia major accumulate body iron over time as a consequence of continuous red blood cell transfusions which cause hepatic, endocrine, and cardiac complications. Despite the availability of three iron chelators, some patients fail to respond adequately to monotherapy with any of them. Combination therapy, consisting in the use of two chelators on the same day, has been introduced to increase the efficacy and to induce negative iron balance in patients with severe iron overload. Extensive long-term experience has shown that combined chelation with deferiprone and deferoxamine (DFO) rapidly reduces liver iron, serum ferritin, and myocardial siderosis, improves cardiac function, reverses and prevents endocrine complications, reduces cardiac mortality, and improves survival. Side effects, though significant, are manageable if properly monitored. Preliminary promising results have been obtained using combined chelation with deferasirox and DFO. As more drug combination regimes are evaluated, it should be possible to better tailor iron chelation to the needs of the patients, minimizing toxicity and maximizing efficacy throughout life.

Keywords: iron chelation; combined therapy; thalassemia and chelators

Patients with thalassemia major accumulate iron in their bodies as a consequence of continuous red blood cell transfusions. Over time this iron causes hepatic, endocrine, and cardiac complications. Deferoxamine (DFO) given by regular subcutaneous infusion is able to reduce and/or prevent iron accumulation, thereby reducing organ dysfunction, morbidity and mortality.[1] Endocrine complications are the most common cause of morbidity in patients with thalassemia major. Hypogonadism has been reported in 35–55% of the patients, hypothyroidism in 9–11%, hypoparathyroidism in 4% and diabetes in 6–10%.[2,3] Cardiac disease occurs in 6–10% of the patients with cardiac failure being the most common cause of death, occurring in more than 70% of the patients.[2–4] Low compliance with the cumbersome DFO infusions is considered a major factor in the occurrence of these complications. Regulatory approval of the oral chelator deferiprone (DFP) in India in 1995 and in Europe in 1999 was a huge step forward in the treatment of iron overload. DFP has been shown to be effective in removing excess iron from the majority of patients receiving regular red cell transfusions.[5,6] Deferasirox (DFX), recently approved for clinical use, is a once-daily oral iron chelator with established dose-dependent efficacy in patients with transfusional iron overload.[7] Unfortunately, some patients, particularly those with severe iron overload, fail to respond adequately to monotherapy with any of the iron chelators noted above at the therapeutic doses used most frequently to induce negative iron balance. This prompted Wonke and colleagues[8] to introduce combination therapy with DFP and DFO in 1998. In principle, the combined use of two chelators has several potential advantages including higher efficacy, accessibility to different iron pools, better tolerability, improved compliance, and better management of potentially toxic non transferrin bound iron (NTBI). Moreover, it should be possible to decrease the dose of chelator so as to reduce toxicity while maintaining a high chelation efficacy.[9] In the literature, the term "combination therapy" has been associated with a

doi: 10.1111/j.1749-6632.2010.05591.x

Table 1. Characteristics of currently available iron chelators

	Deferoxamine	Deferasirox	Deferiprone
Route	parenteral	oral	oral
Denticity	hexadentate	tridentate	bidentate
MW ligand	560	373	139
MW complex with iron	619	798	470
Partition coefficient	0.02	6.3	0.18
Protein Binding	<10%	99%	<10%
Charge	positive	negative	neutral
Volume Distribution	small	small	large
pFe^{3+}	26	22.5	19

wide variety of chelation regimens. For the sake of clarity, the term combination therapy should be limited to the coadministration of two chelators during the same day, either simultaneously or sequentially (e.g., an oral chelator during the day and DFO during the night). Usually the oral chelator is taken every day, while the subcutaneous infusion of DFO varies from 2 to 7 days per week according to the severity of iron overload. In patients with heart failure, DFO can be given intravenously to maximize iron chelation. The term of "alternate chelation" should be reserved for regimens where each chelator is administered on different days (i.e., the oral chelator 3–4 days per week, DFO for the rest of the week).

Combined chelation with DFP and DFO

Iron balance studies

The most relevant pharmacological properties of DFP and DFO are reported in Table 1. The pharmacokinetics of the two chelators differ significantly, because of their physicochemical characteristics. In vitro studies have shown that DFP, like other hydroxypyridones, is able to cross cellular and lysosomal membranes, whereas DFO is incapable of crossing these membranes and enters cells only by endocytosis.[10] Therefore, the two chelators seem to have different tissue distributions and access different iron pools. Metabolic iron balance studies have shown that the concurrent use of DFP and DFO results in an additive or synergistic effect on total (urinary and fecal) daily iron excretion[11,12] (Fig. 1). "Additive" refers to excretion of an amount of iron equal to the sum of that excreted with each agent given separately. In some patients, combination of a chelator (DFP) with lower affinity for iron but a better ability to penetrate cells, with a chelator (DFO) that has a greater affinity but penetrates cells poorly, may result in a "synergistic" effect (i.e., removal of more iron than the sum of that due to each chelator alone) due to iron shuttling between the two compounds. The "shuttle effect," first proposed by Grady,[12] was directly demonstrated by following the fate of chelated plasma iron in thalassemic patients receiving combined DFP and DFO.[13] DFP administration produced a temporary accumulation of chelated iron in the plasma after 2 h whereupon the addition of DFO resulted in the transfer of chelated iron from DFP to DFO with an increase in the total amount of chelated iron in the serum. Shuttling of iron from the bidentate ligand, DFP, to a hexadentate "sink," DFO, at clinically relevant chelator concentrations seems to apply also to iron removal from transferrin.[14] Together, these data suggesting an interaction between DFP and DFO have had important implications for the design of new iron chelation regimens.

Combined chelation with DFX and DFO

Iron balance studies

Now that DFX is used worldwide, it has become quite clear that many patients fail to respond adequately to monotherapy with this drug i.e. they remain in net positive iron balance. Based on the results achieved upon combining DFP and DFO, we have recently undertaken an evaluation of DFX (30 mg/kg, p.o., 30 minutes before breakfast) in combination with DFO (40 mg/kg, s.c., over 8 h at night). Unlike DFP, DFX is almost completely bound to proteins in the circulation so it was not obvious that an additive effect would be achieved or that DFX could shuttle iron to DFO for excretion.

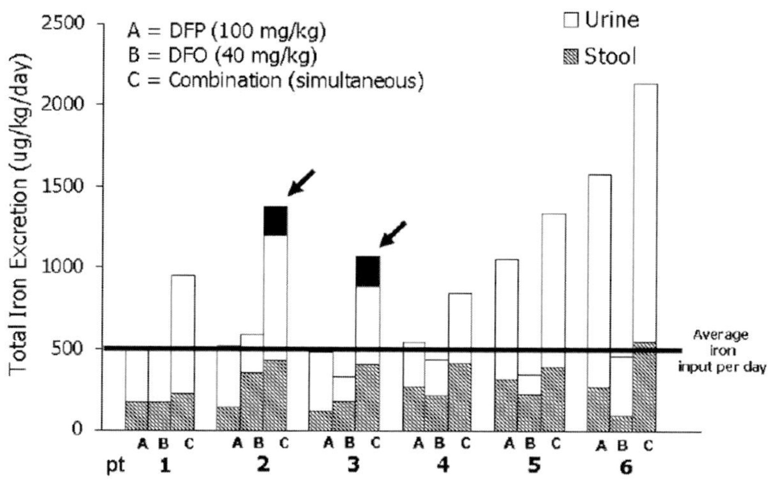

Figure 1. Iron balance studies with DFP+DFO combination therapy. Arrows indicate the two patients in whom combination therapy seems to have a synergistic effect.

Three patients have been studied to date employing the same protocol as that used to evaluate DFP in combination with DFO. Only one patient achieved net negative iron balance on DFX alone while DFO placed all three in negative balance. When the drugs were given in combination, total excretion was synergistic in two patients (35% and 57% more than additive) but less than additive in the third, the patient who responded the best to both drugs individually. Moreover, all of the excess iron appeared in the urine (2.1- and 3.4-fold increase), strongly suggesting that DFX was shuttling extra hepatic iron to DFO. Surprisingly, no increase in urinary iron was seen in the third patient. While only preliminary, these results add to our optimism that combining drugs will prove to be the best approach to iron chelation therapy, a thought reinforced by the results discussed below.

Efficacy of combination with DFP and DFO

Schedule of treatment

One of the most pressing limitations of the clinical studies involving combination therapy is the difficulty of comparing results because of differences in the doses of each drug (DFP, 50–100 mg/kg/day; DFO, 20–60 mg/kg/day), in the number of days that DFO is infused (2–7 days per week), and in the duration of treatment (6–60 months). Usually DFO is given as a subcutaneous infusion, but in patients with cardiac failure intravenous administration is often used. Another limitation is that most of the studies are observational with only a few being prospective and/or randomized (see later).

Cardiac disease

As previously mentioned, a large proportion of patients develop an excessive body iron load despite the availability of DFO because of difficulties in complying with the self-administered subcutaneous infusion of the drug. Therefore, it is not surprising that chelated patients continue to develop iron induced complications, most of them dying from iron-induced cardiac disease.[2,15] Using T2*, a magnetic resonance parameter, to measure organ iron loading, Tanner and colleagues[16] found that myocardial iron overload (T2* below 20 ms) was present in 108 (65%) out of 167 adult patients with thalassemia major on DFO chelation. The cardiac T2* was lower than 8 ms (severe iron overload) in 22 patients (13%). The left ventricular ejection fraction (LVEF) was markedly impaired (<56%) in 62% of them. Fifteen of the patients received combination therapy with subcutaneous DFO (38 ± 10 mg/kg, 5.3 days/week) and daily oral DFP (74 ± 4 mg/kg) for 12 months.[17] Their myocardial T2* improved (from 5.7 ± 0.9 ms to 7.9 ± 2.4, $P = 0.01$), with concomitant improvement in LVEF (from 51.2 ± 10.9% to 65.6 ± 6.7%, $P < 0.001$).

Origa and colleagues[18] also reported an improvement in LVEF (from 49 ± 9% to 57% ± 1%, $P = 0.001$) in 20 patients on combined therapy, no change having been made in their cardiac treatment. Moreover, several authors have described successful recoveries from severe heart failure associated with use of DFP and DFO combination therapy in case reports of patients with thalassemia major as well as with sickle cell anemia and hereditary hemochromatosis.[19–23] In a double-blind, placebo-controlled trial, 65 patients with moderate myocardial iron loading (T2*, 8–20 ms) were randomized to receive subcutaneous DFO and oral DFP (32 patients) or DFO and placebo (33 patients).[24] There were significant improvements in the combined treatment group compared with the DFO/placebo-treated group. Increases were observed in their myocardial T2* (ratio of change in geometric means, 1.50 vs. 1.24, $P = 0.02$), absolute LVEF (2.6% vs. 0.6%, $P = 0.05$) and absolute endothelial function quantified by flow mediated dilatation of the brachial artery (8.8% vs. 3.3%, $P = 0.02$). Iron-mediated endothelial dysfunction has previously been described in patients with thalassemia major and linked to increased arterial stiffness.[25] The improvement associated with combined therapy may be relevant to the management of those patients in whom the interactions between vasculature and ventricle are likely to play a significant role in the development and progression of heart failure.[24]

Liver iron concentration

Liver iron concentration has been evaluated in a few studies. Tanner and colleagues,[17] in their prospective study of patients with severe iron overload and cardiac dysfunction, reported a significant improvement of liver T2* from a baseline of 3.7 ± 2.9 to 10.8 ± 7.3 ms at 12 months ($P = 0.006$). The same authors, in the randomized, placebo-controlled trial, found a significant improvement of liver T2* from a baseline of 4.9 to 10.7 ms at 12 months ($P = 0.001$) in the combined treatment group and from 4.2 to 5.0 ms in the DFO/placebo group ($P = 0.01$). The between-group difference (39%) significantly favored the combined treatment group (95% CI, 20–61%, $P < 0.001$).[24] In a clinical observational study, combination therapy resulted in the most rapid decline of liver iron concentration compared to monotherapy with DFO, DFP, or DFX.[26]

A similar significant reduction in liver iron content has been reported in a randomized prospective study carried out to determine the effectiveness of mild combined therapy (DFP for 7 days and DFO for 2 days per week), in comparison to monotherapy with the individual drugs.[27] In a study of 52 patients transitioned from DFO to combined therapy, 98% of patients had hepatic iron overload (LIC ≥ 5 mg/g dw), and 64% had severe iron overload at baseline (LIC > 12 mg/g dw). After 3 years of intensive combined chelation, these proportions declined to 60 and 10%, respectively. By 5 years, none of the 50 patients remaining on the study had iron overload. This shift toward a normal hepatic iron load over time was highly significant (Fisher's exact test $P < 0.001$).[28]

Serum ferritin

The efficacy of combination therapy as assessed by changes in serum ferritin levels has been reported in many studies, the results from several retrospective studies[8,16,18,29–38] being summarized in Figure 2. A reduction in serum ferritin levels was observed in all studies but one. In the randomized placebo-controlled trial, the mean ferritin level declined from 1574 μg/L at baseline to 598 μg/L at 12 months ($P = 0.001$) in the combined group and from 1379 to 1146 μg/L ($P = 0.01$) in the DFO group after 12 months of therapy. The between group difference was significantly in favor of the combined treatment group (–40%; 95% C.I., –48 to –28%; $P < 0.001$).[24] In a group of 52 thalassemia major patients who were switched from DFO monotherapy to combined chelation, serum ferritin declined at the rate of 85 μg/L per month ($P < 0.001$).[28] After 1 year, 53% of the patients had ferritin levels below 1000 μg/L, this percentage increasing to 85% after 2 years. After 5 years of therapy, 90% of these patients had ferritin values within normal limits (mean 87 ± 25 μg/L).[28]

Urinary iron excretion

Urinary iron excretion (UIE) with combination therapy has been reported in several studies. Kattamis and colleagues[39] observed median UIEs of 0.28 and 0.30 mg/kg/day with DFO and DFP monotherapy, respectively, and 0.65 mg/kg/day upon giving the drugs in combination.

In another study the mean UIE during combined therapy (0.84 ± 0.48 mg/kg/day) was double that during DFO or DFP monotherapy (0.42 ± 0.23 and 0.44 ± 0.37 mg/kg/day, respectively, $P < 0.0001$).[18] In 30 patients with thalassemia major, combination therapy with DFO and DFP resulted in a median 2.3-fold (range 0.28- to 7.35-fold) increase in UIE

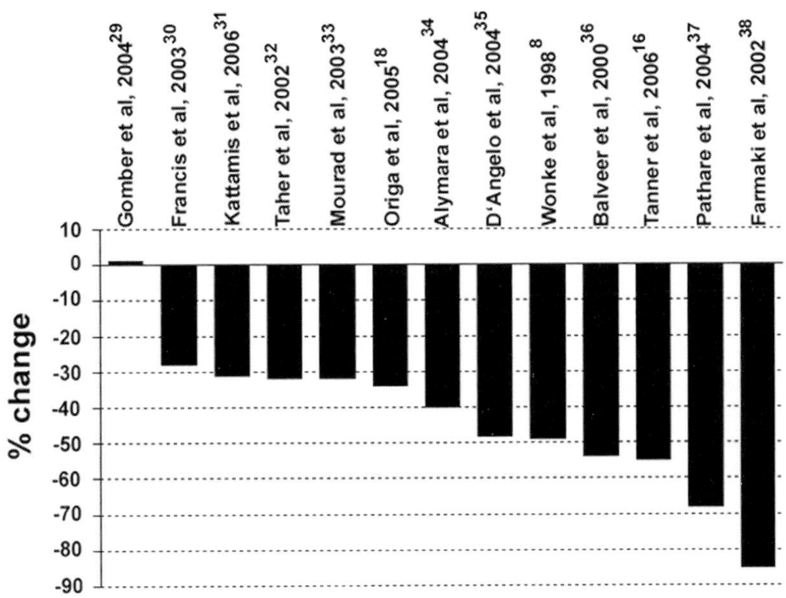

Figure 2. Combination therapy clinical studies: changes in ferritin levels.

compared to monotherapy with DFP.[40] In all of these studies, total absolute iron excretion in response to combination therapy was even higher because fecal iron excretion due to DFO was not accounted for.

Endocrine complications

Endocrine complications are a very common feature of beta-thalassemia.[3,41] In a study from Greece, reversal of endocrine complications with very intensive combined chelation (DFP 75–100 mg/kg/day and DFO 20–60 mg/kg/day) has been reported.[28] In particular, abnormal glucose metabolism was normalized in 17 (44%) of 39 patients. In 18 patients requiring thyroxine supplementation for hypothyroidism, 10 were able to discontinue therapy and 4 others were able to reduce their thyroxine dose. In 14 hypogonadal males on testosterone therapy, 7 stopped treatment and quite remarkably, 6 of 19 females, who were hypogonadal on DFO monotherapy, were able to conceive.[28]

Survival

Two studies have reported on survival in patients on combination therapy. In Cyprus, due to an increasing number of cardiac deaths among patients on standard treatment with DFO, combination therapy was introduced in 1999 for all patients at high risk of heart failure.[42] A multivariate survival analysis was applied to this population to test the hypothesis that survival post-2000 improved relative to that seen between 1980 and 1999. The authors observed a significant upward trend of cardiac deaths between 1980 and 2000 ($P < 0.001$) and a decline after 2000 when the patients were switched from DFO monotherapy to combined chelation ($P = 0.06$). The authors suggested that use of combined chelation explained the decrease in mortality, but could not show this statistically due to insufficient data. For this reason, the question was readdressed after another two years of follow-up.[43] Results of multivariate analysis showed that combined chelation was the only independent factor associated with improved survival. None of the patients on combination therapy died of cardiac disease.

A long-term, multicenter, randomized control trial compared DFO and DFP alone, as well as alternating and combined regimens of DFP and DFO.[44] After more than 7 years of observation, no deaths occurred with DFP-alone or the combined use of DFP and DFO while one death occurred with alternating therapy and 10 with DFO monotherapy.

Safety

Combined therapy with DFP and DFO is generally well tolerated; no new or unanticipated adverse events have been reported as compared to monotherapy with either drug.[18,27,28,45] The adverse events observed in our long-term clinical

Table 2. Adverse events with DFP+DFO combined chelation: clinical experience at thalassemia unit—Cagliari

	Number of events	Occurrence/ 100 Pt-years
Neutropenia	14	2.8%
Agranulocytosis	5	1.0%
ALT (transient increase)*	45	9.0%
Arthropathy	10	2.0%
Gastrointestinal problems	40	8.0%
158 patients/502 patient-years (median = 1.90 years per patient)		

*A large proportion of the patients were HCV positive.

experience (502 patient-years of observation) are reported in Table 2. Their frequency and severity are no different from those observed in patients on DFP monotherapy.[6] As a single study the incidence of agranulocytosis, the most important clinically relevant side effect of DFP, was higher than that reported for DFP alone.[18,31,33] However, the cumulative occurrence of agranulocytosis reported in published studies with combined therapy is not statistically different from that observed during monotherapy trials of DFP sponsored by ApoPharma (2.2% vs. 1.2% in combination vs. DFP monotherapy trials, $P = 0.4659$, Fisher's exact test; Galanello R, unpublished).

Discussion

Iron overload related complications, as a consequence of repeated blood transfusions, are the most important cause of morbidity and mortality in patients with thalassemia major. Although the use of DFO over the past several decades has significantly reduced the occurrence of these complications, cardiac disease is still the main cause of death in these patients due largely to poor compliance over time.[2,15,45] From the cumulative experiences reported to date, combined chelation with DFO and DFP seems to be the treatment of choice in order to achieve a significant decrease in total body iron load, a reduction in iron-related complications and an improvement in survival.

The higher efficacy of combination therapy, as compared to monotherapy, is easily explained by the use of two chelators with different tissue distributions and affinities for iron, and by the increase in the total time that the body is exposed to chelation.[46] However, apart from the expected additive effect, in vitro and metabolic iron balance studies have suggested the possibility of synergy between the two chelators, a "shuttle effect" leading to increased iron excretion.[12] Access of the two chelators to different iron pools would contribute to both additivity and synergy. Strategies and dosing schedules applied to combination therapy have varied widely, making comparison of the results somewhat difficult. Overall, however, the results reported confirm the importance of combination therapy in the management of severe iron overload. A number of clinical studies have concluded that combined therapy offers additional benefits in terms of reducing cardiac iron loading and improving cardiac function.[17,18,20–24,45] The randomized, placebo-controlled study in patients with moderate cardiac iron loading (T2*, 8–20 ms) and the prospective study in patients with severe heart iron load (T2*, less than 8 ms) together with cardiac dysfunction (LVEF below 56%) have shown that the addition of DFP to DFO therapy results in a significant reduction of myocardial siderosis in concert with an improvement in cardiac function. The protective effect on the heart may be due to increased access of DFP to cardiomyocytes rendering toxic labile iron metabolically inactive or causing its removal from the cells. Superior cardiac protection in patients treated with DFP monotherapy, as compared to those on DFO monotherapy, has previously been reported.[4,47,48] Of further interest was the finding of significant relative improvement in endothelial function in patients treated with combined therapy in the placebo-controlled trial.[24] Endothelial dysfunction is likely to play a significant role in the development and progression of heart disease in thalassemic patients and its relief might therefore be beneficial. Favorable changes in other outcome measures have been reported in several clinical studies, including a reduction in liver iron concentrations and serum ferritin levels as well as the reversal of endocrine complications.[16,18,24,26–28] The study by Farmaki and colleagues[28] suggests that intensive chelation may reverse a significant proportion of glucose-related metabolic disorders, hypothyroidism, and hypogonadism in both males and females.

Observational and prospective randomized studies have shown that combined chelation is able to prevent cardiac mortality and improve survival.[42–44]

While this might be due to the cardioprotective effect of DFP, it could also be the result of improved adherence to the combined treatment. The use of questionnaires and close scrutiny of the patients have shown that combination therapy with reduced DFO infusions is accepted by the patients and results in increased compliance (Galanello, unpublished).[49] However, continuous assessment of compliance is recommended because patients actually take DFP regularly, but reduce their use of DFO over time.[45,50] Safety is an issue of major concern for drugs that patients take lifelong. A relatively high dropout rate has been observed in patients on combined therapy because of adverse events.[18,42] However, while the adverse events encountered during combination therapy may be somewhat more severe, they are quite manageable. This highlights the need for supervision by trained specialists. Particular attention should be paid to the monitoring of agranulocytosis. It is recommended that the absolute neutrophil count be checked every 7–10 days, or at least at each transfusion visit, and that DFP should be stopped in case of fever and/or signs of infection, and immediate medical attention be sought. It is recommended that DFP be permanently withdrawn after an episode of agranulocytosis due to the high risk of recurrence (Galanello, unpublished).

Conclusion

Extensive long-term experience has shown that combined chelation with DFP and DFO can successfully be used to treat patients with severe iron overload. Combined chelation rapidly reduces liver iron and serum ferritin, reduces myocardial siderosis, improves cardiac function, reverses and prevents endocrine complications, reduces cardiac mortality and improves survival. Moreover, it offers more flexibility allowing chelation regimes to be tailored to the needs of the patients. It should also be pointed out that combined chelation has significant but manageable adverse effects if properly monitored. As more drug combinations are evaluated, it should be possible to refine the design of individualized chelation regimens so as to minimize toxicity and maximize efficacy throughout life.

Conflicts of interest

Professor Renzo Galanello has received speaker's honoraria and research support from Apotex and Novartis.

References

1. Olivieri, N.F. & G.M. Brittenham.1997. Iron-chelating therapy and the treatment of thalassemia. *Blood* **89:** 739–761.
2. Borgna-Pignatti, C. *et al.* 2004. Survival and complications in patients with thalassemia major treated with transfusion and deferoxamine. *Haematologica* **89:** 1187–1193.
3. Cunningham, M.J. *et al.* 2004. Complications of beta-thalassemia major in North America. *Blood* **104:** 34–39.
4. Borgna-Pignatti, C. *et al.* 2006. Cardiac morbidity and mor tality in deferoxamine- or deferiprone-treated patients with thalassemia major. *Blood* **107:** 3733–3737.
5. Olivieri, N.F. *et al.* 1995. Iron-chelation therapy with oral deferiprone patients with thalassemia major. *N. Engl. J. Med.* **332:** 918–922.
6. Cohen, A.R. *et al.* 2003. Safety and effectiveness of long-term therapy with the oral iron chelator deferiprone. *Blood* **102:** 1583–1587.
7. Cappellini, M.D. & A. Taher. 2009. Deferasirox (Exjade) for the treatment of iron overload. *Acta Haematol.* **122:** 165–173.
8. Wonke, B., C. Wright & A.V. Hoffbrand. 1998. Combined therapy with deferiprone and desferrioxamine. *Br. J. Haematol.* **103:** 361–364.
9. Galanello, R. & S. Campus. 2009. Deferiprone chelation therapy for thalassemia major. *Acta Haematol.* **122:** 155–164.
10. Hershko, C. *et al.* 2003. Objectives and methods of iron chelation therapy. *Bioinorg. Chem. Appl.* **1:** 151–168.
11. Grady R.W. *et al.* 1999. Iron Chelation therapy: a better approach [abstract]. In *Proceedings of the 7th International Conference on Thalassaemia and the Hemoglobinopathies.* Bangkok, Thailand.
12. Grady R.W. *et al.* 2002. Combinations of desferrioxamine and deferiprone markedly enhance iron excretion [abstract]. *Blood* **100:** 241a.
13. Breuer, W. *et al.* 2001. Desferrioxamine-chelatable iron, a component of serum non-transferrin-bound iron, used for assessing chelation therapy. *Blood* **97:** 792–798.
14. Devanur, L.D. *et al.* 2008. Chelator-facilitated removal of iron from transferrin: Relevance to combined chelation therapy. *Biochem. J.* **409:** 439–447.
15. Modell, B., M. Khan & M. Darlison. 2000. Survival in beta-thalassaemia major in the UK: data from the UK Thalassaemia Register. *Lancet* **355:** 2051–2052.
16. Tanner, M.A. *et al.* 2006. Myocardial iron loading in patients with thalassemia major on deferoxamine chelation. *J. Cardiovasc. Magn. Reson.* **8:** 543–547.
17. Tanner, M.A. *et al.* 2008. Combined chelation therapy in thalassemia major for the treatment of severe myocardial siderosis with left ventricular dysfunction. *J. Cardiovasc. Magn. Reson.* **10:** 12.
18. Origa, R. *et al.* 2005. Combined therapy with deferiprone and desferrioxamine in thalassemia major. *Haematologica* **90:** 1309–1314.
19. Wu, K.H. *et al.* 2004. Combined therapy with deferiprone and desferrioxamine successfully regresses severe heart failure in patients with beta-thalassemia major. *Ann. Hematol.* **83:** 471–473.

20. Tavecchia, L. *et al.* 2006. Successful recovery of acute hemosiderotic heart failure in beta-thalassemia major treated with a combined regimen of desferrioxamine and deferiprone. *Haematologica* **91:** 55–57.
21. Tsironi, M. *et al.* 2005 Transfusional hemosiderosis and combined chelation therapy in sickle thalassemia. *Ann. Hematol.* **84:** 353–357.
22. Porcu, M. *et al.* 2006. Effects of combined deferiprone and desferrioxamine iron chelating therapy in beta-thalassemia major end-stage heart failure: a case report. *Eur. J. Heart Fail* **9:** 320–322.
23. Fabio, G. *et al.* 2007. Reversal of cardiac complications by deferiprone and deferoxamine combination therapy in a patient affected by a severe type of juvenile hemochromatosis (JH). *Blood* **109:** 362–364.
24. Tanner, M.A. *et al.* 2007. A randomized, placebo-controlled, double-blind trial of the effect of combined therapy with deferoxamine and deferiprone on myocardial iron in thalassemia major using cardiovascular magnetic resonance. *Circulation* **115:** 1876–1884.
25. Cheung, Y.F. 2002. Arterial stiffness and endothelial function in patients with beta-thalassemia major. *Circulation* **106:** 2561–2566.
26. Berdoukas, V. *et al.* 2009. The efficacy of iron chelator regimes in reducing cardiac and hepatic iron in patients with thalassaemia major: a clinical observational study. *J. Cardiovasc. Magn. Reson.* **11:** 20.
27. El-Beshlawy, A. *et al.* 2008. Iron chelation in thalassemia: combined or monotherapy? The Egyptian experience. *Ann. Hematol.* **87:** 545–550.
28. Farmaki, K. *et al.* 2010. Normalisation of total body iron load with very intensive combined chelation reverses cardiac and endocrine complications of thalassaemia major. *Br. J. Haematol.* **148:** 466–475.
29. Gomber, S. *et al.* 2004. Comparative efficacy of desferrioxamine, deferiprone and in combination on iron chelation in thalassemic children. *Indian Pediatr.* **41:** 21–27.
30. Francis, S. *et al.* 2003. Efficacy of combined chelation therapy with subcutaneous desferrioxamine and oral deferiprone in patients with thalassemia major [abstract]. *Blood* **102:** 517a.
31. Kattamis, A. *et al.* 2006. Iron chelation treatment with combined therapy with deferiprone and deferioxamine: a 12-month trial. *Blood Cells Mol. Dis.* **36:** 21–25.
32. Taher, T.H. *et al.* 2002. Tolerability of statin-fibrate and statin-niacin combination therapy in dyslipidemic patients at high risk for cardiovascular events. *Am. J. Cardiol.* **89:** 390–394.
33. Mourad, F.H. *et al.* 2003. Comparison between desferrioxamine and combined therapy with desferrioxamine and deferiprone in iron overloaded thalassaemia patients. *Br. J. Haematol.* **121:** 187–189.
34. Alymara, V. *et al.* 2004. Effectiveness and safety of combined iron-chelation therapy with deferoxamine and deferiprone. *Hematol. J.* **5:** 475–9.
35. D'Angelo, E. *et al.* 2004. Combined therapy with desferrioxamine and deferiprone: a new protocol for iron chelation in thalassemia. *J. Pediatr. Hematol. Oncol.* **26:** 451–453.
36. Balveer, K. *et al.* 2000. Combined oral and parenteral iron chelation in beta thalassaemia major. *Med. J. Malaysia* **55:** 493–497.
37. Pathare, A.V. *et al.* 2004. Efficient iron chelation resulting in improved myocardial performance with combined desferrioxamine and deferiprone in beta thalassemia major patients [abstract]. *Blood* **104:** 28b.
38. Farmaki, K. *et al.* 2002. Combined chelation therapy in patients with thalassemia major: a fast and effective method of reducing ferritin levels and cardiological complications [abstract]. *Hematol. J.* **3:** 79.
39. Kattamis, K. *et al.* 2003. Combined therapy with desferrioxamine and deferiprone in thalassemic patients: effect on urinary iron excretion. *Haematologica* **88:** 1423–1425.
40. Christoforidis, A. *et al.* 2007. Urinary iron excretion in young thalassemic patients receiving combined chelation treatment with deferoxamine and deferiprone. *J. Pediatr. Hematol. Oncol.* **29:** 598–601.
41. Italian Working Group on Endocrine Complications in Non-endocrine Diseases. 1995. Multicenter study on prevalence of endocrine complications in thalassaemia major. *Clin. Endocrinol.* **42:** 581–586.
42. Telfer, P. *et al.* 2006. Survival of medically treated thalassemia patients in Cyprus,. Trends and risk factors over the period 1980–2004. *Haematoloica* **91:** 1187–1192.
43. Telfer, P. *et al.* 2009. Improved survival in thalassemia major patients on switching from desferrioxamine ro combined chelation therapy with desferrioxamine and deferiprone. *Haemtologica* **94:** 1777–1778.
44. Maggio, A. *et al.* 2009. Improving survival with deferiprone treatment in patients with thalassemia major: a prospective multicenter randomised clinical trial under the auspices of the Italian Society for Thalassemia and Hemoglobinopathies. *Blood Cells Mol. Dis.* **42:** 247–251.
45. Daar, S. *et al.* 2006. Combined therapy with desferrioxamine and deferiprone in beta thalassemia major patients with transfusional iron overload. *Ann. Hematol.* **85:** 315–319.
46. Cabantchik, Z.I. *et al.* 2005. LPI-labile plasma iron in iron overload. *Best Pract. Res. Clin. Haematol.* **18:** 277–287.
47. Anderson, L.J. *et al.* 2002. Comparison of effects of oral deferiprone and subctunaeous desferrioxamine on myocardial iron levels and ventricular function in beta thalassemia. *Lancet* **360:** 516–520.
48. Piga, A. *et al.* 2003. Comparative effects of deferiprone and deferoxamine on survival and cardiac disease in patients with thalassemia major; a retrospective analysis. *Haematologica* **88:** 489–496
49. Telfer, P. *et al.* 2005. Quality of life in thalassemia. *Ann. N.Y. Acad. Sci.* **1054:** 273–282.
50. Kidson-Gerber, G. *et al.* 2008. Adherence to desferrioxamine and deferiprone and the impact of deferiprone co-prescription in thalassaemia major patients. Does the addition of deferiprone improve adherence? *Br. J. Haematol.* **142:** 668–680.

Ann. N.Y. Acad. Sci. ISSN 0077-8923

ANNALS OF THE NEW YORK ACADEMY OF SCIENCES
Issue: *Cooley's Anemia: Ninth Symposium*

Deferasirox—current knowledge and future challenges

John B. Porter
Department of Haematology, University College London, London, United Kingdom

Address for correspondence: Prof. John B. Porter, Department of Haematology, University College London, Paul O'Gorman Cancer Institute, 72 Huntley Street, London WC1E 6DD, UK. j.porter@ucl.ac.uk

Since the last Cooley's symposium in 2005, our knowledge and clinical experience with deferasirox had advanced considerably. This has been based on prospective multicenter clinical trials, on a scale hitherto unprecedented for chelation therapy, now totalling over 7,400 patients. Here, current knowledge about the clinical effects of deferasirox is described in key areas, namely, the pharmacokinetics and its relevance to mechanisms of action; effects on iron balance; effects on serum ferritin; long-term tolerability; and effects on cardiac iron removal. Challenges for future research include a better understanding of the relationship of serum ferritin to iron balance; the optimal target level and rate of decrease in serum ferritin to achieve a "soft landing," as ferritin values fall below 500–1,000 μg/L; the use of surrogate markers, such as mT2*, to infer the likely effects on long-term survival; and the safety and efficacy of deferasirox when combined with other chelators.

Keywords: deferasirox; pharmacokinetics; matabolism; safety; efficacy; efficiency

Pharmacokinetics: relationship to efficacy and clearance of labile plasma iron

Because chelateable iron is both transient and finite at any moment in time, effective and efficient chelation therapy requires continuous exposure of chelators to these iron pools. This is achieved most efficiently when a drug, or combination of drugs, have pharmocokinetics that allow effective concentrations to be present at all times. Previous work with deferoxamine showed that iron excretion was proportional to the area under the curve (AUC) of the chelator[1] and early clinical studies also showed that this was true for deferasirox[2] which has a relatively long plasma half life of 11–19 h[3] achieving steady state trough concentrations of approximately 20 μM at once daily doses of 20 mg/kg/day.[4] Good dose proportionality has also been demonstrated at single doses between 2.5 and 80 mg/kg/day.[3] Interestingly, the current recommendation in the drug labelling of administering deferasirox before meals may not be optimal, as PK single-dose studies have shown increased absorption after meals.[5] Further work is ongoing to determine the relative tolerability and efficacy of repeated administration post-prandially.

There are at least two potential consequences of continuous exposure to effective chelator concentrations: first, increased efficacy of iron chelation and second, improved removal of labile iron pools. There is good evidence of both with deferasirox. The efficiency of iron chelation can be defined as the percentage of the administered dose that is excreted in the iron bound form. The efficiency of deferasirox in 1-year preregistration studies was 27% and remained constant over dose ranges between 10 and 30 mg/kg/day.[6] This compared with 13% (range 10–17%) efficiency with deferoxamine given five nights a week sc in the same study. Reports with deferiprone given at 25 mg/kg/day show low efficiencies with approximately 4% of administered dose eliminated in urine bound to iron.[7] This high efficiency for deferasirox is most likely to be consequent to the prolonged plasma half life which is proportionately linked to AUC values.[2] Additional factors that contribute to this relatively high efficiency are the high iron binding constant and the metabolism of deferasirox mainly to species that retain their ability to bind iron.[8]

Transferrin independent plasma iron species, that are present in iron overload, can be measured in several ways, either as total nontransferrin plasma

doi: 10.1111/j.1749-6632.2010.05582.x

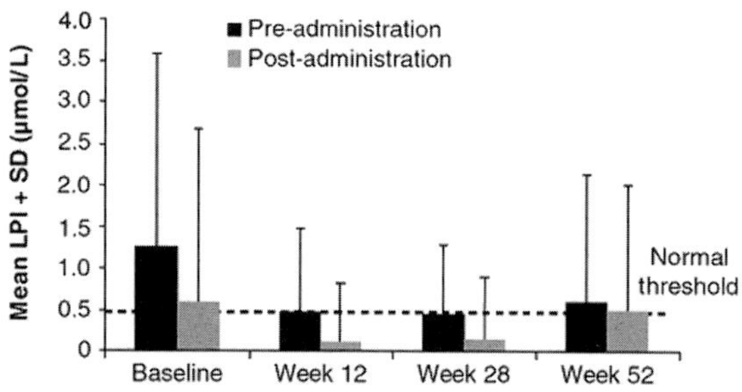

LPI = labile plasma iron; SD = standard deviation.

Figure 1. LPI is shown at baseline 12, 28, and 52 weeks, pre and post daily dosing with deferasirox for thalassemia major patients treated on the EPIC study. The broken line represents the upper limit of "normal" values for LPI. Reprinted from Porter *et al.*,[13] with permission from Elsevier.

bound iron (NTBI) or as a component that is capable of generating oxidative stress namely labile plasma iron (LPI). These are only transiently and incompletely removed while chelators remain present in this compartment.[9,10] Deferasirox has been shown to remove LPI effectively and rapidly after singe doses, but also progressively with longer-term exposure in thalassemia major patients both in the Escalator trial[11] and in the EPIC trial in over 1,000 patients[12,13] (Fig. 1). This contrasts with the intermittent and transient removal, with deferoxamine and deferiprone, that is consistent with their known pharmacokinetics.[10,14]

Probability of iron balance: impact of dose and transfusion rate

Despite clinical experience with deferoxamine and deferiprone going back several decades, it is important to note that knowledge of the impact of dose and transfusional iron loading rates on iron balance had been lacking until now. Short-term formal metabolic iron balance studies previously showed that iron excretion averaged 0.13, 0.34, and 0.56 mg/kg/day at doses of 10, 20, and 40 mg/kg/day, respectively, predicting equilibrium or negative iron balance at daily does of 20 mg and above.[2] Recent prospective studies of iron balance over one year, with a range of doses and transfusion rates[15] have shown that the blood transfusion rate has a key impact on the necessary effective dose of both deferasirox and deferoxamine. This understanding has been made possible by the key findings of Angelucci and colleagues,[16] who previously showed that liver iron concentration (LIC) relates precisely to total body iron stores and hence changes in LIC, together with the iron loading rate from transfusion can be used to derive in iron balance over defined periods of time. One-year studies show that proportion of patients in negative iron balance at 20 mg/kg is 75% at low transfusion rates (<0.3 mg/kg/day) but falls to 55% and 47%, respectively, at intermediate (0.3–0.5 mg/kg/day) and high (>0.5 mg/kg/day) transfusion rates[15] (Fig. 2). This can be increased at 30 mg/kg to 96% in those who have a low transfusional loading, but at intermediate and high transfusional loading rates, the proportion falls to approximately 80% of patients. An important finding here is that at low transfusion rates, 96% of patients are in negative iron balance. This means that so called "nonresponders" at higher transfusion rates are likely to result from relative rather than absolute differences in drug metabolism between patients. In other words, there is unlikely to be a substantial subset of patients whose drug metabolism differs fundamentally from the patient majority. This implies that increased dosing and optimizing of timing of drug administration in relation to meals is likely to maximize the proportion of responders with respect to iron balance.

Effects on serum ferritin

Although body iron load has been estimated to account for only between 30%[17] and 60%[18] of the variability in serum ferritin, this remains the most convenient and repeatedly performed estimate of body iron load. At least six studies have shown a clear effect of long-term control of serum ferritin on prognosis and therefore ferritin trends with deferasirox are important to monitoring response to therapy. A study relating changes in LIC to serum ferritin over a range of underlying anemias, including thalassemia major, has shown a significant correlation ($r = 0.59$) between the serum ferritin trend and LIC trend with deferasirox[19] (Fig. 3). Of interest in this study, the intercept of the delta LIC and ferritin ferritin axes shows that a reduction in LIC over one year (and hence a negative iron balance) of between 4 and 7 mg/day dry wt may not be associated with a decrease in serum ferritin (Fig. 3). This may explain why some patients receiving what appear to be adequate deferasirox doses do not show an early falls in serum ferritin. A mechanistic explanation for this may reside from the preferential removal of iron from the hepatocytes, rather than macrophages

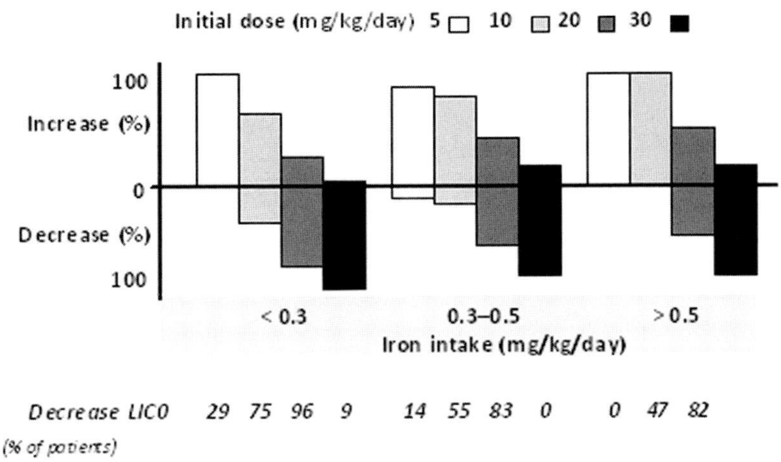

Figure 2. The change in LIC at one year is shown, analysed according to deferasirox dose and the ongoing transfusional iron lading rate. Iron loading rates are divided into low (<0.3 mg/kg/day), intermediate (0.3–0.5 mg/kg/day, representing the majority of patients), and high (>0.5 mg/kg/day). It can be seen that LIC decreases (negative iron balance) in 96% of patients receiving low transfusion and 30 mg/kg/day of deferasirox. At intermediate and high transfusion rates, a lower proportion of patients (82–83%) are in negative iron balance at the same dose. Reproduced with permission of the American Society of Hematology (ASH), from Blood, Cohen AR, *et al.* 111, 2, 2008; permission conveyed through Copyright Clearance Center, Inc.

that was demonstrated in a study of iron distribution taken from liver biopsies taken at baseline (BL) and at one year.[20] Since glycosylated serum ferritin is derived from marcrophages rather than hepatocytes for values up to approximately 4000 μg/L,[17] preferential removal from hepatocytes by deferasirox may not be proportionately reflected by the serum ferritin trend.

It is clear however that with longer-term treatment, the proportion of patients with falling ferritin values increases. Indeed, the percentage of patients achieving serum ferritin levels <1000 μg/L in long term follow up increases gradually from 13.5% in year 1, 18.6% in year 2, 25.7% in year 3, 32.5% in year 4, and 36.7% at 4–5 years.[21] Encouragingly, this has been achieved without signs of decreased drug tolerability in 174 adults and pediatric patients achieving serum ferritin values <1,000 μg/L with increase in the proportion of patients with creatinine increases > 33% above BL and ULN or with ALTs > 10x ULN.[21] Furthermore the large scale one year EPIC study involving >1,700 patients, 937 with thalassemia major, shows that dosing can be adjusted successfully based on baseline ferritin, trends in ferritin and rates of transfusional iron loading.[22] In this study, dose adjustment occurred at a median of 24 weeks of treatment. Based on these findings, as well as the theoretical considerations discussed earlier, dose escalation based on ferritin trends would typically be considered only after at least three months of treatment.

Tolerability profile

Because iron chelation therapy has the potential not only to remove potentially damaging iron species but also potentially useful iron pools that are necessary for synthesis of key metalloenzymes, the potential unwanted effects of over chelation need to be looked for, especially when iron is removed too rapidly or to critically low levels. As experience with deferasirox has now extended to five years, its safety profile is increasingly understood.[23]

In the core pre-registration trials, adverse effects were generally mild, including transient gastrointestinal events in 15%, skin rash in 11% and mild, dose-dependent increases in serum creatinine in 38% of patients which generally remained within the normal range and never exceeded two times the upper limit of normal. Increased liver enzymes, judged to be related to deferasirox were observed in two patients only. No drug-related agranulocytosis was observed. These pre-registration studies (studies 107 and 108) have now been extended, up to 4.5–5 years of treatment with the emergence of important principles for management. Importantly, the incidence of adverse events has gradually decreased over this time in 345 TM patients, at a mean final dose of 22 mg/kg/day.[24] Importantly, the mean

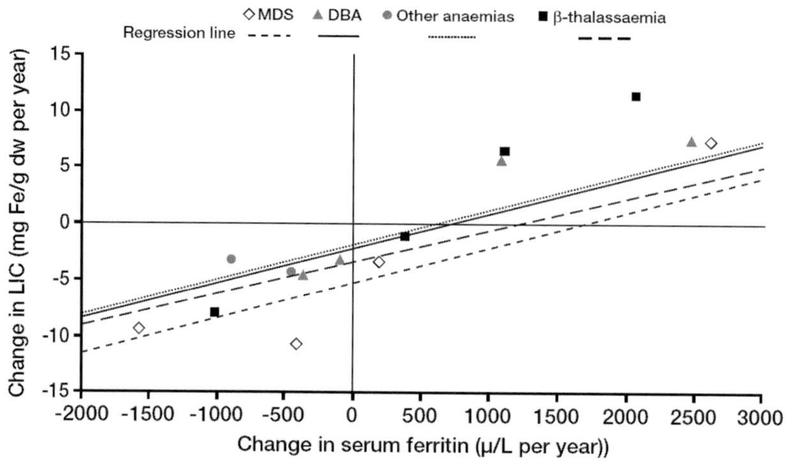

Figure 3. Relationship of changes in ferritin to LIC changes is shown for different disease groups (squares, thalassemia major; diamonds, MDS; triangles, DBA; circles, other anemias). When analyzing the data across combined disease groups (regression line not shown), an overall LIC change over one year is predicted as −3.36 + 0.003 times change in ferritin (Pearson's correlation coefficient = 0.59). Based on the slope of this linear model, a reduction in ferritin of 1000 μg/L predicts a reduction of approximately 6 mg Fe/g dw in LIC. NB: Based on the y axis intercept when there is no change in ferritin ($x = 0$), a decrease in LIC of 4–7 mg/g dw is seen without a decrement in serum ferritin. Based on the x-axis intercept when $y = 0$, a ferritin increase may be seen when LIC is unaltered. (Porter, Galanello *et al.*, EJH (2008) *80*, 168–76). ©2008 John Wiley & Sons, Inc.

serum creatinine has shown no signs of long-term progression. In 137 pediatric patients, followed for a median of 51 months, the mean change in ferritin was 947 μg/L, the frequency of investigator-reported AEs decreased over long-term treatment with no progressive effects on renal or hepatic function and with no negative impact on growth or sexual development.[25]

A further emerging aspect of tolerability is experience at doses >30 mg/kg/day. This has been gained in extension phases of the core studies, as well as with a subset of patients 252 Middle Eastern patients with heavy liver iron loading (mean LIC 19 mg/day dry wt) taking part, in a trial knows as the "Escalator" study.[26] Reported experience totals 228 patients at >30 mg/kg/day for a median of 36 weeks without a trend for increasing serum creatinine but with a clear trend for decreasing serum ferritin after dose escalation.[26] Understanding of the tolerability of deferasirox has also been increased as a result of the large-scale one year EPIC trial.[22] Tolerability was generally in line with preregistration studies: approximately 4% of patients had serum creatinine increases >33% above BL and above the ULN on two consecutive visits but there were no progressive increases. 0.5% of patients had increase in ALT >10 x ULN on two consecutive visits while levels were elevated at BL in four of these patients.[22]

Prevention and removal of cardiac iron deposition

Following initial observational studies of significant improvements in myocardial T2* with deferasirox over one year of treatment,[27] large-scale prospective studies have now been undertaken. In a substudy of the large EPIC trial, in 105 patients with established mild to moderate excess of myocardial iron, a significant reduction in cardiac iron was seen at a mean dose of 32.6 mg/kg/day. For patients with BL T2* values of 10–20 ms, the T2* increased significantly from 14.6 to 17.4 ms, whereas for patients with BL T2* values <10 ms the T2* also increased significantly from 7.4 to 8.2 ms over 1 year[28] (Fig. 4). Experience for up to 2 years now shows further progressive improvement in mT2*.[29] A further sub-study examined trends of mT2* in 75 patients without preexisting myocardial loading. Deferasirox prevented accumulation of cardiac iron in all cases and significantly increased LVEF even though this was within the accepted limits of normal at BL.[30] It is not clear whether this increase in LVEF results from removal of small amounts of myocardial iron that is not detectable by mT2* or is due

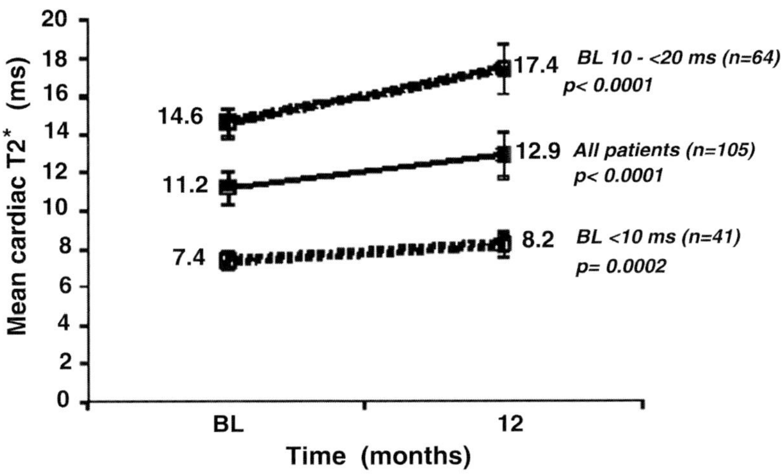

Figure 4. Mycocardial T2* is shown at baseline (BL) and after 12 months of deferasirox treatment for all patients (n = 105, solid line) as geometric mean ± 95% confidence intervals, as well as for patient subsets with BL values 10–20 ms or < 10 m (broken lines). The mean actual dose over one year was 32.6 mg/kg/day. © 2009 Ferrata Storti Foundation. Pennell D, Porter JB, Cappellini MD, Chan LL, El-Beshlawy A, Aydinok Y, *et al.* Efficacy and safety of deferasirox in reducing myocardial siderosis in patients with b-thalassemia major. Haematologica 2009; 94(Suppl 2):abst 193.

to other effects such as those on vascular endothelial function.

Future challenges

Rapid advances in understanding of the efficacy and safety of deferasirox of the last five years, based on large scale prospective trials, mean that evidence-based information about the probability of both response and the probability of side effects are available in a way that has not been previously possible with other chelation therapy regimens. Despite this, there remains important work to do and questions to answer for thalassemia patients.

Further work on the use of serum ferritin to monitor response and to maximise tolerability would be valuable. There may be factors that impact on ferritin trends in addition to those already identified such as dose, compliance, and transfusional loading rates. It is worth noting that such understanding is also required with other chelation regimes. Preliminary work suggesting that deferasirox has a propensity for hepatocellular rather than reticulo-endothelial iron (see earlier), in contrast to deferiprone where the converse occurs, may explain why initial deceases in LIC may not be immediately reflected by changes in serum ferritin (Fig. 3). As the proportion of patients with serum ferritin values <1,000 μg/L increases, there will be a need to understand whether there is a minimum ferritin that can be safely achieved. An important question is whether the principle driver of drug related toxicity is the rate of decrease in body iron and/or the absolute body iron level; in short, how slowly do we need to reduce serum ferritin in order to achieve a "soft landing" as we achieve low serum ferritin values? As the rate of transfusion has been shown to impact on chelation efficiency,[6] it is also possible that the rate of iron loading from transfusion impacts on optimal rate of ferritin reduction and its safe minimal value; an ongoing trial with untransfused thalassemia intermedia is likely to clarify this latter point.

The long-term effects on survival and morbidity are unknown at this time for obvious tautological reasons. However, it is going to be difficult to infer such effects in the very clear way that was previously possible in cohorts of patients treated with deferoxamine, where the comparator to deferoxamine was "no chelation" therapy. Retrospective attempts to ascribe changes in long-term survival to short term changes in chelation regimens or other changes in management are open to a variety of interpretations. On the other hand, a 10 or 20 year prospective study, comparing deferasirox with other forms of chelation in matched populations is unlikely to be practically achievable. Therefore surrogate markers of survival are likely to be the best indicators of long-term effects on mortality for the time being. The most important of these is the recently established link of myocardial T2* to the risk of developing iron mediated heart failure prospectively.[31] The absence of new cases of myocardial iron loading in prospective one year studies is encouraging. Future studies therefore should aim to establish in the long term whether the proportion of patients with increased myocardial iron loading steadily diminishes with deferasirox therapy. Finally there is increasing interest in the use of deferasirox combined with deferoxamine in selected cases. The safety and efficacy of such an approach will need to be tested in well designed prospective trials in order to establish where this might fit in with overall management of transfusional iron overload in thalassemia major.

Conflicts of interest

The author declares no conflicts of interest.

References

1. Porter, J.B. *et al.* 1998. Iron balance and chelation efficiency following single dose depot desferrioxamine. *Blood* **92**(Suppl 1): 325a (Abstract).
2. Nisbet-Brown, E. *et al.* 2003. Effectiveness and safety of ICL670 in iron-loaded patients with thalassaemia: a randomised, double-blind, placebo-controlled, dose-escalation trial. *Lancet* **361:** 1597–1602.
3. Galanello, R. *et al.* 2003. Safety, tolerability, and pharmacokinetics of ICL670, a new orally active iron-chelating agent in patients with transfusion-dependent iron overload due to beta-thalassemia. *J. Clin. Pharmacol.* **43:** 565–572.
4. Piga, A. *et al.* 2006. Randomized phase II trial of deferasirox (Exjade, ICL670), a once-daily, orally-administered iron chelator, in comparison to deferoxamine in thalassemia patients with transfusional iron overload. *Haematologica.* **91:** 873–880.
5. Galanello, R. *et al.* 2008. Effect of food, type of food, and time of food intake on deferasirox bioavailability: recommendations for an optimal deferasirox administration regimen. *J. Clin. Pharmacol.* **48:** 428–435.
6. Porter, J. *et al.* 2005. Iron chelation efficiency of deferasirox (Exjade, ICL670) in patients with transfusional Hemosiderosis. *Blood* **106:** 2690 (Abstract).
7. Hoffbrand, A.V., A. Cohen & C. Hershko. 2003. Role of deferiprone in chelation therapy for transfusional iron overload. *Blood* **102:** 17–24.
8. Waldmeier, F.J. *et al.* 2010. Pharmacokinetics, metabolism and disposition of deferasirox in {beta}-thalassemia patients with transfusion-dependent iron overload who are at pharmacokinetic steady state. *Drug Metab. Dispos.* **38:** 808–816.
9. Porter, J.B. *et al.* 2005. Recent insights into interactions of deferoxamine with cellular and plasma iron pools: implications for clinical use. *Ann. N.Y. Acad. Sci.* **1054:** 155–168.
10. Cabantchik, Z.I. *et al.* 2005. LPI-labile plasma iron in iron overload. *Best Pract. Res. Clin. Haematol.* **18:** 277–287.
11. Daar, S. *et al.* 2009. Reduction in labile plasma iron during treatment with deferasirox, a once-daily oral iron chelator, in heavily iron-overloaded patients with beta-thalassaemia. *Eur. J. Haematol.* **82:** 454–457.
12. Porter, J. *et al.* 2008. Effect of deferasirox (Exjade®) on labile plasma iron levels in heavily iron-overloaded patients with transfusion-dependent Anemias enrolled in the large-scale, prospective 1-year EPIC trial. *Blood* **112:** 3881 (Abstract).
13. Porter, J.B. 2009. Optimizing iron chelation strategies in beta-thalassaemia major. *Blood Rev.* **23**(Suppl 1): S3–S7.
14. Zanninelli, G., W. Breuer & Z.I. Cabantchik. 2009. Daily labile plasma iron as an indicator of chelator activity in thalassaemia major patients. *Br. J. Haematol.* **147:** 744–751.
15. Cohen, A.R., E. Glimm & J.B. Porter. 2008. Effect of transfusional iron intake on response to chelation therapy in -thalassemia major. *Blood* **111:** 583–587.
16. Angelucci, E. *et al.* 2000. Hepatic iron concentration and total body iron stores in thalassemia major. *N. Engl. J. Med.* **343:** 327–331.
17. Worwood, M. *et al.* 1980. Binding of serum ferritin to concanavalin A: patients with homozygous beta thalassaemia and transfusional iron overload. *Br. J. Haematol.* **46:** 409–416.
18. Brittenham, G.M. *et al.* 1993. Hepatic iron stores and plasma ferritin concentration in patients with sickle cell anemia and thalassemia major. *Am. J. Hematol.* **42:** 81–85.
19. Porter, J. *et al.* 2008. Relative response of patients with myelodysplastic syndromes and other transfusion-dependent anaemias to deferasirox (ICL670): a 1-yr prospective study. *Eur. J. Haematol.* **80:** 168–176.
20. Deugnier, Y. *et al.* 2005. Semi-quantitative assessment of hemosiderin distribution accurately reflects reductions in liver iron concentration following therapy with deferasirox (Exjade®, ICL670) or deferoxamine in patients with transfusion-dependent anemia. *Blood* **106**(Suppl 11): 2708 (Abstract).
21. Porter, J.B. *et al.* 2008. Safety of deferasirox (Exjade(R)) in patients with transfusion-dependent anemias and iron overload who achieve serum ferritin levels <1000 Ng/Ml during long-term treatment. *Blood* **112:** 5423 (Abstract).
22. Cappellini, M. *et al.* 2010. Tailoring iron chelation by iron intake and serum ferritin: the prospective EPIC study of deferasirox in 1744 patients with transfusion-dependent anemias. *Haematologica.* **95:** 557–566.
23. Cappellini, M.D. *et al.* 2006. A phase 3 study of deferasirox (ICL670), a once-daily oral iron chelator, in patients with beta-thalassemia. *Blood* **107:** 3455–3462.
24. Cappellini, M. *et al.* 2008. Efficacy and safety of deferasirox (Exjade®) with up to 4.5 years of treatment in patients with thalassemia major: a pooled analysis. *Blood* **112:** 5411 (Abstract).
25. Piga, A. *et al.* 2008. Cumulative efficacy and safety of 5-year deferasirox (Exjade®) treatment in pediatric patients with thalassemia major: a Phase II Multicenter prospective trial. 2008 **112:** 5413 (Abstract).

26. Taher, A. *et al.* 2009. Efficacy and safety of deferasirox doses of >30 mg/kg per d in patients with transfusion-dependent anaemia and iron overload. *Br. J. Haematol.* **147:** 752–759.
27. Porter, J.B. *et al.* 2005. Improved myocardial T2* in transfusion dependent anemias receiving ICL670 (Deferasirox). *Blood* **106:** 3600 (Abstract).
28. Pennell, D.J. *et al.* 2008. Efficacy and safety of deferasirox (Exjade®) in reducing cardiac iron in patients with β-thalassemia major: results from the cardiac substudy of the EPIC trial. *Blood* **112:** 3873 (Abstract).
29. Pennell, D.J. *et al.* 2010. Efficacy of deferasirox in reducing and preventing cardiac iron overload in beta-thalassemia. *Blood* **115:** 2364–2371.
30. Pennell, D. *et al.* 2008. Efficacy and safety of deferasirox (Exjade®) in preventing cardiac iron overload in β-thalassemia patients with normal baseline cardiac iron: results from the cardiac substudy of the EPIC trial. *Blood* **112:** 3874 (Abstract).
31. Kirk, P. *et al.* 2009. Cardiac T2* magnetic resonance for prediction of cardiac complications in thalassemia major. *Circulation* **120:** 1961–1968.

Ann. N.Y. Acad. Sci. ISSN 0077-8923

ANNALS OF THE NEW YORK ACADEMY OF SCIENCES
Issue: *Cooley's Anemia: Ninth Symposium*

Monitoring the efficiency of iron chelation therapy: the potential of nontransferrin-bound iron

R.C. Hider,[1] A.M.N. Silva,[1] M. Podinovskaia,[2] and Yongmin Ma[1]

[1]Division of Pharmaceutical Science, King's College London, London, United Kingdom. [2]London School of Hygiene and Tropical Medicine, London, United Kingdom

Address for correspondence: Robert C. Hider, Pharmaceutical Science Division, 5th floor, Franklin-Wilkins Building, King's College London, 150 Stamford Street, London SE1 9NH, UK. robert.hider@kcl.ac.uk

The major ligands of nontransferrin-bound iron (NTBI) are suggested to be citrate and albumin. The proportion of iron binding to albumin is influenced by the degree of oxidation and glycation of the protein. LC-ICP-MS is demonstrated to be a useful technique for the speciation of NTBI, with unprocessed serum being subjected to analysis. Ferritin iron, citrate iron, and ferrioxamine can be quantified using this technique. This review describes the use of a new fluorescent probe for NTBI quantification.

Keywords: nontransferrin-bound iron; fluorescent reagent

Normally iron is transported between body tissues bound to the serum protein transferrin. Transferrin binds iron with high affinity and delivers iron to cells, which express the transferrin receptor. In clinical treatments centered on regular blood transfusion, for instance thalassemia major and in circumstances of hyperabsorption of iron, for example thalassemia intermedia, transferrin becomes fully saturated with iron. Under these conditions, iron entering the blood supply from intestinal enterocytes and macrophages enters the nontransferrin-bound iron (NTBI) pool; which unlike transferrin lacks an address system. Perfusion of highly vascular tissue, such as heart and endocrine tissue, with blood containing NTBI leads to enhanced iron loading of these tissues. Initially this additional iron is ligated by ferritin, but as this uncontrolled flux of iron continues, the relatively enormous capacity of ferritin is exceeded and excess iron is no longer protected from redox cycling, thereby generating reactive oxygen radicals in sensitive tissues. In addition, the presence of NTBI renders the blood susceptible to invasion by pathogenic bacteria and fungi as the plentiful supply of readily available iron is an essential growth factor for all microorganisms.

The clinical management of patients receiving regular transfusions has been brought into sharp focus recently as a result of the introduction of two orally active iron chelators deferiprone and exjade, in addition to the widely used desferrioxamine.[1] In principle, the monitoring of chelation therapy can be achieved effectively with the regular measurement of NTBI; the dose of the chelator being adjusted to reduce NTBI levels to zero. Unfortunately, there is no such method which is currently widely available for use in clinical laboratories.[2] Typically chelation therapy is monitored using MRI, SQUID, or liver biopsy, but such methods cannot be used on a regular basis for reasons of cost or risk to the patient. The measurement of serum ferritin and transferrin saturation are also employed but both methods have disadvantages.

A problem with the measurement of NTBI is that it is a multicomponent system, consisting of iron bound to ferritin, albumin, and citrate.[3,4] The proportion of NTBI bound to albumin is markedly influenced by the degree of oxidation and glycation of albumin.[4] Not all these components contain redox active iron and so NTBI quantification methods based on the detection of such iron, for instance "labile plasma iron"[5] and "bleomycin-detectable" iron[6] will only measure a proportion of this pool, and this fraction may vary between disease states and with the degree of iron overload.

doi: 10.1111/j.1749-6632.2010.05573.x

To understand more about the nature of NTBI in thalassemia we have developed an LC-ICP-MS system in such a manner that it is possible to quantify components of NTBI, namely iron bound to ferritin, citrate, and chelators. Progress so far is reported in this communication. We also report a newly developed fluorescent-based assay for NTBI measurement, which is user-friendly, robust, and reliable. We are currently applying this new method for monitoring thalassemia patients receiving chelation therapy.

Chemical nature of nontransferrin-bound iron

There are many small molecules in the blood, which are capable of binding iron, for instance acetate, malate, phosphate, citrate, and glutathione. Of these citrate has the highest affinity for iron(III),[7] which is the favored redox state of NTBI. Citrate forms a range of iron(III) complexes,[7,8] but under the physiological conditions provided by serum, only two forms dominate, [Fe(Citrate)$_2$] (Schema 1), and an oligomeric form, which is probably [Fe$_3$(Citrate)$_3$] (Schema 2).[7] The presence of iron citrate in the serum of a nontreated hemochromatosis patient has been directly demonstrated by ^{1}H-NMR.[9] At an iron concentration of 1 μM, the over 100-fold excess of citrate ensures that the mononuclear [Fe(Citrate)$_2$] (Schema 1) dominates, however at higher iron concentrations (10 μM) the proportion of the oligomeric iron citrate species (Schema 2) increases.[7] Surprisingly [Fe(Citrate)$_2$] does not redox cycle in the presence of reduced ascorbic acid to any appreciable extent.[10] In contrast, the oligomeric species [Fe$_3$(Citrate)$_3$] does redox cycle under these conditions, albeit weakly.[11]

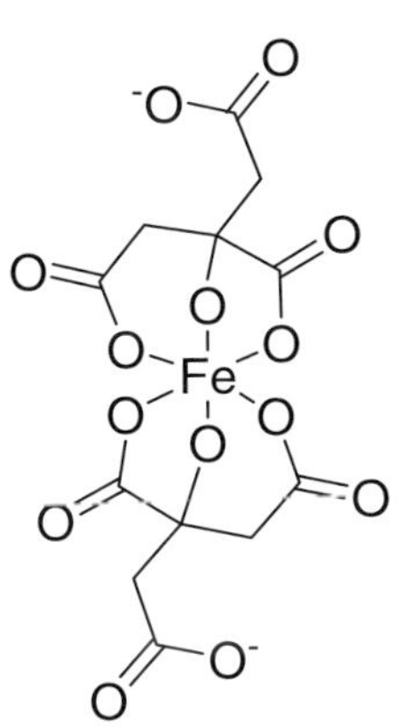

1 [iron (citrate)$_2$]$^{5-}$

Schema 1.

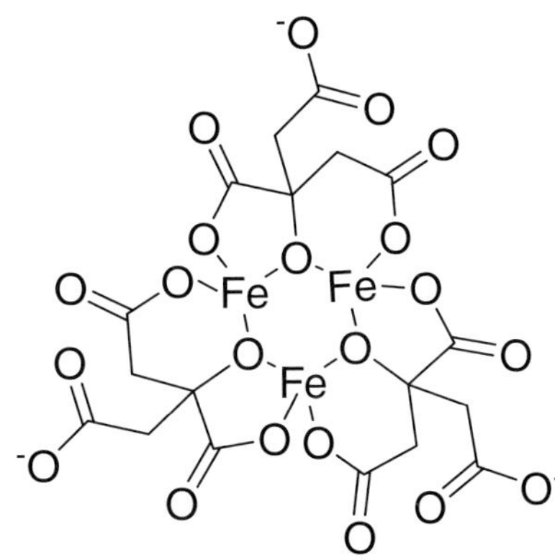

2 [(iron)$_3$(citrate)$_3$]$^{3-}$

Schema 2.

Another important iron-binding component of the serum is albumin, which is present at a relatively high concentration (600 μM). There are many reports relating to the iron binding properties of albumin, some of which are contradictory.[4] These differences are likely to be associated with the fact that albumin is heterogeneous, a proportion of the molecules being partially oxidized and a further proportion being glycated.[4] Albumin carries net charge of 15$^-$, with a large number of carboxylic acids on the surface of the molecule which form potential iron binding sites.[12]

To better understand the nature of NTBI species and to clarify the role of albumin in NTBI speciation, the interaction of iron with human albumin was investigated under plasma-like concentrations of albumin and citrate at physiological values of pH and ionic strength. Gel filtration associated with inductively coupled plasma mass spectrometry (GF-ICP-MS) was used to separate the albumin-bound iron from the small molecular weight iron–citrate complexes and quantitatively determine the concentration of both iron pools. In addition, the ability of nonenzymatic posttranslational modifications to alter the iron binding ability of albumin was assessed.[4] Albumin is one of the most important antioxidants in the serum[13] and as such is exposed to several modifications ranging from the formation of

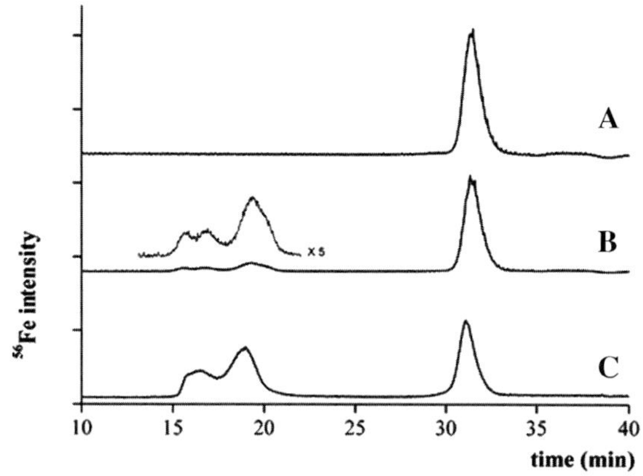

Figure 1. The binding of iron to citrate and albumin. Chromatograms representing the elution of ^{56}Fe after a gel filtration chromatography as detected by ICP-MS. Peaks with elution times between 15 and 22 min correspond to the elution of albumin-bound iron, peaks appearing after 28 min arise from small molecular weight iron–citrate complexes. (A) Solution containing 10 μM Fe, 100 μM citrate, and 150 mM NaCl. (B) Solution containing 40 g/L albumin, 10 μM Fe, 100 μM citrate, and 150 mM NaCl. (C) Solution with 40 g/L oxidized albumin, 10 μM Fe, 100 μM citrate, and 150 mM NaCl. All samples contained 100mM MOPS buffer at pH = 7.4. Research grade recombinant human albumin was used throughout and was a gift from Novozymes Biopharma UK Ltd. Oxidized albumin was prepared as described by Silva *et al.*[4]

mixed disulfides at Cys34, to protein oxidation and glycation. These modifications are known to alter the affinity of albumin for the numerous endogenous and exogenous ligands.[14] The posttranslation modifications that occur with albumin are particularly prevalent in diabetes, but serum markers for oxidative stress are also elevated in iron-overload diseases.[15,16]

Gel filtration allowed the separation of the high molecular weight albumin fraction from the small molecular weight species in solution and coupling to an ICP-MS permitted the quantification of the eluted peaks corresponding to the elution of different iron species. Chromatogram A (Fig. 1) represents the ^{56}Fe elution profile of a solution containing 10 μM iron in the absence of albumin. Under these conditions, there is only a single peak arising from the elution of iron–citrate complexes, this pattern of elution was constant for all the iron concentrations used, demonstrating that under the range of conditions adopted, citrate did not form high molecular weight complexes that could be mistaken as albumin-bound iron. When albumin was introduced into the solutions, three further peaks with retention times between 14 and 22 min could be observed, together with a decrease in the iron-citrate peak area (Fig. 1 – chromatogram B). The appearance of these peaks corresponds to the expected elution profile for albumin, when using a gel filtration chromatography method capable of separating the different aggregates (dimers and hexamers) formed at high albumin concentrations. Albumin was found to bind approximately 20% of the 10 μM iron added to the sample mixture. When 40 g/L (600 μM) oxidized albumin was incubated with 10 μM iron and 100 μM citrate, a larger proportion of the iron present in the sample was found to bind to the albumin fraction, approximately 50% (Fig. 1 – chromatogram C). Similar studies were carried out with glycated albumin, which was shown to possess an even higher affinity for iron.[4] Thus in summary, at an iron(III) concentration of 10 μM, about 50% of the iron is bound to oxidized albumin in contrast to only 20% with the nonoxidized protein.[4] When the iron concentration is reduced to 1 μM, there is a much smaller difference between the amount of iron bound to oxidized and native albumin, 60 and 50%, respectively. In brief, the results demonstrate that albumin-bound iron is an important NTBI species and that albumin modification by oxidation and glycation, increases its iron binding capacity, which may have implications for the pattern of tissue iron distribution. From these *in vitro* experiments it is clear that citrate and albumin are predicted to be major NTBI ligands, and that the proportion of iron bound to albumin depends on its oxidative status and the concentration of iron–citrate complexes. The iron content of serum ferritin will also contribute to this pool, but is less likely to be taken up by the heart and endocrine tissue. Also this portion of NTBI will not be readily scavenged by the iron chelators used clinically.

When the above outlined GF-ICP-MS system was applied to serum samples, the iron content of ferritin and the low molecular weight fraction, presumably iron citrate became apparent (Fig. 2). Unfortunately gel filtration chromatography fails to resolve transferrin from albumin and so the albumin-bound NTBI fraction is swamped by the large transferrin–iron peak. We are currently attempting to resolve this difficulty by using ion exchange chromatography. Normal serum displays iron peaks associated with ferritin and transferrin and only an extremely

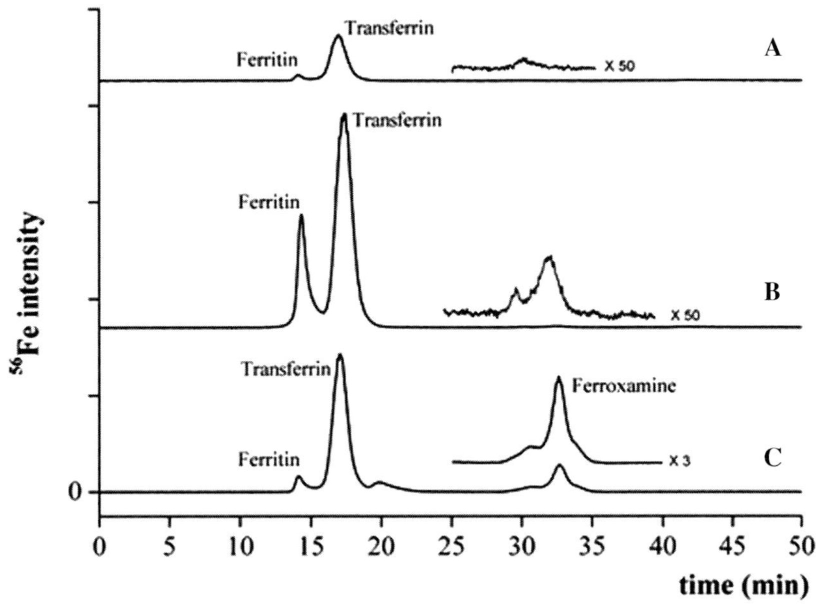

Figure 2. The distribution of iron in serum samples. Chromatograms representing the elution of ^{56}Fe after a gel filtration chromatography as detected by ICP-MS. Peaks with elution times between 14 and 20 min correspond to ferritin and transferrin, peaks appearing after 28 min arise from low molecular weight iron complexes. (A) Normal serum. (B) Thalassemia major serum, patient was not undergoing chelation therapy. (C) Thalassemia major serum, patient receiving subcutaneous desferrioxamine. Serum samples were provided by Professor SweeLay Thein of King's College Hospital.

weak peak due to low molecular weight iron—probably iron citrate (Fig. 2A). In contrast the serum of thalassemia major patients not receiving chelation therapy, displays two appreciable low molecular weight iron peaks in addition to the ferritin and transferrin peaks. The major low molecular weight peak corresponds to [iron(citrate)$_2$] (Schema 1) and the minor low molecular weight peak, possibly corresponds to [(iron)$_3$(citrate)$_3$] (Schema 2) (Fig. 2B). The serum of a thalassemia patient receiving desferrioxamine, shows the presence of a new intense peak in the low molecular weight region which is due to ferrioxamine, together with some nonmobilized low molecular weight NTBI species (Schema 2) (Fig. 2C).

Clearly this system has potential for providing information on the iron states of the patient, for instance the iron content of serum ferritin and the existence of iron–citrate complexes.

The application of fluorescent probes for the measurement of NTBI

Although a wide range of methods have been investigated for the measurement of NTBI, at the present time there is no generally accepted method for the reliable quantification of this pool. In a recent inter-laboratory survey, serum samples of 12 patients were investigated by eight different methods in six laboratories.[2] A poor correlation was found between the methods.[2] In principle, fluorescence-based methods have an advantage of being highly sensitive and relatively easy to use. For these reasons we have

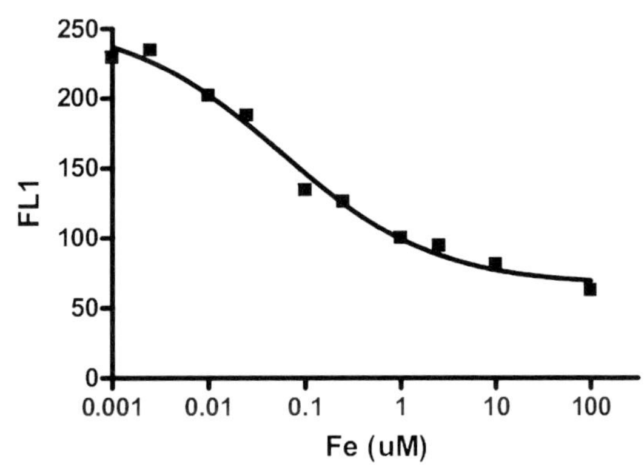

Figure 3. Standard curve of fluorescence quenching by iron in the presence of serum. Iron dextran at indicated concentrations was added to heat-inactivated fetal calf serum (5%) in chelex-treated PBS (pH 7.0). The fluorescence-labeled compound was added to the treated serum samples.

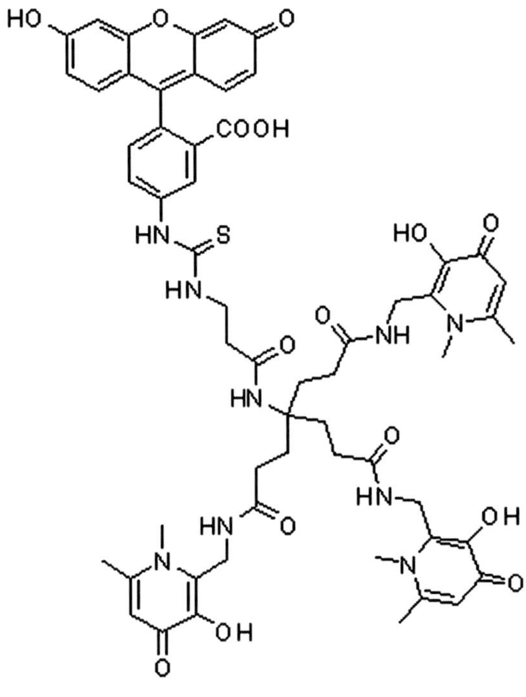

3 CP851

Schema 3.

investigated the potential of several new synthetic probes. We have found that the hexadentate chelator CP851 (Schema 3) is particularly useful. This molecule has a high affinity for iron, is a powerful iron-scavenging agent and yet is essentially unable to mobilize iron from both transferrin and ferritin.[17] In contrast it is able to scavenge iron from iron(III) citrate in a highly efficient manner and much more rapidly than desferrioxamine. When CP851 binds iron, the fluorescence of the attached probe is quenched, the extent of quenching being related to the concentration of iron in the solution under investigation.[17] A standard curve for a related molecule in the presence of serum is presented in Figure 3. This system renders it possible to measure NTBI levels down to 0.1 μM with repeatable accuracy. We are currently using this method to monitor NTBI levels in thalassemia major patients.

Conclusion

NTBI is an important parameter for monitoring the progress of chelation therapy. A reliable quantitative method is urgently required.

LC-ICP-MS is a useful technique, which can provide information on NTBI speciation.

Acknowledgments

The authors would like to thank Novozymes Biophorma UK Ltd. (www.novozymes.com) for the offer of research grade recombinant human albumin used in this study. Andre Siliva would like to acknowledge "Fundacao para a Cienciae Tecnologia" Lisboa Portugal for his PhD grant [SFRH/BD/22633/2005].

Conflicts of interest

The authors declare no conflicts of interest

References

1. Neufeld, E.J. 2006. Oral chelators deferasirox and deferiprone for transfusional iron overload in thalassaemia major: new data, new question. *Blood* **107:** 3436–3441
2. Jacobs, E.M.G., J.C.M. Hendriks, B.L.J.H. van Tits, *et al.* 2005. Results of an international round robin for the quantification of serum non-transferrin-bound iron: need for defining standardization and a clinically relevant isoform. *Anal. Biochem.* **341:** 241–250.
3. Evans, R.W., R. Rafique, A. Zarea, *et al.* 2008. Nature of non-transferrin-bound iron: studies on iron citrate complexes and thalassemic sera. *J. Biol. Inorg. Chem.* **13:** 57–74.
4. Silva, A.M.N. & R.C. Hider. 2009. Influence of non-enzymatic post-translation modifications on the ability of human serum albumin to bind iron: implications for non-transferrin-bound iron speciation. *Biochem. Biophys. Acta* **1794:** 1449–1458.
5. Esposito, B.P., W. Breuer, P. Sirankapracha, *et al.* 2003. Labile plasma iron in iron overload: redox activity and susceptibility to chelation. *Blood* **102:** 2670–2677.
6. von Bonsdorff, L., E. Lindeberg, L. Sahlstedt, *et al.* 2002. Bleomycin-detectable iron assay for non-transferrin-bound iron in hematologic malignancies. *Clin. Chem.* **48:** 307–314.
7. Silva, A.M.N., X.L. Kong, M.C. Parkin, *et al.* 2009. Iron(III) citrate speciation in aqueous solution. *Dalton Trans.* **40:** 8616–8625.
8. Pierre, J.L. & I. Gautier-Luneau. 2000. Iron and citric acid: a fuzzy chemistry of ubiquitous biological relevance. *Biometals* **13:** 91–96.
9. Grootveld, M., J.D. Bell, B. Halliwell, *et al.* 1989. Non-transferrin-bound iron in plasma or serum from patients with idiopathic haemochromatosis. Characterization by high performance liquid chromatography and nuclear magnetic resonance spectroscopy. *J. Biol. Chem.* **15:** 4417–4422.
10. Adam, F.I., R. Kissner & W.H. Koppenol. 2009. Re-evaluating the role of biological ferric citrate in iron overload disease. First international conference on metal chelation in biology and medicin (MCIBAM 2009). Bath, UK. **P1:** 107.
11. Devanur, L.D., H. Neubert & R.C. Hider. 2008. The Fenton activity of iron(III) in the presence of deferiprone. *J. Pharm. Sci.* **97:** 1454–1467.

12. He, X.M. & D.C. Carter. 1992. Atomic-structure and chemistry of human serum-albumin. *Nature* **358:** 209–215.
13. Roche, M., P. Rondeau, N.R. Singh, *et al.* 2008. The antioxidant properties of serum albumin. *FEBS Lett.* **582:** 1783–1787.
14. Oettl, K. & R.E., Stauber. 2007. Physiological and pathological changes in the redox state of human serum albumin critically influence its binding properties. *Br. J. Pharmacol.* **151:** 580–590.
15. Cighetti, G., L. Duca, L. Bortone, *et al.* 2008. Oxidative status and malondialdehyde in beta-thalassaemia. *Eur. J. Clin. Invest.* **32:** 55–60.
16. De Luca, C., A. Filosa, M. Grandinetti, *et al.* 1999. Blood antioxidant status and urinary levels of catecholamine metabolites in beta-thalassemia. *Free Radic. Res.* **30:** 453–462.
17. Ma, Y.M. & R.C. Hider. 2009. The selective quantification of iron by hexadentate fluorescent probes. *Bioorg. Med. Chem.* **17:** 8093–8101.

Ann. N.Y. Acad. Sci. ISSN 0077-8923

ANNALS OF THE NEW YORK ACADEMY OF SCIENCES
Issue: *Cooley's Anemia: Ninth Symposium*

Critical appraisal of growth retardation and pubertal disturbances in thalassemia

Ratna Chatterjee and Rekha Bajoria

Clinical Senior Lecturer/Consultant, Institute for Women's Health, UCL, London, United Kingdom

Address for correspondence: Ratna Chatterjee, M.F.F.P., M.D., Ph.D., Institute for Women's Health, 86-96 Chenies Mews, London WC1E 6HX, UK r.chatterjee@ucl.ac.uk

Growth and pubertal disturbances are the commonest endocrinopathies in homozygous thalassemia, accounting for significant morbidity in 70–80% children and adolescents globally. This review focuses on the pathophysiology of the endocrinopathy from a historical perspective and altered natural history induced by better care due to transfusion and chelation therapy. We have also discussed clinical features, diagnosis, and management strategies of growth retardation, sexual infantilism, pubertal aberrations, and scope of growth hormone, sex steroids, and other endocrine therapies. The article also emphasizes current and future strategies for screening, monitoring of growth and pubertal disturbances, and early intervention for the restoration of fertility potential and bone mass in the affected individuals.

Keywords: growth retardation; hypogonadotrophic hypogonadism; growth hormone; sex steroid; thalassemia

Introduction

Gonadotrophin insufficiency or hypogonadotrophic hypogonadism (HH) resulting from transfusional iron overload continues to be the commonest endocrinopathy in thalassemia patients which affects 70–80% of thalassemic patients worldwide causing sexual infantilism, osteoporosis, and infertility. Growth hormone (GH)—IGF axis is also intertwined with aberrations of growth during childhood and puberty. The diagnosis and management of HH and GH-IGF axis are ill defined and permanent damage may occur with stunted growth with significant embarrassment and poor quality of life. Although the etiology is likely to be iron overload, nutrition, chelation, and hypoxia are all contributors. Patients may be affected as early as 10 years and early diagnosis with prompt intervention can prevent irreversible endocrine damage. We wish to discuss the pathophysiology and management options in this review.

Section A

Pathophysiology: historical perspective

Originally homozygous β-thalassemia was known to affect a significant segment of population in Mediterranean countries,[1] Middle and far East, and West Africa.[2] However, the alteration of migration has changed the geographic distribution and has made it a worldwide health problem in the 21st century. Our understanding of the pathophysiology of growth disturbances of thalassemia has changed significantly in the last five decades with advances in transfusion and chelation treatment as well as the total care. It can be best described in three phases:

Phase 1: 1925–1940

By the beginning of 20th century, European clinicians became aware of the haemolytic anemia syndrome in infancy with massive splenomegaly, pallor, and severe growth retardation.[3] In American literature the first description of growth retardation in thalassemia was attributed to the Detroit physicians Thomas Cooley and Pearl Lee. Cooley and Lee recognized growth retardation as a manifestation of severe haemolysis and ineffective erythropoiesis.[4] Furthermore, bone changes were also reported in the Cooley's triad (severe haemolytic anemia with growth retardation, splenomegaly, and peculiar bone changes of skull and osteoporosis of long bones). As described later by Clegg and

doi: 10.1111/j.1749-6632.2010.05589.x

Weatherall (1976), ineffective erythropoiesis (secondary to depressed β chain synthesis and α chain precipitates with red cell precursor death) was the outstanding feature of thalassemia major.[3] The gross bone marrow expansion to 20 X normal levels with reversal of myeloid: erythroid ratio and maturation arrest (in early polychromatic erythroblasts) was responsible for the clinical picture of growth retardation, increased blood volume, and increased gastrointestinal iron absorption with characteristic bone changes.

Subsequently George Whipple (1935) coined the terminology "thalassemia" and also observed similar growth failure in infants affected with thalassemia.[5] The symptoms of anemia begin at 3–6 months of birth when HbF starts changing into HbA, becoming evident at 1 year of life. Along with anemia children have growth problems and multiple endocrinopathies affecting thyroid, parathyroid, pancreas becoming obvious in early childhood.

In essence, cause of early growth failure in 1920s–1940s was the result of severe anemia and ineffective erythropoiesis, which only occurred with an overactive marrow.[6] Hence, it was called erythroblastic anemia of childhood. The exact prevalence of the growth retardation was not clear-cut but 50–80% are quoted in different series.[6]

The bone changes of thalassemia that contributed to growth retardation during this era included the following, which were appreciated by investigators at a later stage: at birth and childhood bony alterations included hyper-plastic erythropoietic bone marrow. The red marrow is replaced by fatty marrow. Marked porotic hyperostosis of skull with characteristic "hair on end" appearance and facial bones showed frontal bossing and a thickened roughening of maxilla and zygoma led to "mongoloid facies" with malocclusion of jaws. The most severe changes in axial skeleton included widening, reticulation and cortical thinning with porosis and fractures. Decreased height and cupping of end plates can lead to typical "fish vertebrae aspect."[7,8] Compression fractures occurred due to marked lumbo-sacral osteoporosis. Long bones showed a marked widening of medullary cavity with thinning of cortex and a typical flask shaped deformity of metaphyseal area of tubular bones with multiple fragility fracture on Harris lines. Premature and irregular fusion of growth plate can produce deformity with dwarfism.[7,8]

Phase 2: 1960s–early 1990s

In the 1960s a genetic basis of thalassemia was proposed linking it to unbalanced globin chain synthesis.[9] At John Hopkins University, David Weatherall and colleagues used radioactive amino acid *in vitro* and *in vivo* and showed that α and β chain production was defective due to unbalanced globin chain synthesis.[10]

In the 1960s medical awareness and better standard care occurred with the advent of blood transfusion and chelation therapy. It was also appreciated that when the transfusion level was low, bone marrow expansion with hypersplenism was associated with growth retardation from hypoxia. The most striking feature of growth disturbance was lack of muscular tissue, which gave limbs the characteristic "stick- like appearance." In addition, the patients were anorectic due to release of an appetite suppressant by cells dying in bone marrow.

Adequate transfusion corrected the hypoxia and the erythocytic drive and overcame complications of anemia with compensatory bone marrow changes. The picture of chronic illness was reversed by hypertransfusion with complete reversal of bony changes but the children did not attain height velocity. In parallel, transfusions resulted in inexorable accumulations of tissue iron especially in heart and endocrine organs with growth failure and without treatment death was inevitable by the second decade stated that in 1978 the age of death among patients not receiving chelation therapy averaged 21 years.[11,12]

In 1964, Wolman showed that with maintenance of Hb of 10 g/dL the thalassemic children from birth were indistinguishable from normal until the age of 10–12 years, when they showed signs of iron load.[13] At this time growth failure was commonly due to transfusional haemosiderosis rather than ineffective erythropoiesis or anemia.

A decade later desferrioxamine (DFO) gained acceptance as a standard chelation therapy. In the 1970s, transfusion improved and high transfusion became available in 1976.[7] It became apparent that severe growth retardation and failure occurred from iron overload. The progression of organ damage was dependent on rate of progression of transfusional haemosiderosis. The degree of iron load was proportional to severity of endocrinopathy as evident from serum ferritin levels, cardiac dysfunction. Adrenal failure and diabetes and compensated primary hypothyroidism were also documented.[14] In fact, it was shown that at the age of 6 years children had low growth as well as low PTH levels, and reduced insulin secretions.[6] All endocrinopathies were primarily described to be due to iron load.

Chelation was started in the 1960s and IM DFO became available in the 1970s.[15] It was shown that aggressive chelation was equally deleterious for growth if started very early at 2–3 years of age in childhood.[16] Also adverse effects of DFO on bone became apparent which contributed to growth retardation and attainment of future target height.

First report of endocrinopathies in thalassemia

The first report of multiple endocrinopathies in thalassemia was reported in 1967 by Bannerman and colleagues in thalassemia intermedia where the patient had cardiac failure, diabetes, porphyria, and hypopituitarism, all due to due to iron load.[17] After a decade McIntosh suggested that hypoxia and iron load affected internedia patients more than major even in the absence of gross iron load.[14] It is now appreciated that although intermedia patients can be heavily iron loaded from gastrointestinal iron absorption, and have severe osteoporosis, growth retardation and HH are markedly common in transfusion-dependent major patients from an early age.

In subsequent years several authors reported high incidence of growth and pubertal disturbances due to pituitary-gonadal and GH dysfunction.[12,18]

In the 1970s and the 1980s the growth retardation and bony deformities encountered in thalassemics occurred due to combined effects of iron loading and DFO therapy. Most problems became apparent after the age of 10 years.[16] Modell states that before 1967 pattern of growth retardation was difficult to describe, as children were younger. Of the 12 deaths that occurred in older children aged 12–23 years primarily from iron load. All had variable degrees of growth retardation with bone deformity and no patients' attained puberty. Also peak height velocity was absent in all patients. Although the exact age and threshold for iron-induced endocrine damage was not understood, the first observable change around 10–11 years was a change in growth rate when the patients had received an average of 28 g iron.[6] Failed puberty was more common in boys than girls. It was thought to be due to hypothalamic rather than pituitary and gonadal damage.[14] Despite the absence of accurate data about prevalence of growth and pubertal disturbance, it was known that growth failure specially absence of sexual maturation had a significant effect on quality of life due to impact on social rehabilitation. A similar picture was shown in Cyrpus where adolescents had severe behavioral problems due to chronic ill health, delayed puberty, and fear of death.[7] Difficulties included failure to get entrance into Universities and lack of employment, as many employers were prejudiced against employing thalassemics and they felt that patients would take many days off work. Additionally thalassemics were barred from civil service.[7]

In the late 1980s and 1990s growth and pubertal failure became more apparent with improved prognosis of thalassemia and better survival. The expectations of many thalassemics became directed to the same attainments as those of healthy peers: education, employment, well adjusted social and sexual life, and aspiration to have a family. Growth failure and pubertal delay with altered physical appearance and dysmorphic bones present major obstacles to fulfillment of these hopes. Studies in this era describing growth, pubertal disturbances for the most part relate to patients receiving transfusions with low or optimal Hb level with no or sub optimal chelation by Im route.[19]

Comprehensive data on growth and puberty was correlated with haematological data (age at diagnosis, onset of chelation and transfusion therapy, and total units of blood transfused). Compliance with DFO therapy was expressed as chelation index. Bone age, and pubertal maturation was assessed properly by Tanner method.[20] Borgna-Pignatti reported 37% children to be 2SD below the mean for normal height. Most strikingly after the age of 14 years, the percentage of short stature increased to 62% in males and 35% for females. The children were shorter than normal but weight was adequate for height. Seventy-five percent had delayed skeletal maturation. The contribution of ferritin and no of units of transfusion did not reach significance.

Iron load was stated as the main contributor to hypothalamic-pituitary-gonadal (H-P-G) dysfunction and GH dysfunction in many patients. Borgna-Pignetti[20] proposed that perhaps aggressive chelation therapy must be started very early in life around 3 years of age as suggested by De Virgillis and colleagues[16] or even earlier Fargion[21]. Other factors include zinc deficiency, malabsorption, and autoimmune disease.[6] Liver disease[20] and carbohydrate intolerance[22] were also thought to be responsible. Histological evidence of damage to anterior pituitary gland (reduced number of cells and moderate siderosis of pituitary parenchyma), gonads (hyper pigmentation of undifferentiated somniferous tubules with reduced number of Leydig cells in males and thickened stroma of ovaries with reduced number of primordial follicles[23]), and bones were shown by different investigators.[24]

Desferrioxamine toxicity in bones

Interestingly although DFO can limit complications of iron load and improve growth in first decade, it can induce short stature. Intensive chelation with desferrioxamine between the ages of 2–5 years can induce toxicity on body proportion, composition, and complex bony lesions with retarded growth.[25,26] This is probably due to inhibition of cell proliferation, DNA synthesis collagen formation and trace element, such as calcium, copper, and zinc. These complex mechanisms result in platyspondylosis with flattening of vertebral bodies and flattening of spinal height resulting in truncal shortening, also in the presence of normal stature.[27]

Phase 3: 2000–2010

Current picture

Despite these therapeutic progresses, endocrine complications are still commonly found in these patients, HH and impaired growth being the most frequent and account for significant morbidity.[11]

There is a widespread heterogeneity in epidemiological data concerning prevalence of endocrinopathies specially growth and pubertal disturbances due to the following factors:

- Iron load is the major cause in poly-transfused thalassemia major with heart and pituitary being most sensitive to it. The anterior pituitary is particularly sensitive to free radical oxidative stress.
- But anemia, nutritional factors may play permissive roles.
- Widespread variability in treatment protocol of transfusion and chelation, treatment facilities over time (age of transfusion and chelation), compliance with chelation.
- As pituitary is affected at an early age, the age of presentation was important with highest number in adolescents and late childhood.
- Genotypic variations and country of origin played some role as well.[28]
- Bone toxicity, which may be inflicted by DFO. Direct evidence of iron-induced toxicity is also shown to affect bones.[27]

Pathophysiology in relation to stages of life: birth to adulthood

Growth failure in TM has been recognized for many years, and has persisted despite major treatment advances. The child with TM has a particular pattern, which is relatively normal until age 9–10 years; after this age a slowing down of growth velocity and a reduced or absent pubertal growth spurt are observed. The growth plate fusion is usually delayed until the end of the second decade of life.[29] The pathogenesis of growth failure is multifactorial[28,29] and is mainly due to iron overload, chronic anemia and hypoxia, chronic liver disease, zinc and folic acid deficiency, intensive use of chelating agents, emotional factors, endocrinopathies (hypogonadism, delayed puberty, hypothyroidism), and GH-IGF-1 axis dysregulation. The fundamental problem is free iron within expanded labile pool. It is shown that heart and pituitary are especially sensitive to free iron toxicity.[27]

Characteristically three phases of growth according to age of presentation are recognized which have different etiologies (Fig. 1). The first phase of childhood growth disturbance is mainly due to hypoxia, anemia, and nutritional factors. The second phase is due to anemia and iron load affecting GH-IGF axis. The hormonal cause of growth retardation in TM children is complex. It has been apparent that GH-IGF-1 axis plays a role in their abnormal growth besides hypogonadism and hypothyroidism.[29]

However most patients now present after the age of 10–11 years (3rd phase) with peripubertal growth and pubertal disturbance with absence of growth spurt, arrested and absent puberty with growth retardation. This is usually due to iron load affecting H-P-G axis. GH-IGF axis may also be affected. Characteristically, patients frequently present with severe delay/absence of puberty with reduction of final height.

Chronic hypoxia is no longer a contributing factor nowadays in properly treated children. Linear growth in childhood is disrupted only in a small percentage of children due to anemia, ineffective erythropoiesis and iron overload. During the first

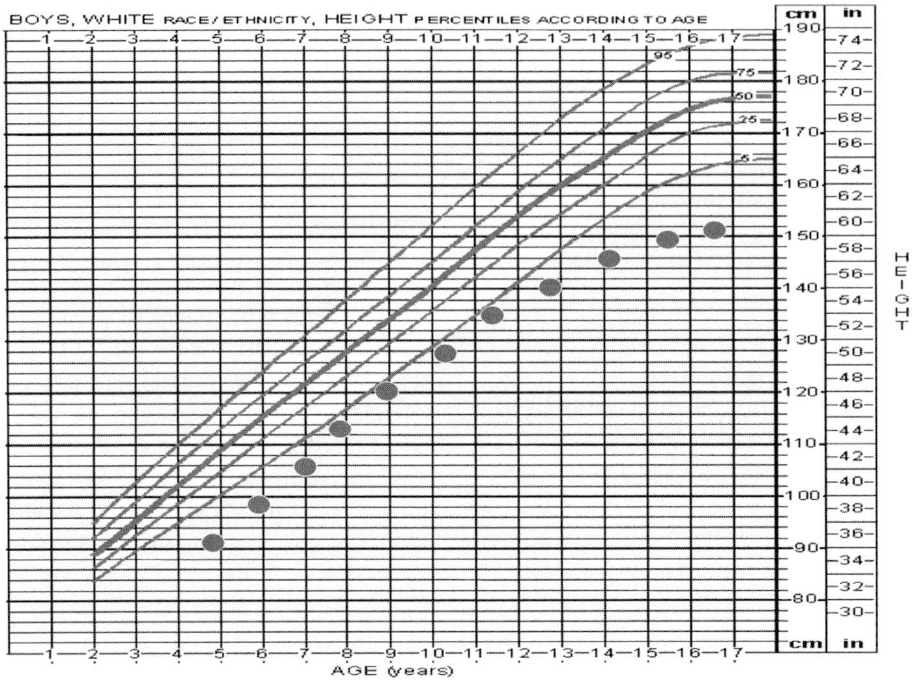

Figure 1. Growth chart of a thalassemia patient, from childhood to adolescence. Note the three phases, which have different causes. (A) First phase of childhood <5 years. This is mainly affected due to hypoxia, nutritional factors, and anemia affecting growth hormone–IGF axis. In the past this type of growth disturbance was common. (B) Second phase: 5–10 years. This is mainly affected due to anemia and iron load affecting growth hormone–IGF axis (C) Third phase: peripubertal years (10–12 years) where growth and pubertal spurt are both affected with disturbance in puberty. Here, the H-P-G axis is mainly affected due to iron load. This is the commonest type in the current years.

decade of life the maintenance of hemoglobin levels above 9 g/dL together with adequate iron chelation therapy makes the children with TM indistinguishable from their non-thalassemic peers.[28]

Zinc deficiency is probably a concomitant factor in growth failure phases 1 and 2. The effects of zinc supplementation on growth velocity were assessed in 22 patients with biochemical evidence of zinc deficiency. The mean height velocity of zinc supplemented children was significantly greater that of normal children.[28] The crucial role of zinc deficiency, however, was not confirmed by other studies.[28]

It is well known that high serum ferritin levels during the first decade of life are associated with final short stature,[20,30,31] indicating that appropriate iron chelation therapy can prevent or limit this complication. However, several studies showed high prevalence of short stature in TM children and adolescents treated intensively with desferrioxamine (DFO).[16,26] It may also contribute in phase 3.

Hypogonadotrophic hypogonadism

Gonadotrophin insufficiency or HH resulting from transfusional iron overload continues to be the commonest endocrinopathy[11,29,32] which affects 70–80% of thalassemic patients worldwide causing sexual infantilism, osteoporosis, and infertility.[32–34] Although it is seldom life threatening, HH phenotype causes severe impairment of quality of life. Early diagnosis and intervention is mandatory to offer best chances of attainment of peak bone mass, growth and puberty with restoration of fertility potential for a better quality of life.

The association of susceptibility to develop HH with the genotype has already been proven.[28] The contribution of the underlying molecular defect in TM to the development of endocrinopathies in TM and particularly HH is significant, because the patients with the more severe defects have a greater rate of iron loading through higher red cell consumption and probably a different vulnerability to free radical damage.[32,35] Hypogonatotrophic hypogonadism in

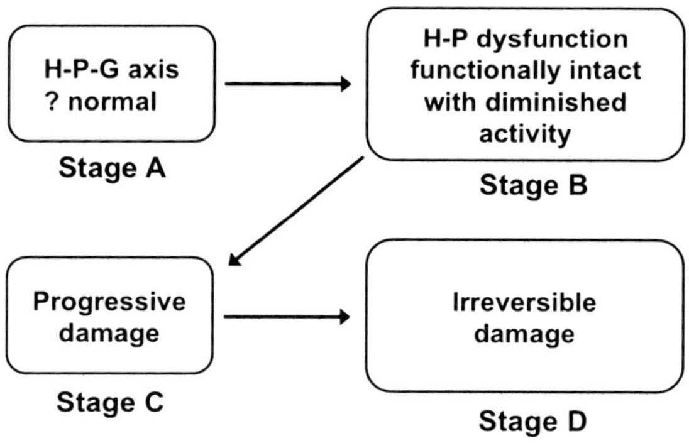

Figure 2. The hypothetical natural history of the H-P-G axis in patients with HH. Stage A: Normal H-P-G axis (patients are usually under 10 years) and have normal gondotrophin reserve and ultradian profile with normal spontaneous gonadotrophin (FSH, LH) pulses. Stage B: H-P axis is functionally intact with diminished gondotrophin reserve and ultradian profile showing sub normal spontaneous gonadotrophin (FSH, LH) pulses. Patients are usually 11–12 years or even younger. Stage C: H-P axis is still functionally intact but has significantly diminished gondotrophin reserve and ultradian profile shows markedly reduced spontaneous gonadotrophin activity. But the HH is reversible by GnRH infusion or sex steroid priming. MRI shows anterior pituitary volume to be normal or slightly reduced. Gonad is unaffected. Patients are usually 16 years or even younger. Stage D: H-P axis is irreversibly damaged with minimal or no gonadotrophin reserve and no gonadotrophin pulsatility (apulsatile HH). This stage is called irreversible HH where MRI shows structural loss to anterior pituitary volume. Gonad may be affected. Patients are usually 18 years or older.

thalassemia is related not only to iron toxicity on gonadotroph cells but also to iron toxicity on the adipose tissue thus changing the physiological role of leptin in sexual maturation and fertility. Leptin is a polypeptide hormone that is produced in fat cells due to the expression of the ob gene. In girls leptin levels increase dramatically as puberty develops and stimulate the H-P-G axis.[28] There is evidence that this hormone acts as a permissive signal allowing puberty to precede. The impaired synthesis of leptin in thalassemic patients seems to be related to transferrin receptor levels and therefore iron toxicity but further research will be required to elucidate this critical issue. Gonadal iron deposition occasionally occurs usually at a late stage when irreversible damage to H-P axis has occurred.[32] The iron deposition on the gonads is a rare condition. In the majority of patients gonadal function is normal as most women with amenorrhea are capable of ovulating with HMG-HCG treatment with successful outcome and similarly men with azoospermia become fathers.[34]

Role of hypogonadism and peak bone mass

The overall frequency of bone disease in hypogonadal patients with TM is increased compared with those of normal gonadal function.[29,33,35] Sex steroids regulate skeletal maturation and preservation in both men and women, therefore the impact of gonadal insufficiency on skeletal integrity has been widely recognized in both genders. BMD normally rises at a steady rate throughout childhood until around the age of 12, and then there is a sudden acceleration of bone mineral accretion that coincides with the onset of puberty and the pubertal growth spurt. Failure to progress normally through puberty is associated with failure of achievement of peak bone mass, which is a contributing factor to the ultimate bone disease in thalassemia.[27,33]

Natural history of HH (Fig. 2)

Although it is well established that transfusional haemosiderosis is the key cause of multiple endocrinopathies, (diabetes, hypothyroidism, hyperparathyroidism) the exact age of onset is unknown. Little is also known about the age of onset and natural history of HH.[36]

Clinical parameters are seldom helpful for understanding of natural history of HH as damage to anterior pituitary affects at an early age and biochemical manifestations may be manifest around 10–12 years. We have shown in a 10 year study that there are two functional subsets of HH: pulsatile (those with gonadotrophin pulses) and apulsatile (those without gonadotrophin pulses) (Fig. 3A and B). In that study we also showed that cycling pulsatile HH patients with thalassemia developed secondary amenorrhoea within 10 years and became apulsatile despite optimal transfusion and chelation therapy indicating progressive damage to H-P axis with development of irreversible HH.[37] In a cross-sectional study using magnetic resonance imaging (MRI) of anterior pituitary we correlated biochemical markers of HH and iron loading of the pituitary.[38]

Our data showed evidence of iron load of the pituitary with structural loss and reduction of anterior pituitary volume in HH thalassemia patients compared with age matched controls (Fig. 4). Interestingly, the apulsatile thalassemia patients had more loss to pituitary height and volume than the pulsatile ones.[38] Christoforidis[39] and Argyropolous[40]

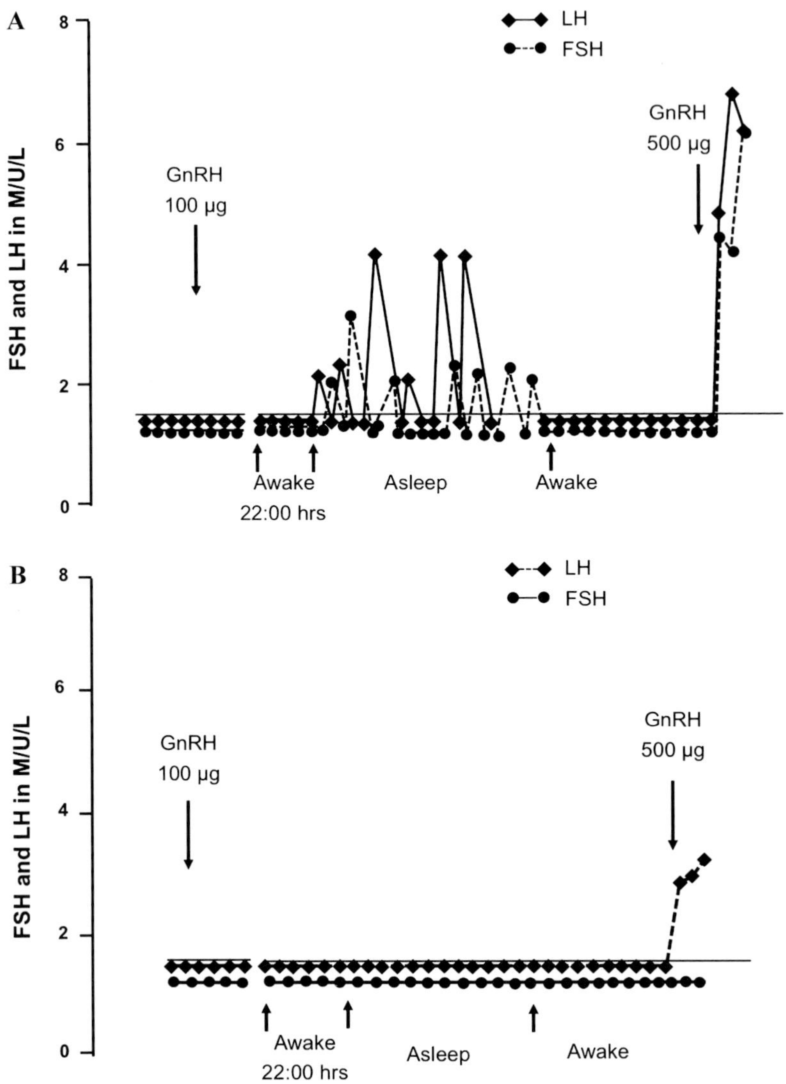

Figure 3. (**A**) The ultradian gonadotrophin profile of an 18-year-old female thalassemia patient with absence of sexual maturation (Tanner stage 1) with biochemical puberty. Note that she has nocturnal sleep entrained LH and FSH pulses (LH > FSH), which disappear when she wakes up. She fails to respond to a standard 100 μg GnRH bolus test, but shows good FSH and LH response to an augmented dose of 500 Ug GnRH IV bolus. This indicates functionally intact gonadotrophs (reversible HH). (**B**) Shows the ultradian gonadotrophin profile of an 18-year-old male thalassemia patient with absence of sexual maturation (Tanner stage 1) with biochemical puberty. Note that he has no nocturnal or LH and FSH pulses both during sleep and wakeful hours (apulsatile HH) (LH > FSH). He fails to respond to a standard 100 μg GnRH bolus test, and shows a very poor FSH and LH response to an augmented dose of 500 Ug GnRH IV bolus. This indicates functionally damaged gonadotrophs (irreversible HH).

have shown that iron is present in the pituitary in thalassemia patients with HH. They showed that T2 relaxation rate of the pituitary gland is a good marker of pituitary siderosis in thalassemic patients with pituitary damage.

It is unknown at what age iron is deposited first and at what stage iron induces H-P dysfunction. Also, presence of iron in an organ does not necessarily suggest that damage has occurred at that time. It is possible that there is a silent period of pituitary siderosis before HH occurs or that HH precedes MRI evidence of pituitary iron at a pre-pubertal age or even earlier if the damage is induced by free toxic iron.

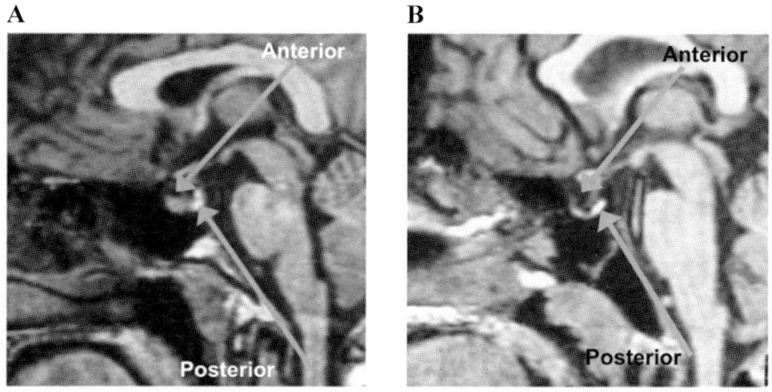

Figure 4. (A) MRI scan of the pituitary of a normal 16-year-old female subject in Tanner stage V. Note posterior pituitary (bright signal) and anterior pituitary are both normal. (B) Shows MRI scan of pituitary of a 16-year-old female thalassemia patient in Tanner stage 1 (absence of puberty). Note posterior pituitary (bright signal) is normal as the control subject. However, she shows volumetric loss to anterior pituitary. This patient is likely to be apulsatile and have irreversible HH.

The ability of MRI to detect and monitor the otherwise silent iron infiltration of cardiac tissue has truly revolutionized the management of transfusional iron overload. Furthermore, intensification of chelation therapy has been shown to reverse cardiac structure and function with removal of iron.[41] Pituitary may mimic cardiac tissue. Specifically, endocrine tissue and heart take up circulating labile iron species that are not bound to transferrin (so-called NTBI), while liver iron uptake is predominantly mediated via transferrin. Unlike heart little or no information is available on the effect of various chelators (desferrioxamine, deferiprone, or deferasirox) on kinetics and uptake of iron by pituitary.

Factors predicting progression of HH[28,32]

- Sex: M > F.
- Degree of serum and tissue iron overload.
- Genotype–phenotype interaction.
- Spontaneous puberty in β0/β0 phenotype.
- Severe clinical endocrinopathy.
- β0/β0 with α deletion, β0/β+, β+/β+ with normal α.

Hematological and related parameters as endocrine disrupters

It is now appreciated that alteration of natural history of hypopituitarism is due to transfusion and chelation as well as genotype. Of the endocrine disrupters described earlier, iron is the key contributor of H-P-G dysfunction with aberrant growth and pubertal phenotypes. However, DFO toxicity is also important. Hypoxia, nutrition, and anemia can also contribute to multiple endocrinopathies. But hypopituitarism, primary hypothyroidism, primary and secondary hyperthyroidism, and vitamin D aberrations must be included in the list of contributors of bone problems. Hypopituitarism can cause low peak bone mass and skeletal dysplasia may also contribute to altered height velocity and reduced target height.

Effect of endocrine disrupters on endocrine system and clinical phenotypes

The following endocrine axes are affected:

(a) H-P-G axis—Anterior pituitary dysfunction with HH and rarely primary hypogonadism.
(b) GH-IGF axis—Anterior pituitary dysfunction with GH deficiency, diminished reserve and GHNSD, and low IGF levels.
(a) + (b) may be affected as well (GH + Hypogonadotrophic hypogonadism + GH-IGF dysfunction).
(c) Leptin-GH-IGF axis may be intertwined with A and B.
(d) CNS- H-P-G axis (including opioids, kisspeptin, Ghrelin.
(e) Endocrine system of bone modulators.
(f) Thyroid- Primary hypothyroidism.
(g) Vitamin D-PTH axis with low vitamin D levels and secondary hyperparathyroidism and sometimes primary hypoparathyroidism.

Clinical phenotypes

(a) Sexual infantilism or pubertal disturbances (absence of puberty, arrested puberty, primary of secondary amenorrhoea, and absence of growth spurt)

(b) Pure growth disturbance – Short stature

(a) + (b) Aberrant growth + delayed/arrested puberty

(c) Other non-growth related effects:

- Bone—Low peak bone mass
- Osteopenia- osteoporosis syndrome ± fractures

Section B: Therapeutic intervention

GH-IGF1 axis: diagnosis of GH deficiency–clinical, biochemical, and other investigations and management

Clinical presentation. The commonest phenotype of growth retardation is stunted growth with reduced height velocity of <2 cm/year. In pubertal years pubertal spurt may be absent. However the latter is mainly due to absence of sex steroids (consequent on HH) rather than GH deficiency although GH and sex hormone deficiency are intertwined.[32,42,43]

GH deficiency can be picked up from growth deceleration (growth chart showing height below 3rd percentile <-2 SDS or -1SDS with retarded bone age (X ray of left hand and wrist) by 2 years behind the chronological age and abnormal GH secretion. Decrease in upper/lower segment ratio has been reported in patients who have been poorly chelated during childhood and adolescence, indicating that other contributing factors include chelation therapy or the disease itself, which can influence spinal growth.[27]

Biochemical diagnosis. GH secretary deficiency due to somatomammotrophic damage of anterior pituitary can be of the following four types:

(a) Pure GH deficiency.

(b) GH deficiency + IGF deficiency.[27]

(c) GH neurosecretory dysfunction where the dynamic reserve is normal but 24 h secretion is subnormal specially with diminished nocturnal secretion and abnormal GH pulses.[29,43] GH peak amplitude may be reduced as well as their nocturnal GH levels.[29,43,44] It is due to hypothalamic or hypothalamic–pituitary dysfunction regulation of GH.[43]

(d) GH deficiency + HH – Defective growth and pubertal development are strictly correlated; the complex interactions between sex steroids through H-P-G axis and GH- IGF axis. This pathway needs to be dissected to identify the exact type of functional hypopituitarism. All patients should have sex steroid priming[43] or GnRH priming prior to GH testing.[31,44]

Evaluation of GH-IGF-1 axis can give contradictory results. So the diagnosis of GH deficiency is difficult. The response to arginine, insulin hypoglycaemia, or GHRH may be normal (>10 ng/L);[44] or reduced with a variable prevalence of short stature.[43,44]

Therefore GH deficiency can be established from subnormal response to at least two dynamic tests (less than 10 ng/L to arginine 0.5 g/kg IV, insulin 0.1 U/kg, GHRH 1.0 ug/kg IV). De Sanctis and colleagues reported 3.1% of thalassemics to have GHRH-GH-IGF axis dysfunction[24] and others have quoted a higher incidence.[44] The presence of GH neurosecretory dysfunction is supported by the impaired 24 h GH secretion due to hypothalamic or pituitary dysfunction.[44]

IGF generation test. IGF generation test has also shown contradictory results with low or normal IGF levels.[44] Several authors have reported normal GH and GHBP levels but low levels of IGF-1 and IGFBP-3 which are not properly increased with IGF-1 generation test, suggesting that insensitivity to GH action may be the cause of abnormal growth.[28,29,44] However, a lack of correlation between IGF-1, IGFBP-3, and height SDS in TM children with growth failure may indicate that growth failure is not specifically related to GH-IGF-1 axis but suggest complete or partial GH resistance.[29] There is also a possibility that DFO and iron loading at the growth plate have a deleterious effect in local IGF-1 production and growth regulation.[43,44]

MRI of pituitary

It is still an experimental/research tool. It may show the following in hypopituitarism:

- Completely empty sella.
- Marked diminution of the anterior pituitary size.
- Thinning of the pituitary stalk with its posterior displacement.
- Evidence of iron deposition in the pituitary gland and midbrain.

- MRI of pituitary can show iron and empty sella in patients with retarded growth.[29] It is shown that even a modest amount of iron deposition within the anterior pituitary can interfere with its function.[29]

Body disproportion between the upper (short) and lower body segment (normal) is observed in approximately 15–40% of TM patients.[27] Spinal growth impairment starts during infancy and deteriorates progressively. Most thalassemics, especially males, do not reach their target height and their sitting height is more severely affected. During puberty hypogonadism aggravates impairment of spinal height and growth. Sex hormones play an important role in the pubertal growth spurt and TM patients with delayed puberty do not exhibit a normal growth spurt; their GH peak amplitude is reduced as well as their nocturnal GH levels.[29,31,43]

Biochemical assessment of H-P-axis is indicated in this group. Basal gonadotrophins are very low. Additionally patients show poor FSH and LH response to GnRH stimulation indicative of HH Women may have primary or secondary amenorrhea and additional endocrinopathies indicating the severity of haemosiderosis. Anterior pituitary function may correlate well with tissue iron deposition in the pituitary gland, as quantitatively determined by MRI measurements (T2*)[38,40] and gonadotrophin pulsatility.[32,38] However, there is no correlation among MRI measurements, the GnRH stimulation test, and the clinical status of the patients.[28,29,38]

Investigations for growth disturbance for thalassemic children under 10 years

1. Current height (both standing and sitting in cm) must be plotted on the growth chart. Target height is based on mid-parental heights. Comparison with previous measurements is done to estimate the growth velocity. Growth and pubertal status (Tanner staging) are noted by the same observer.[32] Bode mass index is calculated (kg/m^2). Physical disproportion (truncal obesity) and waist: hip ratios are also calculated. Nutritional, emotional, and social statuses are also reviewed.
2. Bone maturation is assessed by X ray of left hand and wrist.[32]
3. Routine blood tests include liver function tests, serum ferritin + other markers of iron load (cardiac and hepatic MRI 2*, biochemical profile, and zinc).
4. Urine analysis.
5. Thyroid function test (Free T4, TSH). Vitamin D, PTH must be measured as well.
6. IGF-1 generation test is done in patients with low levels of IGF-1 and IFGBP-3 and normal GH secretion to exclude GH resistance.
7. Stimulation tests to assess GH secretion, where at least two tests are required.

Priming with sex steroids (testosterone depot 100 mg IM in boys and ethinyl estradiol 10 mcg orally for 3 days in girls 72 h before GH testing may be necessary in children who are prepubertal and have a bone age of 10 years. This can differentiate hypogonadotrophic hypogonadism from GH deficiency.[43] GnRH priming may be used as well to differentiate GH deficiency from hypogonadotrophic hypogonadism.[29]

Growth hormone therapy

Indications. Proven GH insufficiency or GH neuro secretary dysfunction with clinical evidence of deceleration of growth velocity (ht SDS <1–2). However patients should be counselled that response might be sub optimal when therapy has to be discontinued after one year. Goal of therapy: to improve growth velocity and attain target height in patients with retarded growth.

Dose and duration of therapy. Treatment with recombinant GH (rhGH) is recommended when GH deficiency is established. Therapeutic response with rhGH administration in cases with GH deficiency, is often non satisfactory. Often supra physiological doses of GH are required to obtain therapeutic response due to partial GH insensitivity.[29]

In poor responders such treatment should be discontinued. Treatment with rhGH for one year seems to be effective in increasing growth velocity, IGF levels without causing adverse effects on bone maturation, glucose tolerance, serum lipids, and blood pressure.[28,44] The encouraging results described during the first year of rhGH treatment do not persist during the second and the third years. This is because increase in bone age with continued treatment is equal to or slightly greater than the height age increase.[44] Prolonged therapy with rhGH might not improve final height; on the contrary a negative effect may be hypothesized.[44]

Growth acceleration is mostly promoted with sex steroids in children with pubertal delay as sexual complications present a significant issue in thalassemics. All patients should be monitored carefully for diabetogenic response (GTT) of GH therapy, especially those with severe iron load.

H-P-G axis and diagnosis and management of disturbances of puberty + growth velocity

Clinical phenotypes of HH. Pubertal complications in TM present the commonest endocrine complication in almost all studies.[29,32,36,44,45] These include:

- Failure in initiation of puberty: Absence of gonadarche in males by 14 years and thelarche in females by 13 years.
- Arrested puberty and hypogonadism. Arrested puberty is defined as the absence of further pubertal progression—once puberty has started—for more than 1 year, where testicular volume in boys never progressed beyond 6–8 mL and breast size in girls remained unchanged.
- Primary amenorrhoea—Failure in menarche by 18 years.
- Secondary amenorrhoea—Absence of periods for >12 months after menarche.

Delayed puberty or failure in initiation of puberty in TM is almost always due to HH, which still remains the most common complication of haemosiderosis.[53] Iron deposition on gonadotrophic cells of the pituitary leads to disruption of gonadotrophin production.

Protocol for investigation of peri pubertal disorder with/without growth disturbance

Clinical

Anthropometry. Assessment of growth: height (sitting and standing), weight, BMI, hip: waist ratio, height velocity, PHV centile chart. Serial monitoring of growth (3–4 monthly) as early as 10 years and puberty (6 monthly) from 12 years must be done. Sitting and standing height (3 monthly) throughout childhood and adolescence is also undertaken, especially those on DFO.

Puberty.

- Clinical signs of puberty: Tanner staging.
- Breast development in girls: thelarche.
- Testicular enlargement in boys: gonadarche.
- Pubic hair: adrenarche (DHEAS) strictly is not a sign of puberty, must be checked as well.

Biochemical: assessment of H-P-G axis includes the following

- Basal FSH, LH, sex steroids, TFT.
- Dynamic testing of the H-P-G axis- GnRH test.
- Spontaneous assessment of H-P axis- Ultradian gonadotropin profile.
- MRI: pituitary (only in selected cases as it is still a research tool).
- GH-IGF axis—see before.
- Dissect gonadotroph from somatotroph damage by sex steroid priming.
- Straight X-ray of spine to exclude micro fracture.
- GnRH test to evaluate the gonadotrophin reserve.
- Gonadal stimulation test to check gonadal reserve – HCG in boys and HMG in girls.[37,38]
- Bone age is helpful for the treatment decision options.

Criteria for intervention for induction/ acceleration of puberty

1. Failure in initiation of puberty or arrest of puberty.
2. CA- Bone age $\geq$ 2 years.
3. Epiphysis–not closed (if growth increment is desired).

Therapeutic approach

Physiological puberty. If H-P-G axis is functionally intact with normal LH and FSH and sex steroid response to GnRH + normal or subnormal LH and FSH pulses (ultradian gonadotrophin profile) options are sex steroid priming, or pulsatile GnRH infusion can be used to induce physiological puberty.[32] Although GnRH infusion is safest with no thrombogenic, hepatic or other metabolic effects, it is often difficult to advocate as H-P axis is irreversibly damaged in many patients. However, we have shown 80% success rate with this therapy if advocated at an early stage of HH.[46] If H-P axis is irreversibly damaged pseudo puberty with sex steroids or gonadotrophins can be given.[32] If there is combined damage to H-P-G axis,[38] sex steroid replacement therapy is the only option to induce pseudo puberty.

Aims of treatment

In delayed puberty the aim is to mimic biological and biochemical pubertal events with promotion of sexual maturation and linear growth as well.[24,29,32]

Induction of physiological puberty in boys for 6 months with sex steroid priming

In boys this can be achieved with testosterone depot IM 25–50 mg monthly for 6 months following reassessment. Pubic hair will appear and penile size will increase. Increase in testicular volume indicates activation of the H-P-G axis and release of gonadotrophins (FSH and LH), where no further treatment is needed except for close observation. GnRH testing and ultradian profile may confirm maturation of H-P-G axis.

Pseudo puberty

In cases where testicular size is unchanged, treatment is continued for 6 months and subsequently the dose is increased to 100 mg monthly for 1 year. The dose may be increased to 250 mg im after Tanner 3–4.

Therapeutic schedule is determined by the growth potential, clinical response and emotional factors. For testicular enlargement, the therapeutic regime is altered to the combination of HCG and HMG or rec FSH, both of which mimic the pituitary gonadotrophins. The final adult dose of testosterone depot is always individualized and usually 50 mg/weekly IM or alternatively trans dermally in patches 5 mg/daily. The oral route (testosterone undeconate) is best avoided in severe iron load to obviate first pass effect.

Induction of physiological puberty in girls

Oral ethinyl oestradiol is preferred at the dose 100 ng/kg/day for 6 months, where increase in breast size and growth acceleration is noted. Maturation of H-P G axis is also assessed from spontaneous and dynamic tests (increased gonadotrophin pulse frequency/amplitude (ultradian gonadotrophin profile) and augmented FSH and LH response to IV bolus GnRH test).

Pseudo puberty

Oral ethinyl oestradiol dose is continued for additional 6 months and is increased to 200 ng/kg/day for the subsequent year. Therapeutic schedule is determined by the same factors as in boys. The adult dose is 400 ng/kg/day, where the uterine size is satisfactorily increased for the induction of menarche. Induction of puberty can be successfully achieved by the transdermal use of estrogens too.

Menarche is achieved by the addition of Medroxyprogesterone 10 mg/day for 10 days (or nor ethisterone 10 mg for 10 days) when the size of the uterus exceeds 5 cm. When menstrual bleeding occurs spontaneously during estrogen treatment, the regime should be adjusted. For maintenance of the menstrual cycle the use of estrogens (conjugated oestrogens 0.625–1.25 mg, ethinyl oestradiol 20 μg) from day 1st to 25th and Progesterone from day 14 to 25 is required. The transdermal use of oestradiol with norethisterone is advantageous in iron-loaded subjects due to decreased liver toxicity and is preferred in most cases as it obviates first pass effect. Ovarian and testicular reserves are usually preserved in HH patients, as they are still able to increase estradiol or testosterone levels following gonadotrophin stimulation test to produce ova or sperms in females and males, respectively.[34,47]

Women with TM who are regularly transfused and are well chelated can have successful pregnancies by gonadotrophins.[34] Males who have normal gonadal function maintain their spermatogenic ability and therefore, frequently become fathers of children with gonadotrophin support.[34]

Other hormone treatment

Other hormonal deficiencies (thyroid, parathyroid, and vitamin D) must be treated with adequate dose of hormone replacement therapy.[24,45]

Other management issues include haematological (transfusion and chelation)

Nutrition-diet, exercise and lifestyle issues and psychological support must be provided adequately.

Special situations

Bone marrow transplantation (BMT) recipients

BMT is a well-recognized recent advancement in thalassemics to offer best chances of disease free survival. To date several thousand bone marrow transplants are done in thalassemics with excellent results.

Patients after successful BMT will be free from further blood transfusion and thus spared from complications of iron overload. DFO may be required after BMT to remove excessive body iron, but long-term use is seldom necessary.[48] On the other hand, the preparative conditioning before BMT and complications of BMT such as graft versus host disease (GvHD) may be life threatening and cause endocrine dysfunction following BMT in children.[48,49]

Data on growth and sexual development in ex thalassemics are now available. Most conditioning regimes used for BMT are strong alkylating gonadotoxic drugs, which are likely to have an effect on puberty and future fertility especially on ovaries with finite supply of oocytes. Busulfan and cyclophosphamide combination are commonly used in children as preparative regimen for both malignant and nonmalignant diseases.

Several series have shown evidence of growth and pubertal aberrations although data are not conclusive.[27] Li and colleagues observed catch-up growth commonly after BMT. However, growth after BMT is also affected by the pre transplant factors.[50] In TM patients, the age at time of transplant has been reported to be an important predictor of growth after BMT who received BMT after 7 years of age were reported to have further worsening of growth delay after BMT.[50] They also failed to achieve their full genetic potential. Some patients were found to have GH deficiency and required GH replacement. Patients transplanted before age of 8 years showed either improvement of growth rate or constant growth rate after BMT. In another study the subjects who received BMT after 7 years of age, failed to achieve their full genetic potential.[51] In conclusion, short stature is present in a significant percentage of transplanted thalassemic children. The studies indicated a close effect of the age at time of transplant on subsequent growth rate, but the growth impairment in these subjects remained multifactorial.

Some studies demonstrated that improvement of growth and bone mineral density after BMT was common.[50] This was probably related to discontinuation of further administration of DFO after BMT. However, cyclophosphamide + busulphan-induced ovarian failure was universal in girls, and some investigators show that boys were spared from gonadal failure if transplant was per formed early.

As iron can induce HH at an early stage and busulphan and cyclophosphamide can compromise future fertility potential, it is important to counsel the thalassemia patients for and against conventional vs. BMT during decision making. Apart from the immediate risks of mortality of BMT, the long-term morbidity of sub fertility is important. This is especially important as the modern oral chelators are improving survival of patients significantly and patients can be expected to live normally up to the 5th decade or even more.

Future advances

This includes the understanding of the pathophysiology of hypogonadotrophic hypogonadism and prevention of irreversible damage with gonadotrophin apulsatility. Use of biochemical and biophysical markers including pituitary MRI may be a way forward for diagnosis and prognostication of HH. The ability of MRI to detect and monitor the otherwise silent iron infiltration of cardiac tissue has truly revolutionized the management of transfusional iron overload. Furthermore, intensification of chelation therapy has been shown to reverse cardiac structure and function with removal of iron. Pituitary may mimic cardiac tissue. Specifically, endocrine tissue and heart take up circulating labile iron species that are not bound to transferrin (so-called NTBI), while liver iron uptake is predominantly mediated via transferrin. Early intervention can reverse HH and induce puberty in thalassemia patients and reduce serum as well as tissue iron load.

Conclusion

In conclusion, despite significant advances in chelation and transfusion therapy growth retardation with pubertal aberrations continues to be a significant challenge in thalassemics due mainly to HH with its consequences on growth and puberty. Although not life threatening improved longevity of thalassemics has brought new challenges of expectation for normal sexual maturation with expected height and a family. Some thalassemics attain optimal growth sexual maturation and can have children without assistance, but many have stunted growth, sexual infantilism, and osteoporosis and are sub fertile due mainly to H-P –G $\pm$ GH – IGF dysfunction, with poor quality of life.

Hypopituitarism is mainly due to iron load and occurs at a very early stage although aggressive and early use of chelators can also induce pituitary damage. The exact cause and its natural history of hypopituitarism are unclear. Early diagnosis and prompt treatment with sex steroid priming for physiological induction of puberty (in reversible HH) or replacement therapy with sex steroids for induction of pseudo puberty is recommended in irreversible hypogonadotrophism. Timely hormonal intervention of patients is mandatory for best chances of attaining optimal growth, sexual maturation with peak bone mass and better reproductive outcome. Supra physiological doses of GH therapy is only required for selected cases with proven GH insufficiency from two dynamic ± low nocturnal pulses. Optimal monitoring of iron load and chelation therapy coupled with the correction of other hormonal deficiency, especially thyroid and vitamin D-PTH axis and nutrients, is mandatory for the best outcome.

Conflicts of interest

The authors declare no conflicts of interest.

References

1. Fawdry, A.L. 1944. Erythroblastic anaemia of childhood (Cooley's anaemia) in Cyprus. *Lancet* **1:** 171–176.
2. Jacsch, R. 1890. Uber Diagnose und Therapie der Erkrankungen des Blutes. *Prager Med. Wochenschr.* **15:** 403–414.
3. Weatherall, D.J. 2001. The thalassemias. In *Williams Hematology*. B. Beutler, M.A. Lichtman, B.S. Coller, T.J. Kipps & S. Seligsohn, Eds.: 562–564, 6th edn. McGraw-Hill. New York.
4. Cooley, T.B. & P. Lee. 1927. A series of cases of splenomegaly in children and peculiar changes in bones; report of cases. *Am. J. Dis. Child.* **34:** 347–363.
5. Whipple, G.H. & W.L. Bradford. 1936. Mediterranean disease— "thalassemia" (erythroblastic anaemia of Cooley); associated pigment abnormalities simulating hemochromatosis. *J. Pediatr.* **9:** 279–311.
6. Modell, B. 1976. Management of thalassaemia major. *Br. Med. Bull.* **32:** 270–276.
7. Angastiniotis, M., S. Kyriakidou & M. Hadjiminas. 1986. How thalassemia was controlled in Cyprus. *World Health Forum* **7:** 291–297.
8. Ortner, D.J. 2003. *Identification of Pathological Conditions in Human Skeletal Remains. Second Edition.* Amsterdam: Academic Press.
9. Nathan, D.G. & R.B. Gunn. 1966. Thalassaemia: the consequences of unbalanced hemoglobin synthesis. *Am. J. Med.* **41:** 815–830.
10. Weatherall, D.J., J.B. Clegg, & M.A. Naughton. 1965. Globin synthesis in thalassaemia: an in vitro study. *Nature* **208:** 1061–1065.
11. Simona, F., A. Albu, F. Vladareanu, *et al.* 2005. Endocrine disorders in thalassaemia. *Acta Endocrinol. (Buc)* **1:** 201–212.
12. Economidou, J. 1982. Problems related to treatment of beta-thalassaemia major. *Paediatrician* **11:** 157–162.
13. Wolman, I.J. 1964. High transfusion treatment of a case of Thalassaemia major. *Ann. N.Y. Acad. Sci.* **119:** 736–747.
14. McIntosh, N. 1976. Endocrinopathy in thalassaemia major. *Arch. Dis. Child.* **51:** 195–201.
15. Letsky, E.A., F. Miller, M. Worwood & D.M. Flynn. 1974. Serum ferritin in children with thalassaemia regularly transfused. *J. Clin. Pathol.* **27:** 652–655.
16. De Virgiliis, S., M. Congia, F. Frau, *et al.* 1988. Deferoxamine-induced growth retardation in patients with thalassemia major. *J. Pediatr.* **113:** 661–669.
17. Bannerman, R.M. 1967. Thalassemia intermedia, with iron overload, cardiac failure, diabetes mellitus, hypopituitarism and porphyrinuria. *Am. J. Med.* **42:** 476–486.
18. Kuo, B., E. Zaino & M.S. Roginsky. 1968. Endocrine function in thalassemia major. *J. Clin. Endocrinol. Metabol.* **28:** 805–808.
19. Canale, V.C., P. Steinherz, M. New & M. Erlandson. 1974. Endocrine function in thalassemia major. *Ann. N.Y. Acad. Sci.* **232:** 333–345.
20. Borgna-Pignatti, C., P. De Stefano, L. Zonta, *et al.* 1985. Growth and sexual maturation in thalassemia major. *J. Pediatr.* **106:** 150–155.
21. Fargion, S., M.T. Taddei, V. Gabutti, *et al.* 1982. Early iron overload in beta-thalassaemia major: when to start chelation therapy? *Arch. Dis. Child.* **57:** 929–933.
22. Lassman, M.N., M. Genel, J.K. Wise, *et al.* 1974. Carbohydrate homeostasis and pancreatic islet cell function in thalassemia. *Ann. Intern. Med.* **80:** 65–69.
23. Costin, G., M.D. Kogut, C.G. Hyman, *et al.* 1979. Endocrine abnormalities in thalassemia major. *Am. J. Dis. Child.* **133:** 497–502.
24. De Sanctis, V. 2002. Growth and puberty and its management in thalassaemia. *Horm. Res.* **58:** 72–79.
25. Caruso-Nicoletti, M., V. De Sanctis, M. Capra, *et al.* 1998. Short stature and body proportion in thalassaemia. *J. Pediatr. Endocrinol. Metabol.* **11:** 811–816.
26. Olivieri, N.F., G. Koren, J. Harris, *et al.* 1992. Growth failure and bony changes induced by deferoxamine. *Am. J. Pediatr. Hematol. Oncol.* **14:** 48–56.
27. De Sanctis, V., M. Roos, T. Gasser, *et al.* 2006. Italian Working Group on Endocrine Complications in Non-Endocrine Diseases. Impact of long-term iron chelation therapy on growth and endocrine functions in Thalassaemia. *J. Pediatr. Endocrinol. Metabol.* **19:** 471–480.
28. Kyriakou, A. & N. Skordis. 2009. Thalassaemia and aberrations of growth and puberty. *Rev.: Mediterr. J. Haematol. Infect. Dis.* **1:** 1–14.
29. Soliman, A.T., M.M. El Zalabany, M. Amer & B.M. Ansari. 2009. Growth and pubertal development in transfusion-dependent children and adolescents with thalassaemia major. *Hemoglobin* **33:** 16–20.
30. Shalitin, S., D. Carmi, N. Weintrob, *et al.* 2005. Serum ferritin level as a predictor of impaired growth and puberty in thalassemia major patients. *Eur. J. Haematol.* **74:** 93–100.
31. Roth, C., A. Pekrun, M. Bartz, *et al.* 1997. Short stature and failure of pubertal development in thalassaemia major: evidence for hypothalamic neurosecretory dysfunction of growth hormone secretion and defective pituitary gonadotropin secretion. *Eur. J. Pediatr.* **156:** 777–783.
32. Chatterjee, R. & M. Katz. 2000. Reversible hypogonadotrophic hypogonadism in sexually infantile male thalassaemic patients with transfusional iron overload. *Clin. Endocrinol. (Oxf.)* **53:** 33–42.

33. Chatterjee, R. & R. Bajoria. 2009. Osteopenia-osteoporosis syndrome in patients with thalassemia: understanding of type of bone disease and response to treatment. *Hemoglobin* **33:** 36–38.
34. Bajoria, R. & R. Chatterjee. 2009. Current perspectives of fertility and pregnancy in thalassemia. *Hemoglobin* **33:** 131–135.
35. Shander, A., M.D. Cappellini & L.T. Goodnough. 2009. Iron overload and toxicity: the hidden risk of multiple blood transfusions. Review. *Vox Sang.* **97:** 185–197.
36. Soliman, A.T. *et al.* 1999. Growth and pubertal development in transfusion-dependent children and adolescents with thalassaemia major and sickle cell disease: a comparative study. *J. Trop. Pediatr.* **45:** 23–30.
37. Chatterjee, R., M. Katz, T.F. Cox & J.B. Porter. 1993. Prospective study of the hypothalamic-pituitary axis in thalassaemic patients who developed secondary amenorrhoea. *Clin. Endocrinol. (Oxf.)* **39:** 287–296.
38. Chatterjee, R., M. Katz, A. Oatridge, *et al.* 1998. Selective loss of anterior pituitary volume with severe pituitary-gonadal insufficiency in poorly compliant male thalassemic patients with pubertal arrest. *Ann. N.Y. Acad. Sci.* **850:** 479–482.
39. Christoforidis, A. *et al.* 2007. MRI for the determination of pituitary iron overload in children and young adults with beta-thalassaemia major. *Eur. J. Radiol.* **62:** 138–142.
40. Argyropoulou, M.I. *et al.* 2001. Pituitary gland height evaluated by MR in patients with beta-thalassemia major: a marker of pituitary gland function. *Neuroradiology* **43:** 1056–1058.
41. Pennell, D.J. 2008. T2* magnetic resonance: iron and gold. *JACC Cardiovasc. Imaging* **1:** 579–581.
42. Chatterjee, R. & M. Katz. 2001. Evaluation of gonadotrophin insufficiency in thalassemic boys with pubertal failure: spontaneous versus provocative test. *J. Pediatr. Endocrinol. Metabol.* **14:** 301–312.
43. Chatterjee, R., M. Katz, T. Cox & H. Bantock. 1993. Evaluation of growth hormone in thalassaemic boys with failed puberty: spontaneous versus provocative test. *Eur. J. Pediatr.* **152:** 721–726.
44. Soliman, A.T. *et al.* 1999. Growth and pubertal development in transfusion-dependent children and adolescents with thalassaemia major and sickle cell disease: a comparative study. *J. Trop. Pediatr.* **45:** 23–30.
45. Vogiatzi, M.G., E.A. Macklin, F.L. Trachtenberg, *et al.* 2009. Differences in the prevalence of growth, endocrine and vitamin D abnormalities among the various thalassaemia syndromes in North America. Thalassemia Clinical Research Network. *Br. J. Haematol.* **146:** 546–556.
46. Chatterjee, R., M. Katz, B. Wonke & A.V. Hoffbrand. 1987. Induction of puberty in patients with beta-thalassemia major. *Birth Defects Orig. Artic. Ser.* **23:** 5A–D.
47. Perera, D., A. Pizzey, A. Campbell, *et al.* 2002. Sperm DNA damage in potentially fertile homozygous beta-thalassaemia patients with iron overload. *Hum. Reprod.* **17:** 1820–1825.
48. Bhatia, M. & M.C. Walters. 2008. Hematopoietic cell transplantation for thalassemia and sickle cell disease: past, present and future. Review. *Bone Marrow Transplant.* **41:** 109–117.
49. Gaziev, J., M. Galimberti, C. Giardini, *et al.* 1993. Growth in children after bone marrow transplantation for thalassemia. *Bone Marrow Transplant.* **12:** 100–101.
50. Li, C.K., K.W. Chik, G.W. Wong, *et al.* 2004. Growth and endocrine function following bone marrow transplantation for thalassemia major. *Pediatr. Hematol. Oncol.* **21:** 411–419.
51. De Simone, M., A. Verotti, L. Lughetti, *et al.* 2001. Final height of thalassaemic patients who underwent bone marrow transplantation during childhood. *Bone Marrow Transplant.* **28:** 201–205.

Ann. N.Y. Acad. Sci. ISSN 0077-8923

ANNALS OF THE NEW YORK ACADEMY OF SCIENCES
Issue: *Cooley's Anemia: Ninth Symposium*

Magnetic resonance assessment of iron overload by separate measurement of tissue ferritin and hemosiderin iron

Ed X. Wu,[1,*] Daniel Kim,[2,*] Christina L. Tosti,[3] Haiying Tang,[4] Jens H. Jensen,[2] Jerry S. Cheung,[1] Li Feng,[5] Wing-Yan Au,[6] Shau-Yin Ha,[7] Sujit S. Sheth,[8] Truman R. Brown,[9] and Gary M. Brittenham[8]

[1]Department of Electrical and Electronic Engineering, University of Hong Kong, Pokfulam, Hong Kong, China. [2]Department of Radiology, New York University, New York. [3]Department of Radiology, Ohio State University Medical Center, Columbus, Ohio. [4]Center for Neuroscience and Regenerative Medicine, Uniformed Services University of the Health Sciences, Henry M. Jackson Foundation, Bethesda, Maryland. [5]Sackler Institute of Graduate Biomedical Sciences, New York University School of Medicine, New York. [6]Department of Medicine, University of Hong Kong, Pokfulam, Hong Kong, China. [7]Department of Pediatrics, University of Hong Kong, Pokfulam, Hong Kong, China. [8]Department of Pediatrics, Columbia University, New York. [9]Departments of Radiology and Biomedical Engineering, Columbia University, New York

Address for correspondence: Gary M. Brittenham, M.D., Department of Pediatrics, Columbia University College of Physicians and Surgeons, CHONY, Room CHN 10-08, 3959 Broadway, New York, NY 10032. gmb31@columbia.edu

With transfusional iron overload, almost all the excess iron is sequestered intracellularly as rapidly mobilizable, dispersed, soluble ferritin iron, and as aggregated, insoluble hemosiderin iron for long-term storage. Established magnetic resonance imaging (MRI) indicators of tissue iron (R_2, R_2*) are principally influenced by hemosiderin iron and change slowly, even with intensive iron chelation. Intracellular ferritin iron is evidently in equilibrium with the low-molecular-weight cytosolic iron pool that can change rapidly with iron chelation. We have developed a new MRI method to separately measure ferritin and hemosiderin iron, based on the non-monoexponential signal decay induced by aggregated iron in multiple-spin-echo sequences. We have initially validated the method in agarose phantoms and in human liver explants and shown the feasibility of its application in patients with thalassemia major. Measurement of tissue ferritin iron is a promising new means to rapidly evaluate the effectiveness of iron-chelating regimens.

Keywords: iron; ferritin; hemosiderin; thalassemia; magnetic susceptibility; magnetic resonance

Introduction

The application of magnetic resonance imaging (MRI) to the study of transfusional iron overload has focused primarily on techniques to determine the total storage (non-heme) iron concentration in tissues and organs.[1–3] We describe here the development of methods to measure separately the two principal types of storage iron, the short-term storage form in ferritin and the long-term deposits in hemosiderin, by using their distinctive effects on MRI signal decay. The unique physiological roles of intracellular ferritin iron[4–6] suggest that measurements of this pool within tissues could provide early warning of iron-induced toxicity, permit rapid monitoring of the effectiveness of iron-chelating regimens, and together with measurements of hemosiderin iron, improve the accuracy of estimates of total storage iron.

Storage forms of iron–ferritin and hemosiderin

Normally, iron entry into cells is meticulously regulated by controlling uptake of the iron-transport protein transferrin from the plasma via the

*E. X. Wu and D. Kim contributed equally to this work.

doi: 10.1111/j.1749-6632.2010.05587.x

transferrin receptor on the cell membrane surface.[7] In patients with thalassemia major and transfusional iron overload, plasma transferrin may become fully saturated with iron and non-transferrin-bound iron (NTBI) may then appear in plasma. This plasma NTBI can bypass physiological controls and enter vulnerable cells (especially hepatocytes, cardiac myocytes, pancreatic beta-cells, and anterior pituitary cells) by routes that are still poorly understood.[7] Within the cytoplasm of cells, metabolically active iron is present physiologically in low-molecular-weight forms[8] destined for incorporation into functional compounds or, if present in amounts exceeding cellular requirements, for storage. A cytosolic iron chaperone, poly (rC)-binding protein 1 (PCBP1), delivers excess iron to ferritin,[9] whose structure maintains large amounts of iron in solution in a compact yet bioavailable form,[4] diffusely distributed within the cytosol.[10] Iron-free ferritin (apoferritin; Mr 440,000) consists of 24 protein subunits arranged in a spherical shell which can house up to 4,000 atoms in an iron core composed of the hydrous ferric oxide mineral *ferrihydrite* with the approximate formula $5Fe_2O_3{\cdot}9H_20$.[4,11] Recent studies have provided compelling evidence that iron entry and exit from ferritin are the result of an equilibrium based on the concentration of cytosolic iron.[5] Both iron incorporation and release seem to be intrinsic, autonomous properties of the ferritin molecule.[5]

With low levels of cytosolic iron, soluble iron-containing ferritin is present in the cytosol as randomly dispersed ferritin particles.[12,13] As cytosolic iron increases, the concentrations of dispersed ferritin increase and small clusters of ferritin particles appear, still soluble and spread throughout the cytosol. With further increases in cytosolic iron, ferritin is collected in lysosomes by fusion of ferritin clusters with lysosomal membranes, by autophagocytosis, or both.[6,12,13] Digestion of ferritin within secondary lysosomes (siderosomes) leads to denaturation of ferritin protein subunits[14] and to aggregation of the ferritin iron cores, processes thought to result in the formation of amorphous, insoluble masses of hemosiderin.[12,13] Under pathological conditions in which the capacity of ferritin to store iron is overwhelmed, ferritin iron may have a pro-oxidant role and contribute to tissue damage.[4] Production of hemosiderin, enclosed within siderosome membranes, seems to sequester the excess iron away from the cytosol and to help protect against iron toxicity. As the total amount of tissue iron increases, the proportion stored as hemosiderin rises, from trace amounts in normal individuals to 90% or more in patients with severe iron overload.[15] Depending upon cellular type, iron supply and use, the half-life of cellular ferritin may range from ~20 to 96 h.[16] Hemosiderin characteristically has a much slower cellular turnover than ferritin.[17] Overall, the available evidence suggests that cytosolic iron is in rapid equilibrium with soluble, dispersed ferritin for short-term storage while exchange with the long-term aggregates of iron within hemosiderin is slow and limited.

The results of recent investigations into the intracellular mechanism of action of iron chelators suggest that measurement of cellular ferritin iron may provide a sensitive means for early assessment of chelator effectiveness. The three iron-chelating agents in clinical use, deferasirox, deferiprone, and deferoxamine, all decrease the intracellular concentration of ferritin iron, although by distinct mechanisms. The membrane-permeable iron chelators, deferasirox, and deferiprone, were found to cause release of iron from ferritin, followed by monoubiquitination of the iron-poor ferritin and its degradation in the proteasome, decreasing the concentration of ferritin iron.[6] By contrast, the poorly membrane-permeable iron chelator deferoxamine, a siderophore produced by *Streptomyces pilosus*, was localized within lysosomes, inducing autophagy and then degradation of ferritin within the lysosome, also decreasing the concentration of ferritin iron.[6] Consequently, measurements of cellular ferritin iron provide a potential means of rapidly monitoring the effectiveness of iron chelators.

Effect of ferritin and hemosiderin iron on MRI signal decay

The differences in solubility and intracellular distribution between ferritin iron (soluble, dispersed, and relatively uniformly distributed) and hemosiderin iron (insoluble and aggregated in irregular micron-sized clusters separated by distances of 10–30 μm[18,19]) produce different effects on MRI signal decay. Ferritin iron affects MRI signal decay principally through molecular spin–spin relaxation mechanisms,[20,21] while hemosiderin aggregates primarily produce magnetic field inhomogeneities that cause spin dephasing.[22,23] MRI methods now in use for estimation of tissue iron levels are intended to measure the *total* storage (ferritin + hemosiderin) iron by determining signal intensity ratios or relaxation rates, such as R_2 ($=1/T_2$) and R_2^* ($=1/T_2^*$).[2,3] Because the microscopic magnetic field inhomogeneities produced by aggregated iron are very efficient in causing spin dephasing at field levels of 1.5 Tesla and above, these ratios and relaxation rates are predominantly determined by hemosiderin iron and will not, in general, accurately reflect ferritin iron concentrations.

Our approach to the use of magnetic resonance for quantitative determination of tissue ferritin and hemosiderin iron is based on the theoretical model of Jensen and Chandra.[24,25] In effect, the physical properties that allow the separation of ferritin (dispersed, soluble iron) from hemosiderin (aggregated, insoluble iron) for biochemical measurements generally correspond to those used in our MRI method. Dispersed, soluble (ferritin-like) iron produces magnetic resonance signal decay with a monoexponential form and the standard transverse relaxation rate R_2 may be derived from monoexponential fitting of a multiple spin echo signal. The R_2 depends linearly on the ferritin iron concentration and increases with the applied field. In contrast, aggregated, insoluble (hemosiderin-like) iron produces magnetic resonance signal decay that is *not* monoexponential and has a strong dependence on the interecho time.[24,25] Non-monoexponential MSE signal decay in liver with iron overload has been demonstrated in a number of earlier studies.[18,26–28] For determination of storage iron concentrations, a "reduced relaxation rate" (RR_2) and an "aggregation index" (A), are determined by fitting the multiple spin echo signal data to this model.[24,25] Subsequently, the ferritin iron concentration can be calculated from RR_2, and the hemosiderin concentration, from A. Overall, this approach may provide an improved characterization of tissue storage iron and potentially lead to more accurate estimates of the total storage iron concentration. Methods based on a single metric, such as R_2 or R_2^*, have an intrinsic uncertainty resulting from variations in the relative amounts of ferritin and hemosiderin iron.

As more fully described elsewhere,[24,25] our approach models the signal decay in iron overloaded tissue by

$$S(t) = S_0 e^{-RR_2 t} \times \exp\left[-A^{3/4}(\Delta t)^{3/4}(t-t_s)^{3/8}\right], \quad (1)$$

where $S(t)$ is the signal amplitude at a time t, S_0 is the initial signal amplitude, RR_2 is the reduced relaxation rate, A is the aggregation index, and t_s is a time shift given by

$$t_s = 2\tau\left[1-\left(\frac{\tau}{\Delta t}\right)^2\right]. \quad (2)$$

It should be noted that Equation (1) only describes the signal decay at the spin echo times. In addition, when $A = 0$ (i.e., in the absence of hemosiderin iron), the signal decay predicted by Equation (1) is monoexponential and RR_2 is simply equal to a conventional R_2 relaxation rate.

Our model assumes that the effect of ferritin iron is entirely reflected in the reduced relaxation rate and similarly that the effect of hemosiderin-like iron is reflected in the aggregation index.[24,25] The reduced relaxation rate is expected to depend linearly on the dispersed, ferritin-like iron concentration according to

$$RR_2 = r_{2,D}C_D + RR_{2,0}, \quad (3)$$

where C_D is the mass of dispersed iron per tissue mass, $r_{2,D}$ is the dispersed iron relaxivity, and $RR_{2,0}$ is the reduced relaxation rate in the absence of dispersed iron. For the aggregation index our model predicts

$$A = kC_A, \quad (4)$$

where C_A is the mass of aggregated (hemosiderin-like) iron per tissue mass and k is a parameter that depends on tissue properties, including the water self-diffusion coefficient, the mean aggregate spacing, and the applied field strength. If we assume that the parameter k is approximately constant, then Equations (3) and (4) imply that the total iron concentration is given by

$$C_T = \alpha_1 + \alpha_2 RR_2 + \alpha_3 A, \quad (5)$$

with

$$\alpha_1 = -\frac{RR_{2,0}}{r_{2,D}}; \quad \alpha_2 = \frac{1}{r_{2,D}}; \quad \alpha_3 = \frac{1}{k}. \quad (6)$$

In addition, we have

$$C_D = \alpha_1 + \alpha_2 RR_2, \quad (7)$$

and

$$C_A = \alpha_3 A, \quad (8)$$

demonstrating explicitly the separate quantification of dispersed and aggregated iron.[24,25]

Validation studies of method with phantoms

To validate our approach with known concentrations of dispersed and aggregated iron, phantoms were prepared with different mixtures of manganese chloride ($MnCl_2$) and iron oxide microspheres designed to mimic the varying amounts of ferritin and hemosiderin found in iron overloaded tissues.[25] $MnCl_2$ was chosen to simulate dispersed iron because it has (longitudinal relaxation time/transverse relaxation time) $T_1/T_2 \approx 10$ at 1.5 Tesla,[29] comparable to the T_1/T_2 ratio of aqueous ferritin solutions[30] as well as many biological tissues. Another convenient property of $MnCl_2$ is that the atomic weight of Mn (54.9) is very close to that of Fe (55.8) so that it is reasonable to define, in analogy to tissue concentration, the total iron concentration (C_T) simply as the sum of the Mn concentration (C_D) and the microsphere Fe concentration (C_A). The iron oxide microspheres consisted of magnetite nanoparticles embedded in a polymer matrix (product code UM3CN/5737, Bangs Laboratories, Fishers, IN, USA). The absolute iron concentrations used in our phantoms are approximately 100 times smaller than hemosiderin iron concentrations in iron overloaded liver but this is compensated by the fact that the specific susceptibility for the microspheres is about 100 times larger (at static magnetic field $B_0 = 1.5$ Tesla) so that the magnetic effects of the microspheres were similar to those of hemosiderin. The phantoms were imaged at room temperature on a 1.5 Tesla whole-body MR scanner (Intera, Philips Medical Systems, Best, the Netherlands) using three different multi-echo spin-echo sequences. Each sequence had a first echo time at $2\tau = 4$ ms but differing values for Δt (2, 4, and 8 ms), and the final echo occurred at 100 ms in each case. The signal decay data for the even order echoes (i.e., $n = 2, 4, 6, \ldots$) were fit globally to the form of Equation (1) using the Levenberg-Marquardt method.[25]

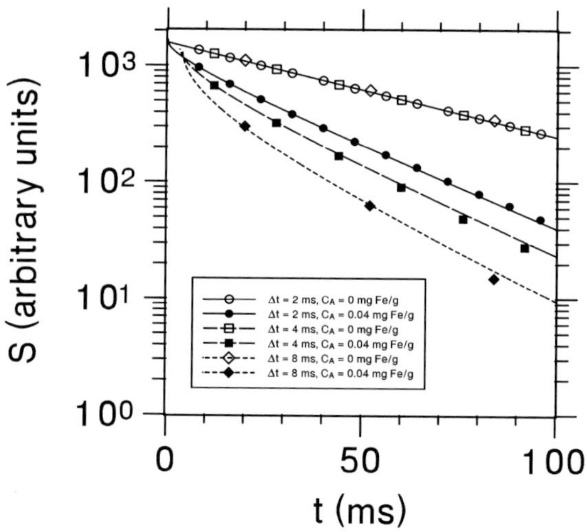

Figure 1. Semilogarithmic graph of representative MSE signal decay data (even echoes only) and fits for phantoms consisting of bottles with agarose gels. The data shown are all from bottles having $C_D = 0.0074$ mg Mn/g. The decay for the bottle with $C_A = 0$ (open symbols) is nearly monoexponential and independent of the interecho time. The decay for the bottle having $C_A = 0.04$ mg Fe/mg (solid symbols) is well fit by the form of Equation (1) with $A = 0.038 \pm 0.001$ ms$^{-3/2}$, indicating a significant degree of non-monoexponentiality and interecho time dependence. Reproduced, with permission, from Jensen *et al.*[25]

Representative signal decay data and fits for the phantom sample bottles are shown in Figure 1, demonstrating that our approach can model the MSE decay.[25] When no microspheres are present ($C_A = 0$), the MSE decay is nearly independent of the interecho time and essentially monoexponential. By contrast, with microspheres, the MSE decay depends strongly on the interecho time and departures from monoexponentiality are apparent. Figure 2 plots the calculated values for the total, aggregated (hemosiderin-like), and dispersed (ferritin-like) iron concentrations ($C_{T,\mathrm{MRI}}$, $C_{A,\mathrm{MRI}}$, $C_{D,\mathrm{MRI}}$) as functions of the actual iron concentrations, along with the linear regression lines.[25] The coefficients of determination are $r^2 = 0.99$, 0.99, and 0.96, respectively, documenting a close correlation between the calculated and actual iron concentrations. For comparison, neither R_2 nor $R_2{}^*$, which are conventionally used for iron estimation, showed a high correlation with the $MnCl_2$ (ferritin-like) concentration, demonstrating a relative insensitivity to the dispersed component.[25]

Related MRI studies of phantoms were conducted using a 7 Tesla Bruker MR scanner with (i) uniform

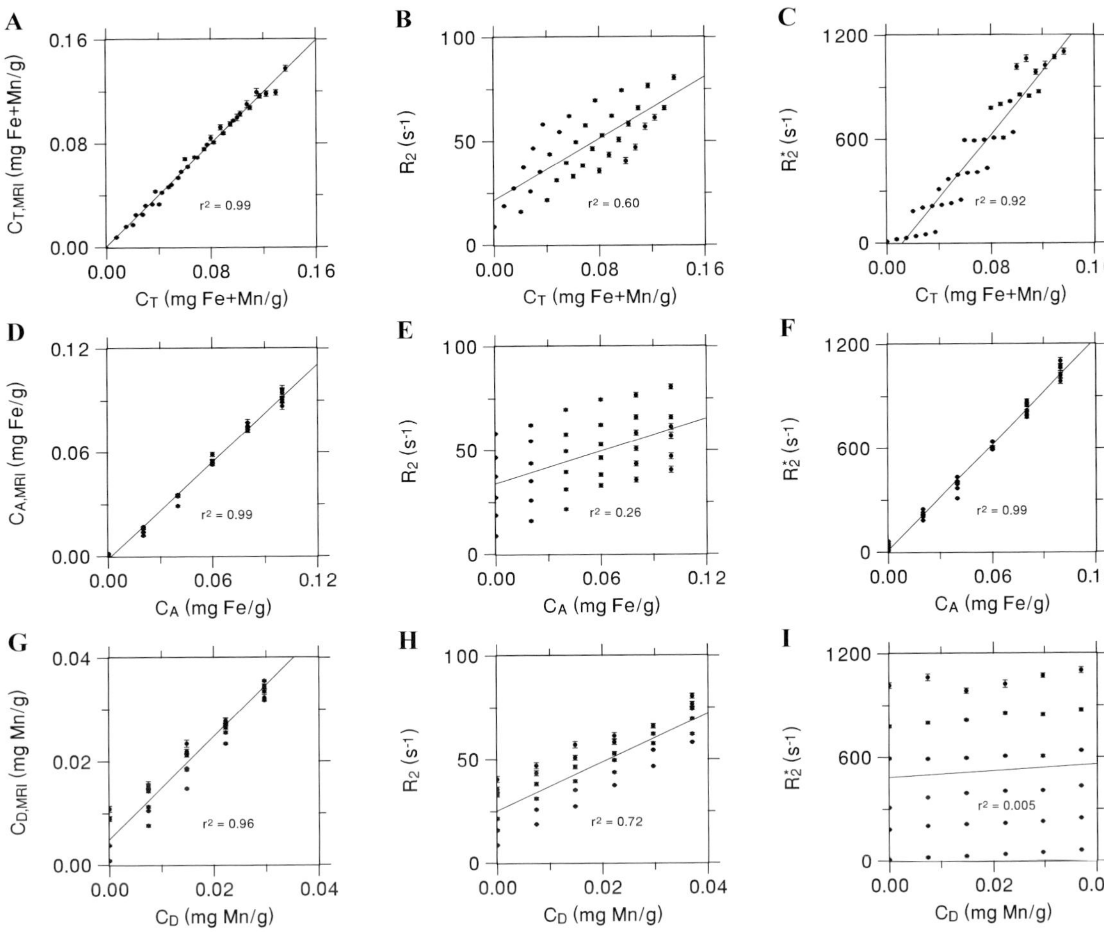

Figure 2. MRI measurements for phantoms as functions of C_T, C_A, and C_D together with linear regression lines. (A) $C_{T,MRI}$ found from Equation (5) with the parameters α_1, α_2, α_3 chosen to minimize the residual sum of squares with respect to C_T, resulting in a coefficient of determination of $r^2 = 0.99$. In comparison, (B) R_2 and (C) R_2^* have $r^2 = 0.60$ and $r^2 = 0.92$ with respect to C_T, suggesting that $C_{T,\text{MRI}}$ is a better predictor of C_T. Both (D) $C_{A,\text{MRI}}$ and (F) R_2^* are strongly correlated with C_A, but (E) $R_2$is not. (G) $C_{D,\text{MRI}}$ correlates much better with C_D than either (H) R_2 or (I) R_2^*. Reproduced, with permission, from Jensen *et al.*[25]

agarose gel suspensions of soluble (ferritin-like) superparamagnetic monocrystalline iron oxide nanoparticles and insoluble (hemosiderin-like) superparamagnetic micron-sized particles of iron oxides and (ii) agarose gel suspensions of iron-loaded cells (mouse embryonic stem cells and human embryonic kidney cells, intracellularly loaded with soluble (ferritin-like) monocrystalline iron oxide nanoparticles or insoluble (hemosiderin-like) micron-sized particles of iron oxides).[31,32] For each set of phantoms, a close correlation ($r^2 > 0.98$) was found between the model calculations and the actual iron concentrations.[31,32] Altogether, these studies provide compelling experimental validation *in vitro* for our approach to the separate measurement of ferritin and hemosiderin iron *in vivo*.

Validation studies of method with human liver explants

To provide further validation for our approach, we have carried out initial studies of samples obtained from diseased livers removed at the time of hepatic transplantation to compare directly our MRI results with biochemical determinations of ferritin, hemosiderin and total storage iron.[33] In brief, we have examined 18 samples (1.5 cm thick) from 9 human liver explants obtained at transplantation for hepatic failure. Each sample was placed in a 50 mL plastic tube filled with saline and immersed in a cylindrical water bath. To better replicate conditions *in vivo*, the experiment was conducted at 37° C by use of circulating heated water and fiber optic temperature probes. MR scanning was performed with a 5-channel phased array cardiac coil in a 1.5 Tesla Philips MR scanner. Three MSE sequences were acquired with different inter-echo times.[33] A region of interest (ROI) was centered on each of the samples in the phantom and propagated over all the images in the echo train. The non-monoexponential fitting computation was performed using the Marquardt method. After MRI, the liver sections were biochemically analyzed for ferritin, hemosiderin, and total non-heme iron. In these livers, the MR model parameters, RR_2 and A, and the corresponding biochemically determined concentrations of ferritin and hemosiderin were closely correlated ($R \sim 0.9$ for both, $P < 0.0001$)[33] over a range of total storage iron concentrations from 19 to 1,147 μg Fe/g liver, wet weight. Studies of additional samples over a wider range of hepatic iron concentrations are needed but these initial results with human liver provide initial evidence of the validity of our MRI method for the separate measurement of ferritin and hemosiderin.

MRI measurement of ferritin and hemosiderin iron in human subjects

We initially examined the feasibility of using our MRI method for separate measurements of ferritin and hemosiderin iron using Carr-Purcell-Meiboom-Gill (CPMG) pulse sequences with electrocardiographic triggering and respiratory navigator gating.[27,34] Using our MRI method, we determined the total hepatic storage iron concentration as the sum of the ferritin iron and hemosiderin iron. The total hepatic storage iron concentration was within the reference range (<1.6 mg Fe/g liver, dry weight) in six healthy volunteers but increased (range 4.3–30.3 mg Fe/g liver, dry weight) in 19 patients with transfusion-dependent thalassemia. The correlation of the MRI-determined total storage (ferrritin + hemosiderin) iron with measurements by biochemical analysis of liver samples by biopsy or by biomagnetic susceptometry was 0.95.[27]

A limitation of the use of such CPMG pulse sequences, or of an alternative, multiple single spin-echo sequences, is that their low data acquisition efficiency generally requires that these studies be performed during free breathing with respiratory gating, making impractical a comprehensive examination of the heart, liver, and other organs during a clinically acceptable examination time.[35] A recent major advance for the potential clinical application of our method has been the development of multi-echo fast spin-echo pulse sequences that permit accurate R_2 measurement in the heart and liver during a single breath hold, both at 1.5 Tesla[35] and at 3 Tesla.[36] Studies to provide an initial assessment of the application of these multi-echo fast spin-echo pulse sequences to the detection of changes in myocardial ferritin iron, as yet reported only in abstract form,[37,38] have yielded encouraging results. In brief, we examined patients with thalassemia major (10 in New York at 1.5 Tesla; 8 in Hong Kong at 3 Tesla), initially after suspending iron-chelating therapy for 1 week and subsequently after restarting oral deferasirox (New York) or parenteral deferoxamine with or without oral deferiprone (Hong Kong) for 1 week. After resuming iron-chelating therapy, our measure of myocardial ferritin iron (mean myocardial RR_2) decreased by approximately 11% ($P < 0.01$) in both sites; R_2* was not changed significantly.[37,38] Further studies in larger numbers of patients with wider ranges of iron loading over longer periods of time are needed but these initial results suggest that measurement of myocardial ferritin iron is a promising investigational method for rapidly evaluating the response of patients with transfusion-dependent thalassemia to new or altered iron-chelating regimens.

Conclusions

Advances in our understanding of intracellular iron metabolism have clarified the physiological roles of ferritin and hemosiderin. Iron incorporation and release seem to be intrinsic, autonomous properties of the ferritin molecule, with iron entry and exit from ferritin the result of an equilibrium based on the concentration of cytosolic iron. Ferritin can safely sequester large amounts of iron in solution in a compact yet bioavailable form. Nonetheless, under pathological conditions, the capacity of ferritin to store iron may be overwhelmed, with ferritin iron acting as a pro-oxidant and contributing to tissue damage. Production of hemosiderin, enclosed within siderosome membranes, seems to sequester the excess iron away from the cytosol and help protect against iron toxicity. This property may help explain the observation that as the total amount of tissue iron increases, the proportion stored as hemosiderin rises, from trace amounts in normal individuals to 90% or more in patients with severe iron overload. Overall, the available evidence suggests that cytosolic iron is in a rapid equilibrium with soluble, dispersed ferritin for short-term storage while exchange with the long-term aggregates of iron within hemosiderin is slow and limited. The three iron-chelating agents in clinical use, deferasirox, deferiprone, and deferoxamine, all decrease the intracellular concentration of ferritin iron, although by distinct mechanisms. Consequently, measurements of cellular ferritin iron provide a potential means of rapidly monitoring the effectiveness of iron chelators.

Established MRI indicators of tissue iron (signal intensity ratios, R_2, $R_2{}^*$) are intended to measure the *total* storage (ferritin + hemosiderin) iron. These ratios and rates are principally influenced by hemosiderin iron, will not accurately reflect ferritin iron concentrations, and change slowly, even with intensive iron-chelating therapy. Moreover, methods to measure the *total* storage (ferritin + hemosiderin) iron based on a single metric, such as R_2 or $R_2{}^*$, have an intrinsic uncertainty resulting from variations in the relative amounts of ferritin and hemosiderin iron.

The physical properties that allow the separation of ferritin (dispersed, soluble iron) from hemosiderin (aggregated, insoluble iron) for biochemical measurements generally correspond to those used in our MRI method. The differences in solubility and intracellular distribution between ferritin iron and hemosiderin iron produce different effects on multiple spin-echo signal decay. Dispersed, soluble (ferritin-like) iron produces signal decay with a monoexponential form while aggregated, insoluble (hemosiderin-like) iron produces signal decay that is not monoexponential and has a strong dependence on the interecho time. For determination of storage iron concentrations, a "reduced relaxation rate" (RR_2) and an "aggregation index" (A), are determined by fitting the multi-echo spin-echo decay data to the model of Jensen and Chandra.[24,25] Subsequently, the ferritin iron concentration can be calculated from RR_2, and the hemosiderin concentration, from A. We have validated this approach with known concentrations of dispersed and aggregated iron in agarose phantoms and in initial studies of samples obtained from explanted livers removed at the time of hepatic transplantation to compare directly our MRI results with biochemical determinations of ferritin, hemosiderin, and total storage iron.

We first showed the feasibility of using our MRI method for separate measurements of ferritin and hemosiderin iron using Carr-Purcell-Meiboom-Gill (CPMG) sequences with electrocardiographic triggering and respiratory navigator gating. A recent major advance for the potential clinical application of our method has been the development of multi-echo fast spin-echo pulse sequences that permit accurate R_2 measurement in the heart and liver during a single breath hold, both at 1.5 Tesla and at 3 Tesla. Our first studies using the breath-hold multi-echo fast spin-echo pulse sequences have suggested that measurement of myocardial ferritin iron could detect short-term changes produced by iron-chelating therapy. While further studies in larger numbers of patients with wider ranges of iron loading over longer periods of time are needed, these initial results suggest that measurement of myocardial ferritin iron is a promising investigational method for rapidly evaluating the response of patients with transfusion-dependent thalassemia to new or altered iron-chelating regimens.

Acknowledgments

This research was supported, in part, by the National Institutes of Health National Institutes of Health (R01-DK069373, R01-DK066251, and R01-DK049108); the American Heart Association; (0730143N); and the Hong Kong Research Grant Council (GRF HKU 7794/07M).

Conflict of interest

The authors declare no conflicts of interest.

References

1. Brittenham, G.M. & D.G. Badman. 2003. Noninvasive measurement of iron: report of an NIDDK workshop. *Blood* **101:** 15–19.
2. Jensen, P.D. 2004. Evaluation of iron overload. *Br. J. Haematol.* **124:** 697–711.
3. Wood, J.C. 2009. History and current impact of cardiac magnetic resonance imaging on the management of iron overload. *Circulation* **120:** 1937–1939.
4. Arosio, P. & S. Levi. 2010. Cytosolic and mitochondrial ferritins in the regulation of cellular iron homeostasis and

oxidative damage. *Biochim. Biophys. Acta* [Epub ahead of print].

5. De Domenico, I., M.B. Vaughn, L. Li, *et al.* 2006. Ferroportin-mediated mobilization of ferritin iron precedes ferritin degradation by the proteasome. *EMBO J.* **25:** 5396–5404.
6. De Domenico, I., D.M. Ward & J. Kaplan. 2009. Specific iron chelators determine the route of ferritin degradation. *Blood* **114:** 4546–4551.
7. Anderson, G.J. & C.D. Vulpe. 2009. Mammalian iron transport. *Cell. Mol. Life Sci.* **66:** 3241–3261.
8. Breuer, W., M. Shvartsman & Z.I. Cabantchik. 2008. Intracellular labile iron. *Int. J. Biochem. Cell. Biol.* **40:** 350–354.
9. Shi, H., K.Z. Bencze, T.L. Stemmler, *et al.* 2008. A cytosolic iron chaperone that delivers iron to ferritin. *Science* **320:** 1207–1210.
10. Bovell, E., C.E. Buckley, W. Chua-anusorn, *et al.* 2009. Dietary iron-loaded rat liver haemosiderin and ferritin: in situ measurement of iron core nanoparticle size and cluster structure using anomalous small-angle X-ray scattering. *Phys. Med. Biol.* **54:** 1209–1221.
11. Chasteen, N.D. & P.M. Harrison. 1999. Mineralization in ferritin: an efficient means of iron storage. *J. Struct. Biol.* **126:** 182–194.
12. Iancu, T.C. 1992. Ferritin and hemosiderin in pathological tissues. *Electron. Microsc. Rev.* **5:** 209–229.
13. Iancu, T.C., Y. Deugnier, J.W. Halliday, *et al.* 1997. Ultrastructural sequences during liver iron overload in genetic hemochromatosis. *J. Hepatol.* **27:** 628–638.
14. Miyazaki, E., J. Kato, M. Kobune, *et al.* 2002. Denatured H-ferritin subunit is a major constituent of haemosiderin in the liver of patients with iron overload. *Gut* **50:** 413–419.
15. Selden, C., M. Owen, J.M. Hopkins, *et al.* 1980. Studies on the concentration and intracellular localization of iron proteins in liver biopsy specimens from patients with iron overload with special reference to their role in lysosomal disruption. *Br. J. Haematol.* **44:** 593–603.
16. Truty, J., R. Malpe & M.C. Linder. 2001. Iron prevents ferritin turnover in hepatic cells. *J. Biol. Chem.* **276:** 48775–48780.
17. Wixom, R.L., L. Prutkin & H.N. Munro. 1980. Hemosiderin: nature, formation, and significance. *Int. Rev. Exp. Pathol.* **22:** 193–225.
18. Ghugre, N.R., T.D. Coates, M.D. Nelson, *et al.* 2005. Mechanisms of tissue-iron relaxivity: nuclear magnetic resonance studies of human liver biopsy specimens. *Magn. Reson. Med.* **54:** 1185–1193.
19. Wood, J.C., C. Enriquez, N. Ghugre, *et al.* 2005. Physiology and pathophysiology of iron cardiomyopathy in thalassemia. *Ann. N.Y. Acad. Sci.* **1054:** 386–395.
20. Gossuin, Y., A. Roch, R.N. Muller, *et al.* 2000. Relaxation induced by ferritin and ferritin-like magnetic particles: the role of proton exchange. *Magn. Reson. Med.* **43:** 237–243.
21. Gossuin, Y., A. Roch, R.N. Muller, *et al.* 2002. Anomalous nuclear magnetic relaxation of aqueous solutions of ferritin: an unprecedented first-order mechanism. *Magn. Reson. Med.* **48:** 959–964.
22. Allen, P.D., T.G. St Pierre, W. Chua-anusorn, *et al.* 2000. Low-frequency low-field magnetic susceptibility of ferritin and hemosiderin. *Biochim. Biophys. Acta* **1500:** 186–196.
23. Brooks, R. A., J. Vymazal, R.B. Goldfarb, *et al.* 1998. Relaxometry and magnetometry of ferritin. *Magn. Reson. Med.* **40:** 227–235.
24. Jensen, J.H. & R. Chandra. 2002. Theory of nonexponential NMR signal decay in liver with iron overload or superparamagnetic iron oxide particles. *Magn. Reson. Med.* **47:** 1131–1138.
25. Jensen, J.H., H. Tang, C.L. Tosti, *et al.* 2010. Separate MRI quantificaiton of dispersed (ferritin-like) and aggregated (hemosiderin-like) storage iron. *Magn. Reson. Med.* **63:** 1201–1209.
26. Bulte, J.W., G.F. Miller, J. Vymazal, *et al.* 1997. Hepatic hemosiderosis in non-human primates: quantification of liver iron using different field strengths. *Magn. Reson. Med.* **37:** 530–536.
27. Tang, H., J.H. Jensen, S. Sheth, *et al.* 2005. MR measurement of ferritin and hemosiderin iron in patients with iron overload. *Proc. Int. Soc. Magn. Reson. Med.* **13:** 1880 (Abstract).
28. Thomsen, C., P. Wiggers, H. Ring-Larsen, *et al.* 1992. Identification of patients with hereditary haemochromatosis by magnetic resonance imaging and spectroscopic relaxation time measurements. *Magn. Reson. Imaging* **10:** 867–879.
29. Ulmer, J.L., V.P. Mathews, C.A. Hamilton, *et al.* 1996. Magnetization transfer or spin-lock? An investigation of off-resonance saturation pulse imaging with varying frequency offsets. *AJNR Am. J. Neuroradiol.* **17:** 805–819.
30. Vymazal, J., O. Zak, J.W. Bulte, *et al.* 1996. T1 and T2 of ferritin solutions: effect of loading factor. *Magn. Reson. Med.* **36:** 61–65.
31. Cheung, J.S., A.M. Chow, J.H. Jensen, *et al.* 2007. MRI characterization of iron in soluble (ferritin-like) and particulate (hemosiderin-like) mixtures. *Proc. Int. Soc. Magn. Reson. Med.* **15:** 1153 (Abstract).
32. Wu, E.X., J.S. Cheung, A.M. Chow, *et al.* 2007. MRI characterization of ferritin-like and hemosiderin-like iron. *Proc. Int. BioIron. Soc.* **78** (Abstract).
33. Tosti, C.L., B.S. Wojczyk, S. Sheth, *et al.* 2010. MR iron quantification of soluble (ferritin-like) and insoluble (hemosiderin-like) iron: a biochemical validation in human liver explants. *Proc. Int. Soc. Magn. Reson. Med.* **18** (Abstract) In press.
34. Sheth, S., H. Tang, J.H. Jensen, *et al.* 2005. Methods for noninvasive measurement of tissue iron in Cooley's anemia. *Ann. N.Y. Acad. Sci.* **1054:** 358–372.
35. Kim, D., J.H. Jensen, E.X. Wu, *et al.* 2009. Breathhold multiecho fast spin-echo pulse sequence for accurate R2 measurement in the heart and liver. *Magn. Reson. Med.* **62:** 300–306.
36. Guo, H., W. Y. Au, J. S. Cheung, *et al.* 2009. Myocardial T2 quantitation in patients with iron overload at 3 Tesla. *J. Magn. Reson. Imaging* **30:** 394–400.
37. Kim, D., J.H. Jensen, C. Tosti, *et al.* 2009. R2 imaging of ferritin iron in thalassemic patients off and on iron-chelation therapy. *Proc. Int. Soc. Magn. Reson. Med.* **17:** 3755 (Abstract).
38. Cheung, J.S., W.Y. Au, S.Y. Ha, *et al.* 2010. Monitoring iron chelation effect in hearts of thalassaemia patients with improved sensitivity using reduced transverse relaxation rate (RR2). *Proc. Int. Soc. Magn. Reson. Med.* **18:** (Abstract) In press.

Ann. N.Y. Acad. Sci. ISSN 0077-8923

ANNALS OF THE NEW YORK ACADEMY OF SCIENCES
Issue: *Cooley's Anemia: Ninth Symposium*

Predicting pituitary iron and endocrine dysfunction

John C. Wood,[1,2] Leila Noetzl,[1] Aleya Hyderi,[1] Mehrdad Joukar,[1] Thomas Coates,[3] and Steven Mittelman[4]

[1]Division of Pediatric Cardiology, Children's Hospital Los Angeles, Los Angeles, California. [2]Division of Pediatric Radiology, Children's Hospital Los Angeles, Los Angeles, California. [3]Division of Pediatric Hematology, Children's Hospital Los Angeles, Los Angeles, California. [4]Division of Pediatric Endocrinology, Children's Hospital Los Angeles, Los Angeles, California

Address for correspondence: John C. Wood, M.D., Ph.D., Divisions of Pediatric Cardiology and Radiology, Children's Hospital Los Angeles, MS#34, 4650 Sunset Blvd, Los Angeles, CA 90027-0034. jwood@chla.usc.edu

Patients with thalassemia major (TM) require lifelong transfusion therapy to survive, leading to toxic iron overload in the endocrine glands and heart. The pituitary gland is one of the most vulnerable targets, leading to irreversible hypogonadotropic hypogonadism in approximately half of patients. Improvements in magnetic resonance imaging (MRI) technology and understanding have allowed earlier recognition of preclinical iron deposition in the heart, pancreas, and liver; prior work also supports a similar role for the pituitary. The purpose of this study is threefold, (1) to develop age-specific nomograms for pituitary iron and volume metrics; (2) to determine the prevalence, severity, and age of onset of pituitary iron deposition and volume loss in TM patients, and (3) to determine whether deferasirox monotherapy can modify the trajectory of pituitary iron accumulation and damage over a two-year period. This article outlines relevant background studies and methodological details as well as providing preliminary results from our first two aims.

Keywords: thalassemia; pituitary; MRI; iron; endocrine

Introduction

Thalassemia and other globin gene defects are among the most common genetic defects in the world. These defects produce a wide clinical spectrum of anemia and other cardiovascular sequelae. Some mutations may be characterized by increased ineffective erythropoiesis, leading to down regulation of hepcidin and increased iron absorption (primary hemochromatosis).[1] If the ineffective erythropoiesis or anemia is too severe, patients may need chronic blood transfusions, producing secondary hemochromatosis. Although the clinical severity and expression is often different in primary and secondary hemochromatosis, iron overload remains a lifelong problem.

Iron overload produces toxic buildup in many organs, including liver, endocrine glands, and heart. Although cardiac toxicity remains the leading cause of death in thalassemia, endocrine dysfunction is the leading cause of morbidity. Table 1 highlights prevalence data from multicenter trials in Italy and the United States.[2,3] Hypogonadotropic hypogonadism was present in more than half of the thalassemia major (TM) population. Hypothyroidism and diabetes mellitus were also quite common.

Growth failure and pubertal delay are among the earliest sequelae of iron toxicity, occurring throughout the first two decades of life. Heavy pancreatic iron deposition occur commonly in the first decade of life but diabetes does not manifest until late adolescence and early adulthood.[4] This suggests a long prodromal state of clinically silent iron deposition. Similar findings are observed in the heart.[5] Cardiac iron becomes detectable by magnetic resonance imaging (MRI) as early as 10 years of age but clinical symptoms often occur much later.[6]

Early identification of cardiac iron through MRI combined with improved chelation strategies appear to be markedly improving survival in thalassemia.[7] As a result, prevention of endocrine complications is becoming increasingly important. Since

doi: 10.1111/j.1749-6632.2010.05545.x

Table 1. Prevalence of endocrine complications in thalassemia

	Borgna-Pignatti *et al.*[3]	Vogiatzi *et al.*[2]
Hypogonadotrophic hypogonadism	54.7	51.3
Hypothyroidism	10.8	12
Diabetes mellitus	6.4	14.1
Hyoparathyroidism	–	2.1

hypogonadotropic hypogonadism is so prevalent and presents early in life, it is a logical and important therapeutic target. By analogy with the heart and pancreas, it is logical that the pituitary gland probably demonstrates a period of clinically silent iron deposition that offers a therapeutic window to prevent irreversible damage. MRI represents the ideal tool for identifying that window and monitoring therapy.

In fact, there has already been excellent work supporting the role of MRI for detection of preclinical pituitary iron deposition. Darkening of the pituitary gland in response to iron deposition has been noted for decades.[8] Numerous studies have demonstrated that pituitary darkening is proportional to ferritin and other somatic iron stores.[9–13] Furthermore, patients with overt hypogonadotropic hypogonadism have higher detectable pituitary iron. Figure 1 demonstrates pituitary R2 levels in 40 control subjects, 14 TM patients without hypogonadotropic hypogonadism (HH), and 15 TM patients with HH (figure drawn from data in reference 9). The diagnosis of HH was confirmed in all subjects by GnRH stimulation test. Roughly 90% of all the TM patients had pituitary iron levels outside the reference range from age-matched controls, but only half exhibited gonadotropic insufficiency. Patients with HH had R2 values that were 50% greater, on average, than asymptomatic TM patients and more than double values seen in control subjects. Sparacia and colleagues, also demonstrated that pituitary iron estimates yield graded risk for HH by clinical and biochemical metrics. By ROC analysis, MRI pituitary signal intensity was able to distinguish HH and non-HH TM patients with an area under the curve of 0.97.

Thus, TM patients with HH demonstrate severe pituitary iron loading, but many TM patients exhibit detectable pituitary iron with no apparent dysfunction. This is analogous to organs such as the heart and pancreas. So are there any other imaging methods for assessing pituitary health? Argyropoulou demonstrated that pituitary height is an important predictor of pituitary function, using the same study population as described in Figure 1.[14] Only 1/15 patients with HH had a pituitary height greater than 4.2 mm while all of the control subjects did. Similarly, only 4/14 of TM patients having normal pituitary function demonstrated a pituitary height less than 4.2 mm. Thus, pituitary height appeared to be a strong predictor of glandular function.

Our current working hypothesis is that pituitary iron develops early in life and is proportional to overall somatic iron balance (as assessed by liver iron concentration [LIC] and serum ferritin). Initially, iron is safely buffered in the cells and glandular volume is maintained, producing a gland that is dark on MRI but functions normally. At this point, aggressive chelation can remove glandular iron with no long-term sequelae. Over time, cumulative iron-mediated oxidative stress triggers apoptosis and the gland shrinks (in adults) or fails to grow appropriately (in children). Ultimately, secretory reserve is exceeded and detectable endocrine abnormalities become apparent. Chelation could potentially improve secretory function in remaining secretory cells but regeneration of dead cells does not occur and some permanent insufficiency is expected.

Thus the motivation of our research is to develop strategies to recognize preclinical iron deposition earlier, to identify predictors of pituitary iron, and to test the ability of iron chelation to prevent primary pituitary iron overload and damage. Specifically, we are determining age-specific normative data for pituitary R2 values and pituitary volume. Second, we are determining the prevalence of pituitary iron and volume loss as a function of age in chronically transfused pediatric and young adult patients. We hypothesize that pituitary iron deposition occurs in the first decade of life. Lastly, we are studying the evolution of pituitary iron and volume over a two-year period in patients using deferasirox monotherapy.

Methods

If pituitary iron deposition is occurring in the first decade of life, than the critical period for therapeutic intervention coincides with the greatest rate of

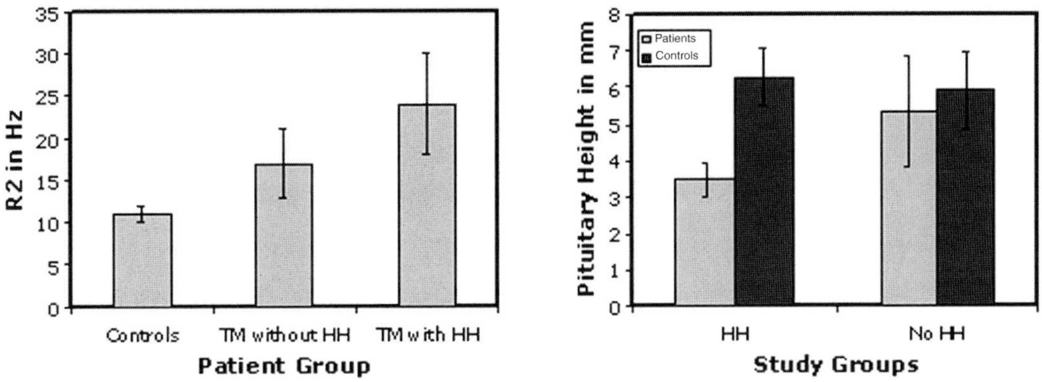

Figure 1. (Left) Plot of pituitary R2 in age-matched normal subjects, TM patients without hypogonadotropic hypogonadism (HH), and TM patients having HH.[9] Nearly all of the patients with HH have increased R2 values. Many of the asymptomatic patients also have increased pituitary R2 compared to control subjects, but average values are less than observed in symptomatic patients. (Right) Bar graph of pituitary height in the same patient population.[14] Patients with HH have significantly smaller pituitary glands than either controls or TM patients having normal pituitary function.

somatic growth. Consequently, it is vital to determine age or body-habitus appropriate metrics of pituitary size. The pituitary gland has a complex, three-dimensional shape. We postulate that high resolution volumetric MRI data will offer more robust metrics of gland health than simple linear height assessments. Pituitary growth grossly parallels somatic growth, thus pituitary volumes will need to be indexed to patient age or body habitus. Small gender differences might also be expected. We are using nonlinear regression, comparing both power law and polynomial relationships, to create pituitary size nomograms. To date, we have scanned 50 normal subjects between the ages of 2–25 years. No gender differences have been observed. Data normalization with respect to age yields the lowest residual error in the corresponding pituitary "growth curves," although height, weight, and body surface area yield satisfactory representations as well.

Pituitary R2 measurements might also be expected to be age dependent. The pituitary becomes increasingly metabolically active as patients enter puberty; iron is essential for many synthetic processes. Furthermore, many organs including liver, heart, and brain, slowly accumulate iron in normal subjects. Figure 2 demonstrates our experimental methodology. We acquire multi-echo, spin-echo images in both coronal and sagittal planes. Imaging parameters include an inplane resolution of 0.8 mm, slice thickness 3 mm, and echo times of 15, 30, 45, 60, 75, 90, 105, and 120 ms. A rectangular region enclosing the entire pituitary is fit to a pixelwise R2 map, using simple exponential functions without offset correction. In the sagittal view, the region of interest is refined to include only R2 values from the pars distalis; the pars intermedia and pars nervosa are excluded. In the coronal view, all visible pituitary tissue is included because the imaging slice is restricted to the pars distalis. The refined ROIs yield a distribution of R2 values; we use the median R2 to represent the pituitary iron concentration.

Relationships between pituitary iron and pituitary size will be assessed by simple linear regression. Pituitary iron will also be compared to iron stores in other compartments including liver, pancreas, and heart. Based upon our normative data, patient pituitary size and volumes can be cast into Z-scores. We hypothesize that both iron and pituitary size Z-scores will be normal in pre-kindergarten children, but that detectable pituitary iron will manifest itself in early school age years. Pituitary volume loss is likely to occur in the second decade because iron toxicity often trails iron deposition by 5–10 years in other organs.

Subject recruitment for our cross-sectional analyses of pituitary iron and volume draw from all chronically transfused patients who are willing to participate. The primary goal is to determine the prevalence, severity, and age of onset of pituitary iron/volume loss as well as to determine their major predictors. The second arm of our study is limited to chronically transfused patients (excluding sickle

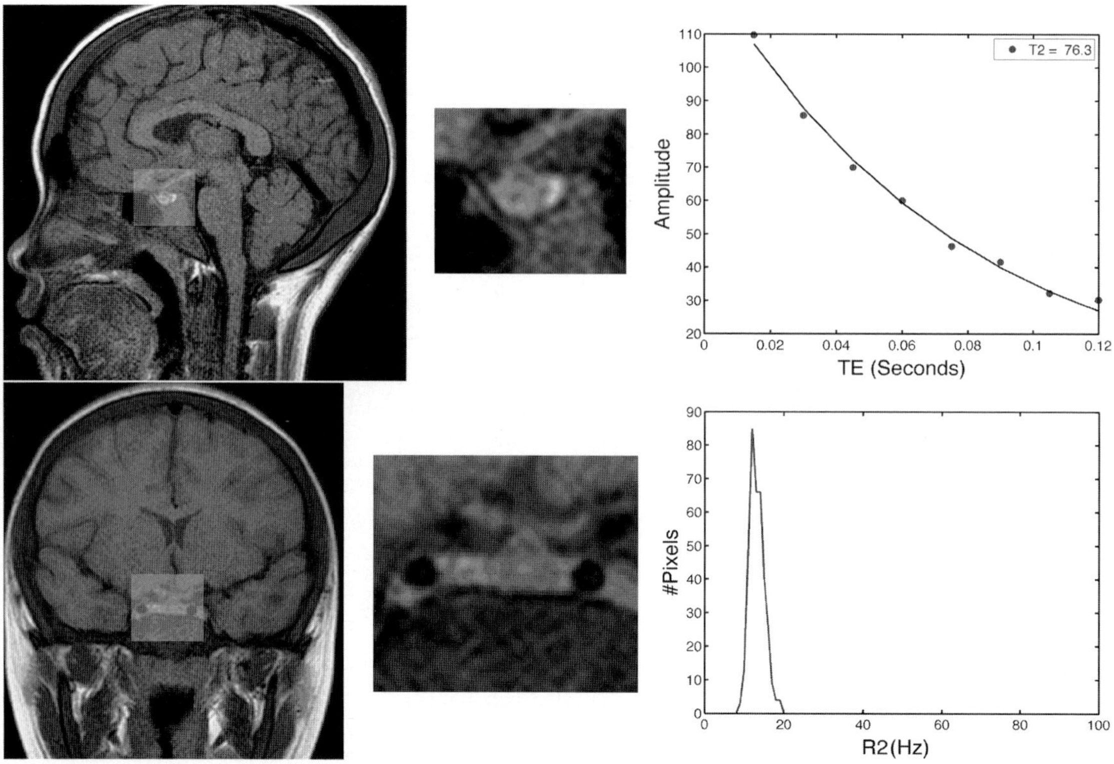

Figure 2. Representative sagittal and coronal images in an adolescent normal control patient (left). Middle panes represent zoomed up views of the pituitary gland depicting the relevant regions of interest. Top right panel demonstrates a monoexponential fit to data averaged from the whole ROI; calculated T2 is 76.3 (R2 of 13.1 Hz). Bottom panel depicts a histogram of R2 values calculated from a pixelwise fit to the data. Data are unimodally and symmetrically distributed with comparable mean R2.

cell disease) who are currently taking deferasirox monotherapy. The goal is to determine whether deferasirox iron chelation, as used in standard clinical care, can stabilize or reverse pituitary iron deposition and damage over a two-year period. Trends in pituitary Z-scores will be used as the primary outcome variable.

Results

The study is currently enrolling and definitive data are not yet available. Nonetheless, some of the preliminary findings may be useful to other investigators in the field. First, pituitary R2 is not identical when measured in the coronal and sagittal planes, even when attempting to "match" the regions of interest. The differences are small and it does not appear that one measurement is "superior" to another but the data should not be used interchangeably. Pituitary R2 also rises with age in normal controls; age-specific norms should improve diagnosis of pituitary iron overload in young subjects.

In patients, pituitary R2 is closely correlated to LIC and pancreatic iron but not to cardiac iron metrics. This suggests that the kinetics of pituitary iron loading are relatively rapid. As a result, pituitary iron loading is common in the first decade of life and was observed in children as young as 4 years of age. Pituitary volumes are mildly diminished ($\sim$1 standard deviation below the mean) in our study subjects, independent of pituitary iron concentration. However, pituitary iron loading was associated with additional volume loss, with striking changes seen in the second decade of life. Only one patient had documented hypogonadotropic hypogonadism. Figure 3 demonstrates pituitary R2 and volume in this patient compared to an age-matched TM patient having normal pituitary size and iron. The pituitary from the HH patient is truncated anteriorly posteriorly as well as superiorly–inferiorly, having a volume approximately half of normal (Z-score of -5.0). The R2 value was 25 Hz (Z-score $+$ 15), compared with 12.3 Hz (Z-score $+$ 0.3)

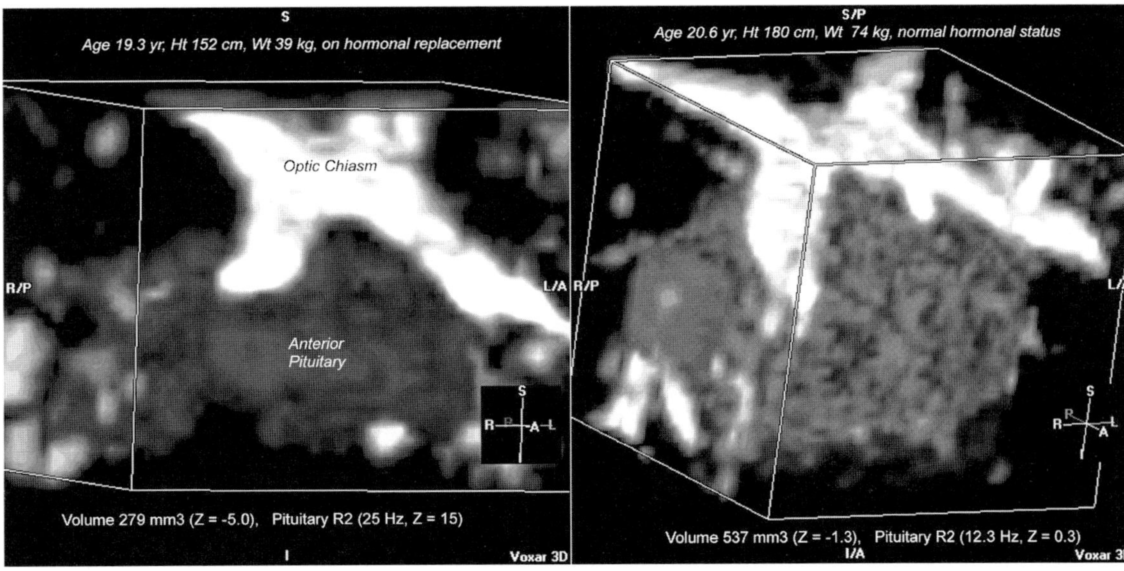

Figure 3. (Left) Volume rendering of pituitary gland in a 19-year-old TM patient with HH; patient was growth impaired and required sex hormone replacement. The gland is heavily iron loaded (mean R2 of 25 Hz, Z score +15) and shrunken (pituitary volume 279 mm^3, Z score of −5.0). (Right) Age-matched TM patient with normal growth and sex hormone parameters. No pituitary iron was detected (pituitary R2 of 12.3 Hz, Z score 0.3). Pituitary volume is in the low normal range (537 mm^3, Z = −1.3) but visibly larger than the previous patient.

in the age-matched patient with normal pituitary function.

Discussion

Our current works-in-progress will improve the utility of pituitary MRI by defining age-specific norms for pituitary volume and R2, allowing earlier recognition of relevant iron deposition and damage. The use of pituitary R2, rather than signal intensity ratios, will improve the inter-center transferability of our technique. Despite some methodology and machine differences, we are obtaining quite similar R2 values as published by Argyropoulou in control subjects, TM patients without HH, and TM patients having HH.[9] At some point, formal characterization of inter-study, inter-machine, and inter-institution differences are warranted, but these studies are expensive and unlikely to demonstrate novel information given the proven robustness of MRI tissue-iron methods.

The development of pituitary iron overload in patients as young as 4 years of age is a novel and concerning finding. While the toxicity of this iron is not yet known, it bears careful study. Longitudinal analyses will allow us to determine whether the presence of pituitary iron attenuates somatic or pituitary growth trajectories. It will also be critically important to determine whether routine deferasirox therapy can stabilize or improve pituitary iron and growth curves.

Preliminary data also suggests that our chronically transfused patients have smaller pituitary glands than age-matched controls, even if they do not have pituitary iron. Since it was impossible to ethnically match our control and patient populations, there are undoubtedly ethnic biases with respect to patient size, diet, and socioeconomic status that contribute to this difference. However, iron is not the only stressor on the hypothalamic-pituitary-gonadal axis. Longstanding anemia, ineffective erythropoiesis, and nonspecific stress from chronic illness all could contribute to changes in pituitary volume.

In summary, pituitary MRI is a powerful tool for characterizing pituitary size and iron concentration. Our results-to-date reinforce prior work in the field and extend the techniques for children in the first decade of life. We postulate that appropriate recognition and treatment of preclinical pituitary iron can prevent the pan-endocrine dysfunction that currently troubles so many TM patients.

Acknowledgments

This work is supported by an investigator-initiated research grant from Novartis, USA.

Disclosure statement

Drs. Wood and Coates have research funding from Novartis for basic and clinical research studies.

Conflicts of interest

The authors declare no conflicts of interest.

References

1. McLaren, G.D., W.A. Muir & R.W. Kellermeyer. 1983. Iron overload disorders: natural history, pathogenesis, diagnosis, and therapy. *Crit. Rev. Clin. Lab. Sci.* **19:** 205–266.
2. Vogiatzi, M.G., E.A. Macklin, F.L. Trachtenberg, *et al.* 2009. Differences in the prevalence of growth, endocrine and vitamin D abnormalities among the various thalassaemia syndromes in North America. *Br. J. Haematol.* **146:** 546–556.
3. Borgna-Pignatti, C., S. Rugolotto, P. De Stefano, *et al.* 2004. Survival and complications in patients with thalassemia major treated with transfusion and deferoxamine. *Haematologica* **89:** 1187–1193.
4. Noetzli, L.J., J. Papudesi, T.D. Coates & J.C. Wood. 2009. Pancreatic iron loading predicts cardiac iron loading in thalassemia major. *Blood* **144:** 4021–4026.
5. Wood, J.C., J.M. Tyszka, N. Ghugre, *et al.* 2004. Myocardial iron loading in transfusion-dependent thalassemia and sickle-cell disease. *Blood* **103:** 1934–1936.
6. Wood, J.C., R. Origa, A. Agus, *et al.* 2008. Onset of cardiac iron loading in pediatric patients with thalassemia major. *Haematologica* **93:** 917–920.
7. Modell, B., M. Khan, M. Darlison, *et al.* 2008. Improved survival of thalassaemia major in the UK and relation to T2∗ cardiovascular magnetic resonance. *J. Cardiovasc. Magn. Reson.* **10:** 42.
8. Fujisawa, I., M. Morikawa, Y. Nakano & J. Konishi. 1988. Hemochromatosis of the pituitary gland: MR imaging. *Radiology* **168:** 213–214.
9. Argyropoulou, M.I., Z. Metafratzi, D.N. Kiortsis, *et al.* 2000. T2 Relaxation rate as an index of pituitary iron overload in patients with beta-thalassemia major. *AJR Am. J. Roentgenol.* **175:** 1567–1569.
10. Sparacia, G, M. Midiri, P. D'Angelo & R. Lagalla. 1999. Magnetic resonance imaging of the pituitary gland in patients with secondary hypogonadism due to transfusional hemochromatosis. *Magma* **8:** 87–90.
11. Sparacia, G., A. Iaia, A. Banco, *et al.* 2000. Transfusional hemochromatosis: quantitative relation of MR imaging pituitary signal intensity reduction to hypogonadotropic hypogonadism. *Radiology* **215:** 818–823.
12. Lam, W.W., W.Y. Au, W.C. Chu, *et al.* 2008. One-stop measurement of iron deposition in the anterior pituitary, liver, and heart in thalassemia patients. *J. Magn. Reson. Imaging* **28:** 29–33.
13. Christoforidis, A., A. Haritandi, V. Perifanis, *et al.* 2007. MRI for the determination of pituitary iron overload in children and young adults with beta-thalassaemia major. *Eur. J. Radiol.* **62:** 138–142.
14. Argyropoulou, M.I., D.N. Kiortsis, Z. Metafratzi, *et al.* 2001. Pituitary gland height evaluated by MR in patients with beta-thalassemia major: a marker of pituitary gland function. *Neuroradiology* **43:** 1056–1058.

Ann. N.Y. Acad. Sci. ISSN 0077-8923

ANNALS OF THE NEW YORK ACADEMY OF SCIENCES
Issue: *Cooley's Anemia: Ninth Symposium*

Better survival and less cardiac morbidity in female patients with thalassemia major: a review of the literature

Maria Marsella,[1] Alessia Pepe,[2] and Caterina Borgna-Pignatti[1]

[1]Department of Clinical and Experimental Medicine (Pediatrics), Ferrara, Italy. [2]MRI Laboratory, Institute of Clinical Physiology, "G. Monasterio" Foundation/CNR, Pisa, Italy

Address for correspondence: Caterina Borgna-Pignatti, Department of Clinical and Experimental Medicine (Pediatrics), via Savonarola no. 9, 44100 Ferrara, Italy. c.borgna@unife.it

Female patients with thalassemia and other hemoglobinopathies enjoy a longer survival when compared to males. We report data from the literature and from our own studies on gender differences in survival of thalassemia patients, and also examine this phenomenon in animals and in the general population. Some of the more widely accepted hypotheses that try to explain the differences in longevity between males and females are reviewed. The oxidative stress hypothesis is commonly accepted by the researchers on ageing, although further support for it is needed. In conclusion, it appears that male and female patients with transfusion-dependent thalassemia major are at the same risk of accumulating iron, but females survive longer and develop less cardiac disease because they tolerate iron toxicity better, possibly as an effect of increased tolerance to chronic oxidative stress.

Keywords: thalassemia; survival; oxidative stress; gender; MRI T2*

Introduction

Regular blood transfusion and iron chelation have improved the survival of patients with thalassemia major, mainly as a consequence of a reduction in cardiac deaths due to iron overload. This favorable trend continues, thanks to the introduction of new oral iron chelators and imaging methods, which allow better management of iron overload. Unfortunately, the prevalence of complications is still high and cardiac disease remains the leading cause of death in these patients, amounting to 71% of all deaths.

All the studies have been concordant in documenting significantly better survival and less cardiac complications in female than in male patients.[1–3]

Role of iron

It has been known for several decades, since the original studies by Buja,[4] that the heart of thalassemic patients dying of cardiac disease is replete with iron. More recently, it has been demonstrated that iron is deposited more abundantly in the ventricular walls and in the epicardium, while the atria and the conduction system are less affected. The degree of cardiac dysfunction is proportional to the amount of iron deposited in individual myocardial fibers and to the number of fibers affected.[5]

Initially, the iron derived from the transfused red blood cells and in part absorbed from the gut, is stored in intracellular lysosomes in the form of ferritin and hemosiderin (the end-product of the degradation of ferritin). Ferritin is characterized by a highly conserved three-dimensional structure similar to a spherical shell, designed to accommodate large amounts of iron in a safe, soluble, and bioavailable form. The iron, stored in ferritin and hemosiderin, is nontoxic. Normally iron circulates bound to transferrin. However, when the amount of iron exceeds the iron-binding capacity of transferrin, it appears in plasma as non-transferrin-bound iron, whose toxicity is much greater than that of transferrin-iron because of its ability to promote hydroxyl radical formation, via the Fenton reaction, resulting in peroxidative damage. The damage to membrane lipids and proteins is mediated by reactive oxygen species, including the hydroxylic radical (OH°), the superoxide anion (O^{2-}), and hydrogen

doi: 10.1111/j.1749-6632.2010.05588.x

peroxide (H_2O_2).[6] In the heart, this results in impaired function of the mitochrondrial respiratory chain and abnormal energy metabolism.

Thalassemia

An Italian cooperative study that has been going on for the past 30 years, including over 1,000 thalassemia patients born since 1960, has demonstrated that, in 2003, 68% of the patients were alive at age 35 years, with significantly better survival rates for patients in younger birth cohorts and for females ($P = 0.0014$).[2]

Among patients for whom reliable data on complications were available, females had a lower incidence of heart failure (9.2% vs. 4.1%) and arrhythmias (8.1% vs. 3%). Of the patients with heart failure 71% were males.[2] Other complications such as diabetes, HIV infection, thrombosis, hypothyroidism, and hypogonadism were frequent, but, contrary to what observed for overall-survival, no association between sex and complication-free survival was found. In a Greek study, thalassemic women had 23% longer life expectancy than men[1] and in a large report from Cyprus, including the entire population born after 1974, a multivariate analysis demonstrated that the risk of death in women was less than half of the risk in men.[3] In all reported series, females live longer because of a lower prevalence of cardiac failure and arrhythmias.

To directly measure iron accumulation in the vital organs, we compared, by means of T2* MRI, cardiac and hepatic iron overload in males and females, enrolled in the Myocardial Iron Overload in Thalassemia (MIOT) project. MRI T2* has become a widely used, accurate, and noninvasive technique for monitoring iron overload in thalassemia patients.[5]

The MIOT project is a network involving 57 Italian thalassemia centers and six Italian MRI sites where cardiac magnetic resonance is performed using homogeneous, standardized and validated procedures.[7] All centers are linked by a web-based network, configured to collect and share patients' anamnestic, clinical, and diagnostic data.[8]

The method that we adopted measures the global heart iron and therefore is apt at identifying areas of iron deposition in different parts of the heart. This can be important in thalassemic hemosiderosis, where the distribution of iron in the heart is heterogeneous.[9]

In our study, all the patients were transfusion dependant and had been chelated with deferoxamine for the majority of their lives, without significant difference in compliance between males and females

We found that global heart T2* values were significantly lower in patients with heart failure, compared to those without heart failure, but males and females were at the same risk of accumulating iron in their hearts. Also, liver T2* was not different in males and females.[10]

We concluded that the increased survival of female patients could not be attributed to lower cardiac iron overload.

A better life expectancy in females is not exclusive of thalassemia. In fact, it has been observed also in other hemoglobinopathies and it is the rule in the general population and even in animals.

Other hemoglobinopathies

Several epidemiological studies on sickle cell disease and sickle cell-hemoglobin C have documented increased longevity in females.

In a prospective study conducted in the United States, the median age at death among patients with sickle cell disease was 42 years for males and 48 years for females. For patients with sickle cell-hemoglobin C disease median age at death was 60 years for males and 68 years for females.[11] Similar results have been reported from Tennessee.[12] Also studies from Jamaica[13] and Nigeria[14] have found that females with sickle cell disease have an age-related survival advantage over males, with better survival rates in adulthood. Patients with these hemoglobinopathies, contrary to patients with thalassemia, do not die of iron overload, but, for the most part, during an acute episode of pain, chest syndrome, or stroke.[11] Most authors, on the basis of recent studies, consider sickle cell anemia an inflammatory disease. They hypothesize that the sticky, stiff, oxidizing sickle red cell is an irritant that provokes an inflammatory response as it obstructs flow. The tissues are not only under-perfused, but also exposed to inflammatory cytokines, growth factors, and the actions of the activated cells that respond to and produce them.[15] In addition, studies on transgenic mice have suggested that part of the damage in sickle cell anemia could be due to reperfusion injury. The implication is that once oxygen is restored to ischemic tissues, oxygen radicals are formed, and inflammatory endothelial and tissue injury occurs.[16]

Survival by gender in the animal and in the population at large

Superior female longevity is quite widespread in the animal world. Female tarantulas commonly live into their thirties, whereas male tarantulas die after five years. Male honeybees live only weeks, while queens live years. Among mammals one could cite numerous examples, starting from male Wistar rats, who have an average life span of 24 months whereas the females' median life span is 29 months, that is, 14% more than in males. Female macaques live an average of eight years longer than males. And longer survivals have been documented for female bats, chimpanzees, and whales.[17]

A population census has existed in Sweden since 1749, making it one of the oldest reliable registers of this kind. Already at that time, a sex difference existed in terms of life expectancy. Between 1751 and 1790, in fact, the average life expectancy at birth was 36.6 years for women and 33.7 years for men. In the most recent update of life expectancy and mortality in 2002–2004 in the modern European Union, life expectancy was 75.1 years for men and 81.3 years for women.[18] Of the known supercentenarians (>110 years) 90% are women.

As pointed out by Austand,[17] the fact that this difference occurs in animals as well as in humans, indicates that the difference cannot be attributed to sociological differences but rather to specific biological characteristics of both genders.

So what are the possible explanations of better survival and reduced cardiac morbidity in patients with thalassemia, as well as in other hemoglobinopathies and in the population at large?

Hypotheses

In thalassemia patients, more scrupulous compliance with chelation therapy has been proposed as an explanation for the better results obtained. In fact, if females were more adherent than males to therapy, they would accumulate less iron in their heart and liver. However, in our series, ferritin levels were not significantly lower in females, suggesting that the iron control was no better than in males. Indeed, in a previous work we have found ferritin levels of females to be higher than that of males, both for patients alive and for patients who died the year after the ferritin measurements, suggesting a relative greater resistance of females to the damaging effects of iron. In addition, the magnetic resonance study performed in our large population of thalassemia patients does not support a preferential accumulation of iron in the hearts or in the livers of males.

One very popular hypothesis is that females live longer because of a more efficient immune system. It is difficult, however, to imagine how the immune system could protect female thalassemia patients against cardiac disease.[17]

Estrogens are also considered an important factor in protecting females at the cellular level. Recent research purports that high levels of estrogens in females protect them against ageing by up-regulating the expression of antioxidant, longevity-related genes, such as that of selenium-dependent glutathione peroxidase (GPx) and Mn-superoxide.[19] Again this hypothesis does not fit well in a population of female patients who, especially in the past, had delayed or absent puberty, and whose estrogen supplements are a relatively recent adjunct to their therapy.

The balancing effects of testosterone and estrogens in regulating the blood levels of LDL and HDL cholesterol, are also considered among the factors contributing to longer survival in females. However, our patients, both male and female, tend to have very low levels of total cholesterol.[20]

Recent ageing research in fruit flies, in *Caenorhabditis elegans*, a roundworm, and in mice has shown that a reduced activity of growth hormone and of the insulin-like growth factor 1 signaling cascade favors longevity.[17] However, patients with thalassemia have often growth hormone problems, both in males and females and, according to this hypothesis they should be protected from early death.

Another hypothesis is the so-called heterogametic sex hypothesis, according to which it is the lack of a second X chromosome that decreases longevity.[17] In practice, the theory goes, any deleterious alleles on the X chromosome could be compensated by the second X chromosome in females, but not in males.

Finally the most convincing, even if not all-explaining, is the oxidative stress hypothesis according to which oxygen radicals, produced as a consequence of metabolism, damage the cells and their machinery. The free radical theory of ageing was first proposed in the 1950s.[21,22] In 1980, Miquel introduced a further development of this theory, pointing to the role of mitochondria as source of free radicals and as a target of oxidative damage in the ageing cell.[23]

The differences in longevity between genders seem to be related to free radical production. In fact, females produce less radicals only in animal species in which they live longer than males. It has been observed that oxidative damage to key mitochondrial components is significantly greater in males than in females. Mitochondria from females produce approximately half the amount of H(2)O(2) than males. And, in addition, they overexpress both superoxide dismutase and glutathione peroxidase and, in general, have more efficient antioxidant defenses. A study comparing oxidative damage to DNA in males and females demonstrated significantly higher levels of modified DNA bases in males.[24] It has been proposed that this is due to estrogens that act by binding to the estrogen receptors and subsequently activating the mitogen activated protein (MAP) kinase and nuclear factor kappa B (NF-κB) signaling pathways.[19]

The damage due to reactive oxygen species can be limited by the administration of antioxidants. Glutathione is a major intracellular antioxidant, whose intracellular levels are considered a biological marker of ageing and mitochondrial glutathione is related to the damage associated with ageing.[19]

As mentioned earlier, in patients with iron overload, hydroxyl radicals, notoriously implicated in vascular damage, especially in the presence of iron overload, are ubiquitous and very damaging. The better survival and reduced cardiac morbidity of females could, according to this hypothesis, be explained by the fact that, probably in addition to other factors, females are better equipped in quenching the damage due to reactive oxygen species generated by non transferrin bound iron. Further research is needed in this field.

If we could clearly understand the reasons for the better survival of female patients with thalassemia and the mechanisms at the base of the protection against reactive oxygen species, we could, hopefully, increase the longevity of males whether affected or not by thalassemia.

Acknowledgments

We wish to thank Ms. Cinzia Tonioli for helpful secretarial assistance.

Conflicts of interest

The authors declare no conflicts of interest.

References

1. Chouliaras, G., C.T. Yiannoutsos, V. Berdoukas & V. Ladis. 2009. Cardiac related death in thalassaemia major: time trend and risk factors in a large Greek Unit. *Eur. J. Haematol.* **82:** 381–387.
2. Borgna-Pignatti, C., S. Rugolotto, P. De Stefano, *et al.* 2004. Survival and complications in patients with thalassemia major treated with transfusion and deferoxamine. *Haematologica* **89:** 1187–1193.
3. Telfer, P.T., F. Warburton, S. Christou, *et al.* 2009. Improved survival in thalassemia major patients on switching from desferrioxamine to combined chelation therapy with desferrioxamine and deferiprone. *Haematologica* **94:** 1777–1778.
4. Buja, L.M. & W.C. Roberts. 1971. Iron in the heart. Etiology and clinical significance. *Am. J. Med.* **51:** 209–221.
5. Cohen, A.R., R. Galanello, D.J. Pennell, *et al.* 2004. Thalassemia. *Hematol. Am. Soc. Hematol. Educ. Program* 14–34.
6. Breuer, W., C. Hershko & Z.I. Cabantchik. 2000. The importance of non-transferrin bound iron in disorders of iron metabolism. *Transfus. Sci.* **23:** 185–192.
7. Ramazzotti, A., A. Pepe, V. Positano, *et al.* 2009. Multicenter validation of the magnetic resonance T2* technique for segmental and global quantification of myocardial iron. *J. Magn. Reson. Imaging* **30:** 62–68.
8. Meloni, A., A. Ramazzotti, V. Positano, *et al.* 2009. Evaluation of a web-based network for reproducible T2* MRI assessment of iron overload in thalassemia. *Int. J. Med. Inf.* **78:** 503–512.
9. Pepe A, V. Positano, M.F. Santarelli, *et al.* 2006. Multislice multiecho T2* cardiovascular magnetic resonance for detection of the heterogeneous distribution of myocardial iron overload. *J. Magn. Reson. Imaging* **23:** 662–668.
10. Marsella, M, C. Borgna-Pignatti, A. Meloni, *et al.* 2010. Cardiac iron loading measured by multislice multiecho T2* MRI and cardiac disease in male and female patients with thalassemia major. In Press.
11. Platt, O.S., D.J. Brambilla, W.F. Rosse, *et al.* 1994. Mortality in sickle cell disease. Life expectancy and risk factors for early death. *N. Engl. J. Med.* **330:** 1639–1644.
12. Shankar, S.M., P.G. Arbogast, E. Mitchel, *et al.* 2005. Medical care utilization and mortality in sickle cell disease: a population-based study. *Am. J. Hematol.* **80:** 262–270.
13. Wierenga, K.J., I.R. Hambleton & N.A. Lewis. 2001. Survival estimates for patients with homozygous sickle-cell disease in Jamaica: a clinic based population study. *Lancet* **357:** 680–683.
14. Kotila, T.R. & W.A. Shokunbi. 2001. Survival advantage in female patients with sickle cell anaemia. *East Afr. Med. J.* **78:** 373–375.
15. Platt, O.S. 2000. Sickle cell anemia as an inflammatory disease. *J. Clin. Invest.* **106:** 337–338.
16. Kaul, D.K. & R.P. Hebbel. 2000. Hypoxia/reoxygenation causes inflammatory response in transgenic sickle mice but not in normal mice. *J. Clin. Invest.* **106:** 411–420.

17. Austad, S.N. 2006. Why women live longer than men: sex differences in longevity. *Gend. Med.* **3:** 79–92.
18. Bonneux, L.G., C.C. Huisman & J.A. de Beer. 2010. Mortality in 272 European regions, 2002–2004. An update. *Eur. J. Epidemiol.* **25:** 77–85.
19. Vina, J., C. Borràs, J. Gambini, *et al.* 2005. Why females live longer than males? Importance of the upregulation of longevity-associated genes by oestrogenic compounds. *FEBS Lett.* **579:** 2541–2545.
20. Shalev, H., J. Kapelushnik, A. Moser, *et al.* 2007. Hypocholesterolemia in chronic anemias with increased erythropoietic activity. *Am. J. Hematol.* **82:** 199–202.
21. Gerschman, R., D.L. Gilbert, S.W. Nye, *et al.* 1954. Oxygen poisoning and X irradiation: a mechanism in common. *Science* **119:** 623–626.
22. Harman, D. 1956. Aging: a theory based on free radical and radiation chemistry. *J. Gerontol.* **11:** 298–300.
23. Miquel, J., A.C. Economos, J. Fleming & J.E. Johnson. 1980. Mitochondrial role in cell aging. *Exp. Gerontol.* **15:** 575–591.
24. Proteggente, A.R., T.G. England, A. Rehman, *et al.* 2002. Gender differences in steady-state levels of oxidative damage to DNA in healthy individuals. *Free Radic. Res.* **36:** 157–162.

Ann. N.Y. Acad. Sci. ISSN 0077-8923

ANNALS OF THE NEW YORK ACADEMY OF SCIENCES
Issue: *Cooley's Anemia: Ninth Symposium*

A preclinical approach for gene therapy of β-thalassemia

Laura Breda,[1] Dorothy A. Kleinert,[1] Carla Casu,[1] Laura Casula,[1] Luca Cartegni,[2] Eitan Fibach,[3] Irene Mancini,[4] Patricia J. Giardina,[1] Roberto Gambari,[4] and Stefano Rivella[1]

[1]Department of Pediatrics, Division of Hematology-Oncology, Weill Cornell Medical College, Children's Blood and Cancer Foundation Laboratories, New York, New York. [2]Department of Molecular Pharmacology and Chemistry, Memorial Sloan Kettering Cancer Center, New York, New York. [3]Department of Hematology, Hadassah – Hebrew University Medical Center, Jerusalem, Israel. [4]Department of Biochemistry and Molecular Biology, Division of Molecular Biology, University of Ferrrara, Ferrara, Italy

Address for correspondence: Stefano Rivella, 515E 71 Street Room S-702, New York, NY 10021. str2010@med.cornell.edu

Lentiviral-mediated β-globin gene transfer successfully treated β-thalassemic mice. Based on this result, clinical trials were initiated. To date, however, no study has investigated the efficacy of gene therapy in relation to the nature of the different β-globin mutations found in patients. Most mutations can be classified as β^0 or β^+, based on the amount of β-globin protein produced. Therefore, we propose that a screening *in vitro* is necessary to verify the efficacy of gene transfer prior to treatment of individual patients. We used a two-phase liquid culture system to expand and differentiate erythroid progenitor cells (ErPCs) transduced with lentiviral vectors. We propose the use of this system to test the efficiency of lentiviral vectors carrying the human β-globin gene, to correct the phenotype of ErPCs from patients preparing for gene therapy. This new approach might have profound implications for designing gene therapy and for understanding the genotype/phenotype variability observed in Cooley's anemia patients.

Keywords: β-thalassemia; β-globin; gene therapy; lentiviral vectors; hemoglobin; erythroid progenitor cells

Introduction

β-Thalassemia alleles that are associated with lacking or limited β-globin chain synthesis are classified as β^0 or β^+, respectively. Based on the combination of these two alleles, thalassemic patients are classified as $\beta^{0/0}$, $\beta^{+/0}$, or $\beta^{+/+1}$. This classification, however, falls short of describing the various mechanisms that cause each mutation to interfere with the synthesis of the β-globin chain. The majority of the more than 200 mutations leading to thalassemia affect globin gene transcription, mRNA processing or translation.[1] For instance, the point mutations $\beta^0$39 and β^+IVS1–110 represent the most common alleles in the Mediterranean area. $\beta^0$39 introduces a termination codon in position 39 and triggers a rapid degradation of the mutant mRNA by nonsense mediated decay (NMD) resulting in low accumulation of β^0-globin mRNA and absence of β-globin chains.[2,3] β^+IVS1–110 activates an aberrant 3′ cryptic splice site without completely abolishing normal splicing.[4] In this case, some normal mRNA and protein are made.

Our long-term objective is to investigate how mutations in the human β-globin gene influence the outcome of gene transfer in β-thalassemia. Our research,[5–9] along with that of others reviewed in Rivella and Rachmilewitz[10] and Breda and colleagues,[11] showed that it is possible to rescue β-thalassemia mice by lentiviral-mediated transfer of the human β-globin gene, its promoter, introns and large portions of the locus control region (LCR). The original studies, however, used β-globin knocked out mice,[12,13] which do not carry the large spectrum of mutations observed in patients. Based on the studies successfully completed in mice, clinical trials have been proposed or are underway,[14] but so far only a limited amount of information is available from these endeavors.[15] We believe that there is a gap between our knowledge of the primary mutation, the corresponding phenotype, and the therapeutic approach required to correct the phenotype, based on

doi: 10.1111/j.1749-6632.2010.05594.x

the individual's genotype (i.e., our understanding of the disease and its treatment by genetic modalities). We hypothesized that the sequence, timing and differential expression of endogenous globin mRNA in patients could influence the ability of a transgenic β-globin mRNAs to correct the thalassemic phenotype. If this were confirmed, it would suggest the desirability of performing an *in vitro* test to assess the potential outcome of β-globin gene transfer prior to treatment.

Lentiviral vector design and production

To investigate our hypothesis, we generated a protocol to correlate (A) the number of viral integrants, e.g., vector copy number (VCN), (B) the amount of β-globin mRNA, and (C) the hemoglobin (Hb) production in erythroid progenitor cells (ErPCs) following *in vitro* β-globin gene transfer and erythroid differentiation.[16] Our ultimate goal is to compare these parameters with those from untransduced ErPCs obtained from patients, carriers and normal donors processed in the same fashion. A scheme of the procedure and analyses is shown in Figure 1A. For our experiments we used a vector named T9W,[16] (Fig. 1B), which is a modified version of TNS9, a lentiviral vector carrying the human β-globin gene and large elements of the LCR that was able to improve the anemia in thalassemic mice.[5,6,17,18] To increase the safety and efficiency of TNS9, we disarmed the 3′ long terminal repeat (3' LTR) by deleting the U3 region (self inactivating-LTR or SIN-LTR, Fig. 1B).[18] This deletion, which includes the TATA box and all the major determinants responsible for regulating the HIV-1 promoter, abolished the promoter activity of the LTR,[19–22] but did not affect vector titers or transgene expression *in vitro.*[16] We also introduced the *cis*-acting woodchuck post regulatory element (WPRE)[23] between the LCR and the 3' SIN-LTR. WPRE has been shown to increase transcription and stability of lentiviral RNA as well as virus production, but not of the β-globin mRNA, because it is not included in its transcript. An additional vector, named pPeGW (Fig. 1C), was initially used to verify the ability of our lentiviral system to infect human ErPCs (Fig. 1D).[16] This vector was generated by replacing the whole β-globin expression cassette in T9W with the housekeeping human-phosphoglycerate (PGK) promoter driving expression of the enhanced-green fluorescent protein (eGFP).[16,18] Viral stocks were generated by co-transfection into 293T cells of the gene transfer plasmid T9W together with the envelope plasmid (VSV-G), the packaging plasmid (pMDLg/p RRE) and pRSV-REV vector, which expresses the Rev protein. Rev binds the Rev responsive element (RRE) and is essential for posttranscriptional transport of the unspliced viral mRNAs from nuclei to cytoplasm.[22,24,25] Twenty-four hours prior to transfection, 5×10^6 293T cells were seeded onto 10-cm cell culture dishes in 10 mL of Iscove's modification of Eagle's medium containing 10% fetal calf serum, 100 U/mL penicillin and 100 mg/mL streptomycin. The cells were incubated at 37° C under a 5% CO_2. The culture medium was changed 2 h prior to transfection. The precipitate was formed by adding 50 uL of 2M $CaCl_2$ to a suspension of the plasmids in 450 uL of $0.1 \times$ TE ($0.1\times$ TE is 10 mM Tris plus 1 mM EDTA), followed by adding 500 uL of $2\times$ HEPES-buffered saline (281 mM NaCl, 100 mM HEPES, 1.5 mM Na_2HPO_4) drop-wise while vortexing. The viral precipitate was immediately added to the 293T cultures. The culture medium was replaced after 16 h. The viral supernatant was collected at 24 and 48 h from the washing step, cleared by low speed centrifugation, and filtered through 0.2 um cellulose acetate filters. Viral concentration was then achieved by ultracentrifugation.

Two-phase liquid culture and cells transduction

We modified the protocol described by Fibach and Rachmilewitz.[18,26] Consented normal individuals and patients with β-thalassemia major donated 20–30 mL of peripheral blood, which was collected into EDTA-treated sterile tubes.[16] The mononuclear cell fraction, containing erythroid precursors, was obtained by Ficoll-Hypaque density gradient centrifugation. The mononuclear cells were then seeded into α-modified essential medium (α-MEM), containing 10% fetal calf serum, 10% conditioned medium from the 5637 bladder carcinoma cell line, 10 ng/mL stem cell factor, cyclosporine A, streptomycin and glutamine (phase 1). After 5–7 days, the nonadherent cells were harvested, washed, and transferred into fresh media with 30% fetal calf serum, 10% deionized bovine serum albumin, 10^{-5}M β-mercaptoethanol and 10^{-6}M dexamethasone.[18,26] Erythropoietin was added (2 U/mL) to stimulate erythroid differentiation (phase 2).[18,26] Cells were infected at the beginning of phase 2 with the viral

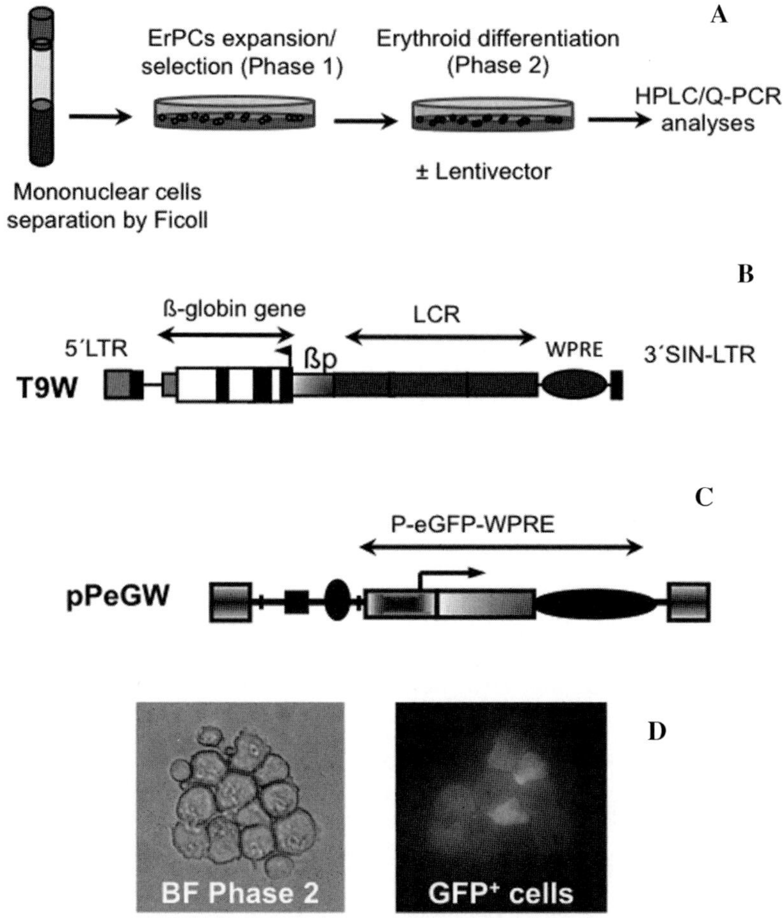

Figure 1. (A) Schematic representation of the isolation, expansion, and differentiation of erythroid progenitor cells (ErPCs). Cells were infected at the beginning of phase 2. (B) The lentiviral vector used in this study (T9W) is improved by the insertion of the CMV promoter in the 5′LTR, a partial deletion of the 3′LTR, and the inclusion of the woodchuck hepatitis virus posttranscriptional regulatory element (WPRE) to increase safety and production, respectively. Black rectangles represent exons of the **β**-globin gene (in B). We initially tested the ability of our lentiviral system to infect ErPCs using a lentiviral vector, named pPeGW, encoding the enhanced fluorescent protein (C). (D) GFP positive ErPCs infected with pPeGW are photographed in bright field (left) or with a fluorescent filter (right).

solution, starting from a multiplicity of infection (MOI) of 0.3 and up to sixfold higher MOI. Cells were harvested on day 10 of phase 2 for analyses. The pPeGW construct was initially used to optimize the conditions for infecting ErPC, including the number of viral molecules integrated into the genome. A low VCN (between 0.2 and 3) is required to minimize genotoxicity from the prospective of using the lentiviral system in a clinical setting. pPeGW was also used to confirm that viral integration *per se* does not alter the amounts or percentages of Hbs in either healthy or thalassemic cells.[16] In Figure 1C representative, normal cultured ErPCs infected with pPeGW are shown. These cells expressed eGFP as shown by fluorescence microscopy (Fig. 1D) and FACS analysis.[16] Cell morphology and hemoglobin content were analyzed by light microscopy on cytocentrifuged smears stained with O-tolidine followed by May–Grunwald–Giemsa staining. Hemoglobin-containing cells were identified in the culture by benzidine staining. For all staining procedures we followed standard methods already described in the literature.

Analysis of β-globin mRNA and protein synthesis

Retrotranscription of total mRNA was followed by real-time PCR (RT-PCR) assays using specific

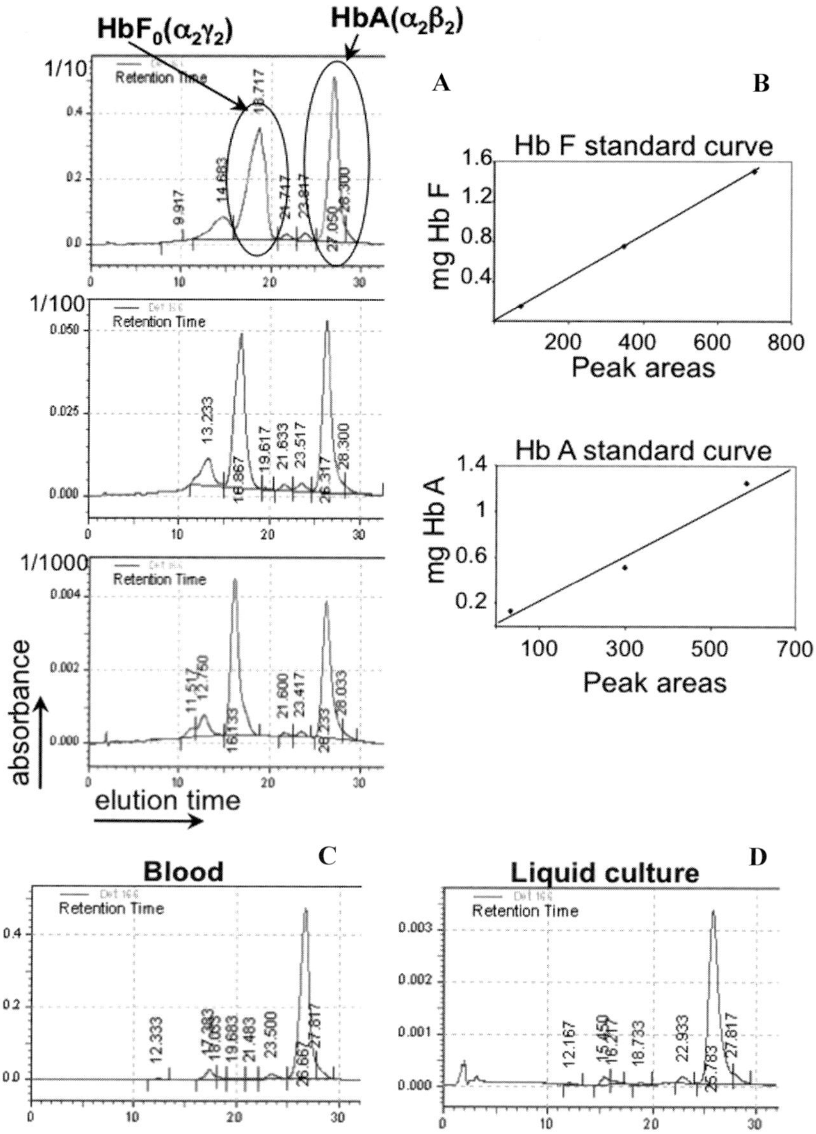

Figure 2. (A) shows the HPLC profiles of three different amounts (from top to bottom: 0.22, 0.022, and 0.0022 mg total Hb, respectively) with known proportions of HbA and HbF. (B) Standard curves obtained by plotting the quantities of HbA or HbF and the areas under the respective peaks, using the serial dilution shown in (A). The HPLC hemoglobin profiles of the blood (C) and cultured ErPCs of the same healthy individual (D) are shown. HbF and HbA peaks correspond to elution times of 16 and 26 min, respectively.

oligonuclotides for β-globin and α-globin, and the human glyceraldehyde-3-phosphate dehydrogenase (GAPDH) and human 18S ribosomal as endogenous controls.[16] The number of integrations (VCN) was quantified by RT-PCR using oligos for a specific sequence present in the vector (WPRE) and compared to an endogenous control present in two copies in the genome (ID1 gene).[16] Moreover, we infected murine erythroleukemia cells and clones bearing one, two, or three copies of T9W were isolated as described in Rivella and colleagues,[17] DNA from these clones was used to quantify the VCN in transduced ErPCs using the oligonucleotides for WPRE and ID1. The oligonucleotides for ID1 were designed so that they could amplify both the human and murine versions of the gene.[18] Cells pellets were lysed with HPLC grade water and loaded into an Akta Purifier instrument. Hbs were separated on a cation-exchange Synchropak CM300 column and detected at wavelength of 415 nm. The Hbs were bound to the column while dissolved in mobile phase B (10 mmol/L Bis-Tris, 1 mmol/L KCN, pH 6.15) and then gradually eluted with mobile phase A (10 mmol/L Bis-Tris, 1 mmol/L KCN containing sodium acetate trihydrate, pH 6.3) in a gradient ranging from 90 to 10% of mobile phase B over 40 column volumes. Serial dilutions of a solution with known concentrations of HbA and HbF were used to generate a calibration curve, where the area under the curve was plotted against the concentrations. The Hb content of the samples was then calculated from the standard curve. The types of Hbs were determined by elution time. To identify the peaks corresponding to the different Hbs in ErPCs and their concentrations, we used standard Hb solutions. In Figure 2A standard curves generated using purified hemoglobin A and F are shown. We analyzed the HPLC profiles of three serial dilutions derived from HbA and HbF solution, with known concentration. We then correlated the concentrations of HbA and HbF with with their respective peak areas, generating two calibration curves (Fig. 2B). The peak areas can be used to quantify Hbs concentration in normal or patients HPLC profiles.

Analysis of ErPCs from β-thalassemic patients

A large fraction of ErPCs from thalassemic patients might be lost during the last period of differentiation due to accumulation of α-aggregates and subsequent apoptosis. For this reason, we compared the percentages and absolute amounts of HbA in cultured at day 10 of phase 2. To control for the level of differentiation and to use a very stringent cutoff for each sample, we analyzed only cultures that exhibited ≥95% positivity to benzidine staining. Comparing the results on day 14 to those on day 10, we observed only a slight increase in the percentage of HbA (roughly 2.5%) and a 1.5-fold increase in the absolute Hb content. This indicates that, although the total amount of hemoglobin is increased on day 14, the percentage of HbA is relatively stable from day 10 and day 14. Thus, we routinely analyzed cells on day 10, although on many occasions we also analyzed cells on day 14 to exclude major differences in HbA during differentiation.

To assess the validity of the culture system, we compared its Hb profile to that of peripheral blood

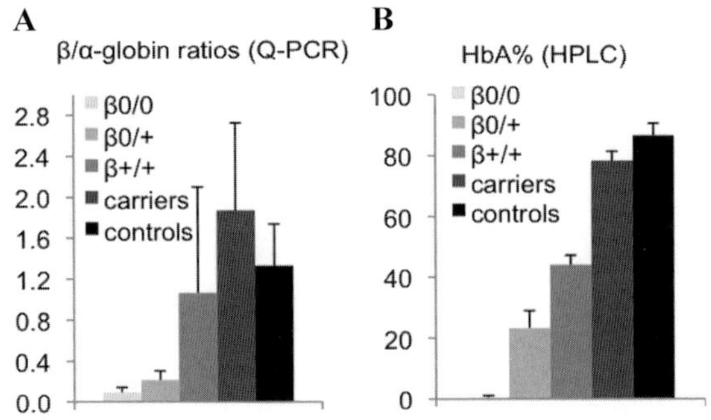

Figure 3. The β/α-globin mRNA ratios of ErPCs from control donors, carriers, and three patients groups ($\beta^{+/+}$, $\beta^{+/0}$, and $\beta^{0/0}$) were analyzed by Q-PCR (A) and HPLC (B).

of the same individual (Fig. 2C and D). The results showed that the cultured cells achieved a percentage of HbA (88.82%) comparable to that observed in the blood (86.56%), indicating that cultured ErPCs recapitulated very closely the relative proportion of HbA observed *in vivo*. To determine the baseline of α- and β-globin mRNA and Hb levels in ErPCs from healthy controls, carriers and thalassemic patients, we analyzed more than 40 specimens.[16] In each group of patients, the baseline α- and β-globin mRNA values were compared to those found in cells from healthy controls ($N = 8$) and asymptomatic carriers ($N = 6$), having only one allele affected by β-thalassemic trait. The average β/α-globins mRNA was 1.32 ± 0.38 in the healthy controls, 1.80 ± 0.85 in the carriers, and 0.01 ± 0.05, 0.22 ± 0.09, and 0.91 ± 1.04 in the three thalassemic groups (classified as $\beta^{0/0}$, $\beta^{0/+}$, and $\beta^{+/+}$, respectively) (Fig. 3A). The percentages of HbA were 85.5 ± 4.1 in normal donor cells, 77.0 ± 3.6 in the cells of carriers, 44.3 ± 4.9 in $\beta^{+/+}$ cells, 25.6 ± 8.9 in $\beta^{0/+}$ cells, and 0.8 ± 1.1 in $\beta^{0/0}$ cells (Fig. 3B).[16] We then transduced (VCN = 1) ErPCs from a $\beta^{0/0}$39 homozygous patient with T9W and subsequently analyzed the untreated and treated samples for differentiation by benzidine staining, for globin mRNA content by Q-PCR and for Hbs by HPLC. Compared to healthy cells, $\beta^{0/0}$39 ErPCs do not produce any HbA, as indicated by the arrow in Figure 4A. After transduction with T9W, the HbA (consisting of α- and β-globin chains) increased from 0 to 42% (Fig. 4B). Furthermore, compared to untreated cells, ErPCs treated with T9W were more differentiated as shown by the O-tolidine staining and morphological analysis (Fig. 4C and D).[18]

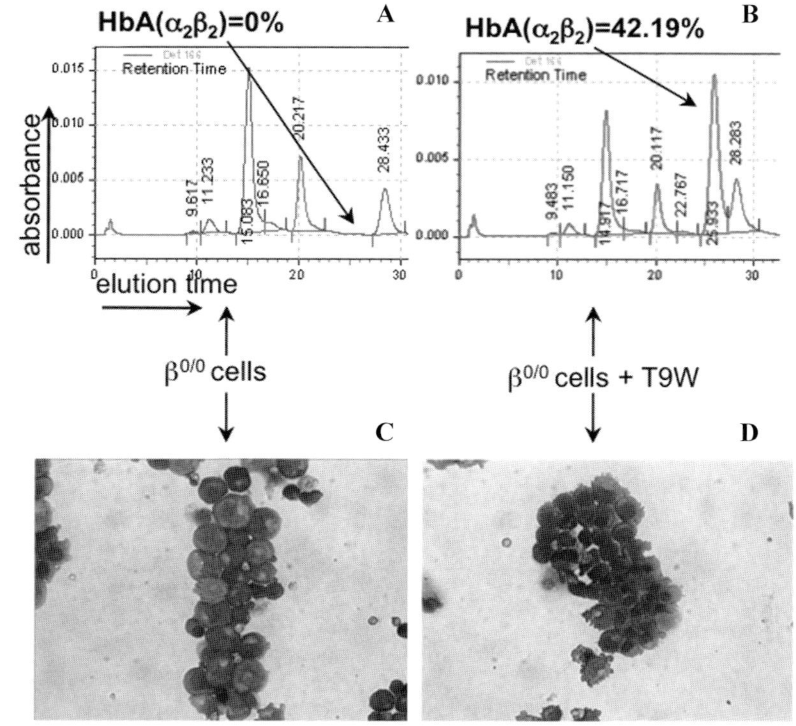

Figure 4. The HPLC profile of $\beta^{0/0}$39 homozygous ErPCs is shown at baseline (A) and after integration of T9W (B) with VCN = 1. The same cells were observed after O-tolidine-Giemsa staining for erythoid stage analysis and hemoglobin quantification (C and D).

Future prospects

Our analyses confirmed that the two-phase liquid culture is a reliable *in vitro* model that replicates *in vivo* erythroid differentiation. Based on our observations, we propose that this approach could be used to predict the outcome of gene transfer *in vivo*. Blood and cultured ErPCs were found to exhibit a similar proportion of HbA. Both the total and relative Hb types were determined by comparison with a solution of HbA and HbF of known concentration. We assessed the baseline levels of β- and α-globin mRNA and their imbalance by quantitative Q-PCR in $\beta^{+/+}$, $\beta^{0/+}$, and $\beta^{0/0}$ ErPCs. As expected, we found aggravated imbalance in samples with the β^0 phenotype, in accordance with the amount of HbA produced. Following treatment with T9W, a lentiviral vector carrying the human β-globin gene and regulatory elements of the human LCR, $\beta^{0/0}$ ErPCs carrying the mutation β°-39 in homozygosity, showed a remarkable amelioration of their thalassemic phenotype as indicated by significant accumulation of HbA, observed by HPLC analysis. Following infection with VCN = 1, HbA increased from 0 to more than 40% of the total Hb. This result is encouraging and supports the findings reported in mice either homozygous or heterozygous for a β^0 mutation. Moreover, this preliminary data suggests that a single copy of T9W might produce 50% as much HbA as produced in normal cells. This level of HbA content might even improve *in vivo*, where HbA-producing cells might have selective growth/survival advantages. Further analyses are necessary to verify the ability of gene therapy in the β-thalassemia population at large, the main reason being that the β^0 mutation represents only a limited subset of the mutations found in patients.

In conclusion, our goal is to use the methodology described here to determine the efficacy of gene therapy $\beta^{+/+}$, $\beta^{\ 0/+}$, and $\beta^{0/0}$ thalassemia patients with different mutations. We believe that this study will facilitate the translation process of effective gene therapy for β-thalassemia into the clinical setting and more generally will help in our understanding of the complexity involved in genotype/phenotype variability.

Acknowledgments

This work was supported by the Cooley's Anemia Foundation (L.B.), by the Associazione Veneta per la Lotta alla Talassemia (AVLT) of Rovigo (C.C.), by the Associazione Regionale Sarda per la Lotta Contro la Thalassemia e per l'Assistenza dei Talassemici (L.C.), by Telethon (contract GGP07257) (R.G.), by Fondazione CARIPARO (R.G.), by the NIH grant 5K01DK063992, Clinical and Translational Science Center (CTSC; NIH grants UL1RR024992), and the Carlo and Micol Schejola Foundation (S.R.). We thank Dr. Michel Sadelain for providing us the TNS9 vector.

Conflicts of interest

The authors declare no conflicts of interest.

References

1. Steinberg, M.H. *et al.* 2001. *Disorders of hemoglobin: Genetics, Pathophysiology and Clinical Management*. Cambridge University Press. Cambridge, UK.
2. Maquat, L.E. *et al.* 1981. Unstable beta-globin mRNA in mRNA-deficient beta o thalassemia. *Cell* **27:** 543–553.
3. Romao, L. *et al.* 2000. Nonsense mutations in the human beta-globin gene lead to unexpected levels of cytoplasmic mRNA accumulation. *Blood* **96:** 2895–2901.
4. Spritz, R.A. *et al.* 1981. Base substitution in an intervening sequence of a beta+-thalassemic human globin gene. *Proc. Natl. Acad. Sci. USA* **78:** 2455–2459.
5. May, C. *et al.* 2000. Therapeutic haemoglobin synthesis in beta-thalassaemic mice expressing lentivirus-encoded human beta-globin. *Nature* **406:** 82–86.
6. May, C. *et al.* 2002. Successful treatment of murine beta-thalassemia intermedia by transfer of the human beta-globin gene. *Blood* **99:** 1902–1908.
7. Rivella, S. & M. Sadelain. 2002. Therapeutic globin gene delivery using lentiviral vectors. *Curr. Opin. Mol. Ther.* **4:** 505–514.
8. Breda, L. & S. Rivella. 2003. Development of new mouse models to study globin gene regulation. *Minerva Biotecnologica.* **15:** 107–121.
9. Rivella, S. *et al.* 2003. A novel murine model of Cooley anemia and its rescue by lentiviral-mediated human beta -globin gene transfer. *Blood* **101:** 2932–2939.
10. Rivella, S. & E. Rachmilewitz. 2009. Future alternative therapies for β-thalassemia. *Expert Rev. Hematol.* **2:** 685–697.
11. Breda, L., R. Gambari & S. Rivella. 2009. Gene therapy in thalassemia and hemoglobinopathies. *Mediterr. J. Hematol. Infect. Dis.* **1**.
12. Ciavatta, D.J. *et al.* 1995. Mouse model of human beta zero thalassemia: targeted deletion of the mouse beta maj- and beta min-globin genes in embryonic stem cells. *Proc. Natl. Acad. Sci. USA* **92:** 9259–9263.
13. Yang, B. *et al.* 1995. A mouse model for beta 0-thalassemia. *Proc. Natl. Acad. Sci. USA* **92:** 11608–11612.
14. Bank, A., R. Dorazio & P. Leboulch. 2005. A phase I/II clinical trial of beta-globin gene therapy for beta-thalassemia. *Ann. N.Y. Acad. Sci.* **1054:** 308–316.
15. Kaiser, J. 2009. Gene therapy. Beta-thalassemia treatment succeeds, with a caveat. *Science* **326:** 1468–1469.
16. Breda, L. *et al.* 2009. *Following Beta-Globin Gene Transfer, the Production of Hemoglobin Depends upon the -Thalassemia Genotype: The Traffic Jam Hypothesis*. American Society of Gene Therapy (ASGT). San Diego.
17. Rivella, S. *et al.* 2000. The cHS4 insulator increases the probability of retroviral expression at random chromosomal integration sites. *J. Virol.* **74:** 4679–4687.
18. Breda, L. *et al.* 2009. Following beta-globin gene transfer, the production of hemoglobin depends upon the beta-thalassemia genotype. *Blood* **114:** 978.
19. Liu, J. *et al.* 1992. Specific NF-kappa B subunits act in concert with Tat to stimulate human immunodeficiency virus type 1 transcription. *J. Virol.* **66:** 3883–3887.
20. Ross, E.K. *et al.* 1991. Contribution of NF-kappa B and Sp1 binding motifs to the replicative capacity of human immunodeficiency virus type 1: distinct patterns of viral growth are determined by T-cell types. *J. Virol.* **65:** 4350–4358.
21. Zeichner, S.L., J.Y. Kim & J.C. Alwine. 1991. Linker-scanning mutational analysis of the transcriptional activity of the human immunodeficiency virus type 1 long terminal repeat. *J. Virol.* **65:** 2436–2444.
22. Zufferey, R. *et al.* 1998. Self-inactivating lentivirus vector for safe and efficient in vivo gene delivery. *J. Virol.* **72:** 9873–9880.
23. Zufferey, R. *et al.* 1999. Woodchuck hepatitis virus post-transcriptional regulatory element enhances expression of transgenes delivered by retroviral vectors. *J. Virol.* **73:** 2886–2892.
24. Miyoshi, H. *et al.* 1998. Development of a self-inactivating lentivirus vector. *J. Virol.* **72:** 8150–8157.
25. Dull, T. *et al.* 1998. A third-generation lentivirus vector with a conditional packaging system. *J. Virol.* **72:** 8463–8471.
26. Fibach, E. & E.A. Rachmilewitz. 1993. The two-step liquid culture: a novel procedure for studying maturation of human normal and pathological erythroid precursors. *Stem Cells* **11**(Suppl 1): 36–41.

Ann. N.Y. Acad. Sci. ISSN 0077-8923

ANNALS OF THE NEW YORK ACADEMY OF SCIENCES
Issue: *Cooley's Anemia: Ninth Symposium*

The role of reduced intensity preparative regimens in patients with thalassemia given hematopoietic transplantation

Alice Bertaina,[1] Maria Ester Bernardo,[1] Angela Mastronuzzi,[1] Giorgio La Nasa,[2] and Franco Locatelli[1]

[1]University of Pavia, Department of Paediatric Haematology/Oncology, Ospedale Bambino Gesù, Rome, Italy. [2]Unità Operativa Centro Trapianti Midollo Osseo, Ospedale R. Binaghi, Cagliari, Italy

Address for correspondence: Prof. Franco Locatelli, M.D., Dipartimento di Scienze Pediatriche, Università di Pavia, IRCCS Ospedale Bambino Gesù, Piazzale Sant'Onofrio 4, 00165-I Rome, Italy. f.locatelli@opbg.net

Allogeneic hematopoietic stem cell transplantation (HSCT) still remains the only curative treatment for patients with thalassemia major (TM). However, HSCT is associated with a non-negligible risk of both transplantation-related mortality (TRM) and morbidity. Great interest and relevant expectations have been raised by the introduction in the clinical practice of reduced-intensity preparative regimens, which may represent an effective strategy to reduce the toxicity of transplantation and may also help reduce the incidence of late effects. Although some reports have documented the feasibility of using reduced-intensity preparative regimens for successfully treating patients with TM, a high incidence of graft failure has been frequently reported. Recently, treosulfan-based myeloablation has been demonstrated to be associated with limited extra-medullary toxicity and a high rate of sustained donor engraftment. This novel approach is a promising alternative for reducing the risk of life-threatening complications and increasing the number of TM patients successfully cured with an allograft.

Keywords: thalassemia; allogeneic hematopoietic stem cell transplantation; reduced-intensity preparative regimens; cord blood; unrelated donors

Introduction

There is no doubt that the last two decades have witnessed a dramatic improvement in both survival and quality of life of patients with thalassemia major (TM).[1–3] Indeed, especially in Western countries, the optimization of blood transfusion regimens and iron chelation therapy, as well as the availability of new iron-chelating agents which can be taken by mouth and allow better compliance with chelation,[4,5] have changed a previously fatal disease with early death, to a chronic, although progressive, disease compatible with prolonged survival.[2,3,6] Despite the improvements in conservative treatment that have considerably ameliorated the life-expectancy of patients with TM, hematopoietic stem cell transplantation (HSCT) still remains the only curative treatment for this disorder.[7–10] Since the first allograft performed almost 30 years ago,[11] hundreds of patients with TM have been cured after having received HSCT, in most cases performed using an HLA-identical sibling as donor and bone marrow (BM) as stem cell source.[7–10] More recently, the use of BM from an unrelated volunteer, selected using high-resolution molecular typing of class I and II HLA loci and stringent criteria of immunogenetic compatibility, has proved to be a valuable alternative for patients lacking a compatible family donor.[12–15] In fact, the proportion of patients successfully cured with HSCT from an unrelated volunteer approaches that reported in patients transplanted from an HLA-identical relative.[12–15] In terms of alternative stem cell sources, the Eurocord cooperative group has reported that patients with TM can be safely transplanted with cord blood cells from a sibling, no patient out of the

doi: 10.1111/j.1749-6632.2010.05590.x

33 analysed having died for transplantation-related complications.[16]

The risk of fatal complications and of graft failure after HSCT

Although HSCT is the only treatment able to definitively cure TM, as well as other severe hemoglobinopathies, it is associated with a consistent risk of complications that can dramatically shorten the life duration of some patients. Indeed, in different reports on TM patients given HSCT, transplantation-related mortality (TRM) has been reported to range between 5% and 35% and it has been demonstrated to be mainly dependent on patient age, iron overload and liver viral infections, especially when they result into active chronic hepatitis or liver cirrhosis.[7,9,10,17,18] Among pediatric patients (i.e., those with an age younger than 18 years) with TM, three classes of risk have been identified by the Pesaro group on the basis of regularity of previous iron chelation, liver enlargement and presence of portal fibrosis.[9,10,17] The best results in terms of probability of thalassemia-free survival and risk of dying due to transplantation-related complications can be obtained in patients with limited iron overload and without severe organ damage.[17,18] These patients, belonging to the class 1 and 2 of the Pesaro classification, have a probability of survival with transfusion independence in the order of 85%[9] and are the "ideal" candidates for an allograft, whereas older, heavily iron-overloaded patients (i.e., class 3 patients who are those having low compliance with iron chelation and showing signs of severe liver damage) run a considerable risk of transplantation-related life-threatening complications.[7,9,10] The risk of experiencing fatal complications for patients with TM given the allograft during adulthood has been reported to be comparable (in the order of 20–30%) to that of children belonging to the class 3 of the Pesaro classification.[8] Although adult patients with reduced compliance to iron chelation and children belonging to the class 3 of the Pesaro classification are those at greater risk of dying for transplantation-related complications, it is also to be mentioned they are those, whenever the transplant is successful, who receive the maximum benefit from it, given their much reduced life expectancy.

Another relevant impediment to the success of allogeneic HSCT for the cure of TM is represented by graft rejection, whose incidence is considerably higher than that observed in patients transplanted for leukemia, since up to 10% of TM patients have been reported to experience either early or late graft failure.[7,9,10] Interestingly, in TM patients transplanted from an HLA-identical sibling, the incidence of rejection is directly correlated with the patient's class of risk, defined according to the Pesaro criteria, an incidence of 4%, 8%, and 12% being observed in patients belonging to risk class 1, 2, and 3, respectively.[9,19] In general, several factors are known to influence the probability of engraftment (see also Fig. 1 for further details); among them, for what specifically concerns TM patients, pretransplantation exposure to blood products, having not received any chemotherapy treatment before HSCT and expanded erythropoietic marrow, together with the presence of splenomegaly, may contribute to explain why these patients have an increased risk of graft failure as compared to subjects with haematological malignancies (in particular those with acute leukemia). In comparison to patients transplanted from an HLA-identical sibling, an increased incidence of graft rejection has been observed when an unrelated donor (UD) is used, this being an argument that may discourage the application of UD-HSCT to thalassemia patients.[14,15] A recent study has demonstrated that the risk of rejection in UD-HSCT for TM is associated with the presence of nonpermissive HLA-DPB1 mismatches in the host-versus-graft (HVG) direction, as defined by a

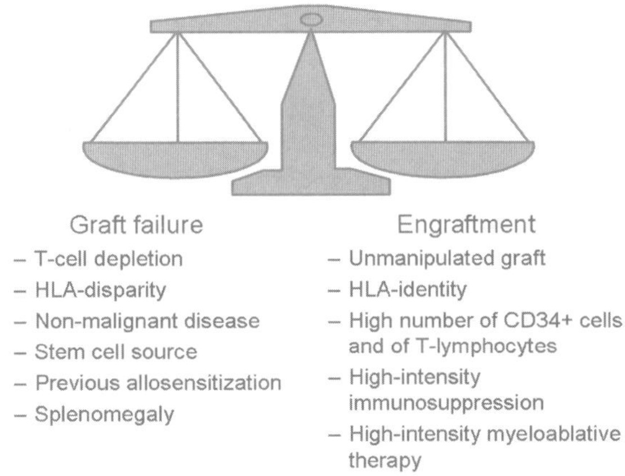

Figure 1. Factors influencing the probability of graft failure (on the left-hand side) and of sustained engraftment of donor hematopoiesis (on the right-hand side) after allogeneic hematopoeitic stem cell transplantation.

previously published algorithm,[20] regardless of the patient's class of risk.[14] These results, underlining once more that immunogenetic factors play a crucial role for the occurrence of complications due to alloreactivity in HSCT, are potentially useful for selecting the most suitable unrelated volunteer, as the incidence of graft failure after HSCT in TM can be reduced by appropriate selection of UD, performed taking into account functional rules of immunogenetics.

Mixed chimerism after HSCT and new transplant strategies for patients with hemoglobinopathies

Previously reported data indicate that the detection at a certain time point of hematopoietic and immune cells of host origin, commonly referred to as donor/recipient mixed chimerism (MC), is not uncommon in patients receiving bone marrow transplantation (BMT) for TM.[21,22] The majority of these patients exhibiting MC convert to full donor chimerism (FDC) weeks/months after BMT; among the remaining patients, some have MC stable over time even after discontinuation of immune-suppressive therapy, while a not negligible proportion of them develop secondary graft failure, in particular when increasing proportions of recipients' cells are observed in serial monitoring. A recent study clearly demonstrated that a sustained donor/recipient MC of circulating leukocytes can be found in the majority of patients with TM given CBT from an HLA-identical relative and it is associated with a favorable transplantation outcome, as all the 27 patients investigated were alive and transfusion independent.[23] These data suggest that, while early MC is associated with an increased risk of graft failure in BMT recipients, MC sustained over time can be found in a large proportion of patients given CBT, without predicting the occurrence of graft failure and that CBT, more than BMT, promotes the development of a state of reciprocal tolerance between recipient and donor cells.[23] More importantly, patients with hemoglobinopathies developing stable chimerism, even with a low percentage of donor marrow progenitors (20–30%), have been reported to experience marked enrichment of donor cells in the mature red blood cell compartment (i.e., a different donor/recipient distribution between erythroid and other hematopoietic lineages), which makes them clinically asymptomatic and transfusion independent.[21,24] The presence of residual host cells may also contribute to reduce the incidence and severity of graft-versus-host disease (GvHD), as, in animal models, MC is associated with reduced susceptibility to GvHD, probably through mechanisms of central tolerance, with negative selection of host-reactive donor T cells.[25,26]

The observations that: (i) patients with TM given an allograft and having a sustained MC with a percentage of donor cells as low as 20–30% remain disease-free;[22–24] (ii) reduced-intensity preparative regimens are associated with lower morbidity and mortality after transplantation;[27] and (iii) patients with malignancies who are not eligible to standard allograft either because of age or poor medical conditions can be safely transplanted using nonmyeloablative regimens,[28,29] has provided the rationale for using this type of preparation in the context of thalassemia. This approach to transplantation, introduced in the clinical practice in the last decade, is based on immune suppression (mainly achieved with the use of purine-analogues like fludarabine) with minimal or limited host myeloablation. This immune suppression is, however, sufficient to achieve donor chimerism, and may also have the advantage of reducing the incidence of late effects, in particular those concerning growth and fertility, resulting from high-dose chemotherapy used for conventional HSCT.

Some reports have unquestionably demonstrated the feasibility of using reduced-intensity preparative regimens for successfully treating patients with hemoglobinopathies.[30–33] However, results of well-controlled, large clinical trials on minimal-intensity conditioning regimens by centers experienced in HSCT are not available. Moreover, and more importantly, the available evidence indicates that the barrier to stable partial donor engraftment after minimally toxic regimens employed for transplantation in patients with hemoglobinopathies seems much more difficult to be overcome than in adults with hematological malignancies.[34,35] Indeed, in the largest cohort of patients (six with sickle cell disease and one with thalassemia), reported by Iannone and colleagues, the use of a nonmyeloablative regimen before the allograft produced minimal toxicity, but resulted in only transient donor engraftment followed by late graft failure.[35] As already mentioned, previous alloimmunization to blood products (facilitating the generation of host immune competent cells able to interfere with donor engraftment), no chemotherapy treatment before HSCT and expanded erythropoietic marrow together with splenomegaly may all contribute to promote graft rejection in patients with TM.

Despite these important obstacles still not overcome, the scenario of identifying novel schemes of preparation to the allograft able to reduce the morbidity and mortality associated to the procedure is in great evolution. Indeed, some recent reports prove that pretransplantation therapy can be optimized in terms of reduction of the risk of both graft failure and TRM. As paradigmatic example, a preliminary study, although enrolling a limited number of class 3 TM patients, has suggested that the adoption, during the two months preceding HSCT, of a hypertransfusion regimen, intended to reduce the expansion pressure on the erythron, together with the use of azathioprine and hydroxyurea to suppress hematopoiesis and fludarabine for reducing the risk of rejection, may lower the probability of treatment failure and improve posttransplant outcome.[36] The addition of thiotepa to the preparative regimen and the substitution of cyclophosphamide with fludarabine, a drug displaying comparable immune suppression with lower extra-medullary toxicity, were also shown to improve the outcome of patients with thalassemia transplanted from an unrelated volunteer or with cord blood progenitors.[12,16]

In recent years, a new agent, treosulfan, has progressively emerged as a valid alternative to busulfan in terms of both efficacy and safety for obtaining profound myeloablation and immune suppression without inducing severe extra-medullary toxicity. Treosulfan (L-treitol-1,4-bis-methanesulphonate) is a prodrug of a bifunctional alkylating agent, in which the introduction of two hydroxyl groups in the molecule and the different mode of alkylation are responsible for the differences with busulfan. Preclinical and clinical data have produced evidence supporting the use of treosulfan in regimens for both autologous and allogeneic HSCT.[37,38] In particular, treosulfan, besides being effective against different types of malignant cells displays pronounced killing of both committed and more immature haematopoietic progenitors.[37,39] Moreover, treosulfan is easily administered even in young children, has limited extra-medullary toxicity and its pharmacokinetics is linear, with

Table 1. Patient, donor, and transplantation characteristics

Number of patients	39 (100%)
Gender	
Males	24 (62%)
Females	15 (38%)
Age at HSCT (years, median, range)	8 (1–29)
Pesaro class at time of HSCT	
Class 1	16 (41%)
Class 2	11 (28%)
Class 3/adults	12 (31%)
Type of donor employed	
Matched family donor	8 (21%)
Matched unrelated donor	31 (79%)
Stem cell source	
Bone marrow	35 (90%)
Cord blood	2 (5%)
Peripheral blood	2 (5%)
Number of BM cells infused (nucleated cells $\times 10^8$/kg; median, range)	5 (2–13)
Conditioning regimen	
Thiotepa + Treo + Flu	8 (21%)
Thiotepa + Treo + Flu + ATG	31 (79%)
GvHD prophylaxis	
CsA + MTX[a]	8 (21%)
CsA + MTX + ATG[b]	31 (79%)
Number of days to PMN recovery[c] (median, range)	21 (14–30)
Number of days to PLT recovery[d] (median, range)	22 (11–32)
Graft failure[e]	3 (8%)
Chimerism[f] (median, range)	100% (60–100)

HSCT, haematopoietic stem cell transplantation; Treo, Treosulfan; Flu, Fludarabine; ATG, anti-thymocyte globulin; GvHD, graft-versus-host disease; CsA, cyclosporine; MTX, Methotrexate; PMN, polymorphonuclear neutrophils; PLT, platelets.

[a]Recipients of HLA-identical sibling HSCT.

[b]Recipients of unrelated donor HSCT.

[c]Defined as the first of three consecutive days with an absolute neutrophil count equal to or greater than 0.5×10^9/L.

[d]Defined as the first of 7 consecutive days with an unsupported platelet count equal to or greater than 20×10^9/L.

[e]Defined according the criteria reported in the text.

[f]Haematopoietic chimerism was evaluated, starting from DNA obtained either from peripheral blood and/or BM mononuclear cells and T-cell subsets, by microsatellite analysis.

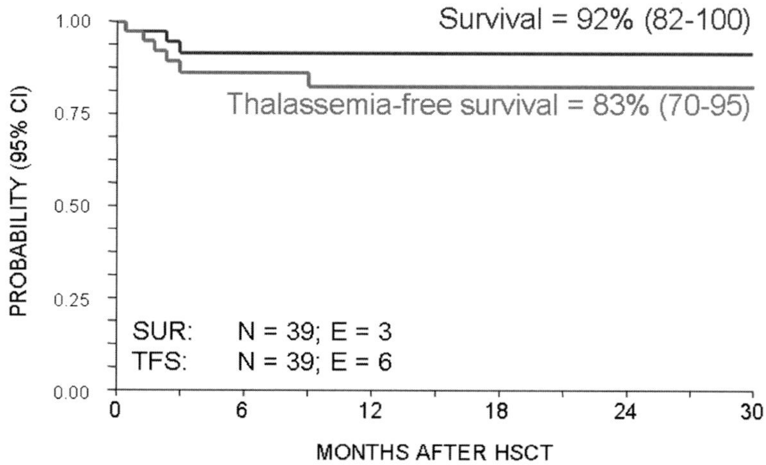

Figure 2. Kaplan-Meier estimate of survival and survival with transfusion independence in patients given the combination of thiotepa, treosulfan, and fludarabine in preparation to the allograft.

reliable systemic exposure and low inter-patient variability.[37,40]

We have recently published the results of allogeneic HSCT in TM patients given a combination of Thiotepa/Treosulfan/Fludarabine as conditioning regimen.[40] In detail, patients received intravenous thiotepa (8 mg/kg on day −7), treosulfan (14 g/m^2 for 3 consecutive days, from day −6 to −4), and fludarabine (40 mg/m^2 for 4 consecutive days, from day −6 to −3). GvHD prophylaxis was based on the use of Cyclosporine (given for 12 months after transplantation), together with short-term methotrexate (10 mg/m^2 on day +1, +3, +6, +11). Pretransplantation anti-thymocyte globulin (10 mg/kg/day for 3 consecutive days, from day −5 to −3) was administered in the 17 UD-HSCT recipients. In that report, the probability of thalassemia-free survival was 85%, while the cumulative incidence of TRM and graft failure was 5% and 11%, respectively.

The updated analysis of this study now involves 39 patients (see also Table 1 for details on patient, donor, and transplantation characteristics). This treosulfan-based preparative regimen confirms to be well tolerated, limited organ toxicity having been observed and no patient having died for causes directly attributable to the toxicity of the cytotoxic drugs. Only five patients developed grade I and II liver toxicity (i.e., transient elevation of liver enzymes), respectively; no case of veno-occlusive disease was diagnosed. All patients engrafted; details on neutrophil and platelet recovery are reported in Table 1. Three patients (both transplanted from a UD) experienced secondary graft failure after transient engraftment of donor cells, this leading to a cumulative incidence of graft failure of 9% (95% confidence interval, CI, 3–27%). Only three patients died of transplantation-related complications (namely acute GvHD in two patients and viral pneumonia in one), the cumulative incidence of TRM being 7% (95% CI, 3–25%).

The 30-month Kaplan-Meier estimates of overall survival and thalassemia-free survival are 92% (95% CI, 82–100%) and 83% (95% CI, 70–95%), respectively (see also Fig. 2). All surviving patients have a Karnofsky/Lansky score of 100%. Also in this updated analysis, we did not observe any difference in terms of outcome between patients belonging to class 1/2 of the Pesaro classification and those allocated to class 3, the probability of thalassemia-free survival being 86% (95% CI, 71–100%) and 74% (95% CI, 49–99%), respectively (see also figure 3). In view of these findings, treosulfan-based myeloablation might find elective application in adult patients or in those with poor performance status and/or organ dysfunction, all predicting a high risk of life threatening complications if busulfan is employed. The thalassemia-free survival probability of the 31 patients given a UD-HSCT is 78% (95% CI, 63–94%), while all patients transplanted from an HLA-identical sibling are alive and transfusion independent.

These results provide further support to the preliminary observation[40] that, in addition

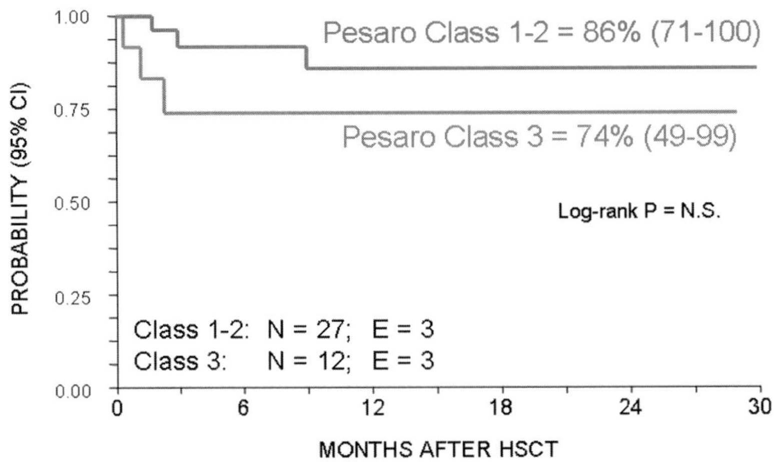

Figure 3. Kaplan-Meier estimate of survival with transfusion independence in patients given the combination of thiotepa, treosulfan, and fludarabine in preparation to the allograft according to the class of risk at time of the allograft. Adult patients and children belonging to the class 3 of the Pesaro classification are grouped together.

to mild extra-medullary toxicity, the combination thiotepa/treosulfan/fludarabine is an effective myeloablative regimen for allogeneic HSCT. It is reasonable to speculate that the limited non-haematopoietic toxicity, with the associated cytokine storm, contributed also to the low incidence of grade II-IV acute and chronic GvHD we observed, the cumulative incidence of these alloreactive-mediated complications being 18% (95% CI, 9–39%) and 7% (95% CI, 2–28%), respectively.

Future prospective, randomized trials comparing this treosulfan-based and the busulfan-based regimens in patients with TM given allogeneic HSCT are warranted.

Conclusions

Although the optimization of blood transfusion support and iron chelation therapy have dramatically improved both survival and quality of life of TM patients over the last two decades, allogeneic HSCT still remains an important treatment option and the only radically curative one. Transplant strategies based on the use of reduced-intensity preparative regimens and the induction of MC are attractive options for rendering safer allogeneic HSCT. Reduced intensity preparative regimens may find their appropriate application in older patients or in those with poor performance status and/or organ dysfunction, predicting a high risk of life-threatening complications if a fully myeloablative regimen is employed. In this regard, a preparation with treosulfan/thiotepa/fludarabine appears to be particularly promising.

Acknowledgments

This work has been partly supported by grants from Associazione Italiana Ricerca sul Cancro (AIRC), Consiglio Nazionale delle Ricerche (CNR), and Ministero dell'Istruzione, Universitàe della Ricerca (MIUR) to F.L.

Conflict of interest

The authors declare no conflicts of interest.

References

1. Olivieri, N.F. 1999. The β-thalassemia. *N. Engl. J. Med.* **34:** 99–109.
2. Borgna-Pignatti, C., S. Rugolotto, P. De Stefano, *et al.* 1998. Survival and disease complications in thalassemia major. *Ann. N.Y. Acad. Sci.* **850:** 227–231.
3. Modell, B., M. Khan & M. Darlison. 2000. Survival in beta-thalassaemia major in the UK: data from the UK Thalassaemia Register. *Lancet* **355:** 2051–2052.
4. Cappellini, M.D., A. Cohen, A. Piga, *et al.* 2006. A phase 3 study of deferasirox (ICL670), a once-daily oral iron chelator, in patients with beta-thalassemia. *Blood* **107:** 3455–3462.
5. Borgna-Pignatti, C., M.D. Cappellini, P. De Stefano, *et al.* 2006. Cardiac morbidity and mortality in deferoxamine- or deferiprone-treated patients with thalassemia major. *Blood* **107:** 3733–3737.
6. Borgna-Pignatti, C., S. Rugolotto, P. De Stefano, *et al.* 2004. Survival and complications in patients with thalassemia major treated with transfusion and deferoxamine. *Haematologica* **89:** 1187–1193.

7. Locatelli, F. & P. De Stefano. 2004. New insights into haematopoietic stem cell transplantation for patients with haemoglobinopathies. *Br. J. Haematol.* **125:** 3–11.
8. Lucarelli, G., R.A. Clift, M. Galimberti, *et al.* 1999. Bone marrow transplantation in adult thalassemic patients. *Blood* **93:** 1164–1167.
9. Storb, R.F., G. Lucarelli & P.A. McSweeney. 2003. Hematopoietic cell transplantation for benign hematological disorders and solid tumors. *Hematol. (Am. Soc. Hematol. Educ. Program)* 372–397.
10. Giardini, C. & G. Lucarelli. 1999. Bone marrow transplantation for beta-thalassemia. *Hematol. Oncol. Clin. North Am.* **13:** 1059–1064.
11. Thomas, E.D., C.D. Buckner, J.E. Sanders, *et al.* 1982. Marrow transplantation for thalassemia. *Lancet* **2:** 227–229.
12. La Nasa, G., C. Giardini, F. Argiolu, *et al.* 2002. Unrelated donor bone marrow transplantation for thalassemia: the effect of extended haplotypes. *Blood* **99:** 4350–4356.
13. La Nasa, G., F. Argiolu, C. Giardini, *et al.* 2005. Unrelated bone marrow transplantation for beta-thalassemia patients: the experience of the italian bone marrow transplant group. *Ann. N.Y. Acad. Sci.* **1054:** 186–195.
14. Fleischauer, K., F. Locatelli, M. Zecca, *et al.* 2006. Graft rejection after unrelated donor hematopoietic stem cell transplantation for thalassemia is associated with non-permissive HLA-DPB1 disparity in host-versus-graft direction. *Blood* **107:** 2984–2992.
15. Hongeng, S., S. Pakakasama, A. Chuansumrit, *et al.* 2006. Outcomes of transplantation with related- and unrelated-donor stem cells in children with severe thalassemia. *Biol. Blood Marrow Transplant.* **12:** 683–687.
16. Locatelli, F., V. Rocha, W. Reed, *et al.* on behalf of the Eurocord Transplant Group. 2003. Related umbilical cord blood transplantation in patients with thalassemia and sickle cell disease. *Blood* **101:** 2137–2143.
17. Lucarelli, G., M. Galimberti, P. Polchi, *et al.* 1990. Bone marrow transplantation in patients with thalassemia. *N. Engl. J. Med.* **322:** 417–421.
18. Lucarelli, G., M. Galimberti, P. Polchi, *et al.* 1993. Marrow transplantation in patients with thalassemia responsive to iron chelation therapy. *N. Engl. J. Med.* **329:** 840–844.
19. Lucarelli, G., R. Clift, M. Galimberti, *et al.* 1996. Marrow transplantation for patients with thalassemia: results in Class 3 patients. *Blood* **87:** 2082–2088.
20. Zino, E., G. Frumento, S. Marktel, *et al.* 2004. A T cell epitope encoded by a subset of HLA-DPB1 alleles determines non-permissive mismatches for hematological stem cell transplantation. *Blood* **103:** 1417–1424.
21. Andreani, M., M. Manna, Lucarelli, G., *et al.* 1996. Persistence of mixed chimerism in patients transplanted for the treatment of thalassemia. *Blood* **87:** 3494–3499.
22. Li, C.K., K.W. Chik, K.S. Tsang, *et al.* 2002. Mixed chimerism after bone marrow transplantation for thalassemia major. *Haematologica* **87:** 781–782.
23. Lisini, D., M. Zecca, G. Giorgiani, *et al.* 2008. Donor/recipient mixed chimerism does not predict graft failure in children with beta-thalassemia given allogeneic cord blood transplantation from an HLA-identical sibling. *Haematologica* **93:** 1859–1867.
24. Wu, C.J., E.P. Hochberg, S.A. Rogers, *et al.* 2003. Molecular assessment of erythroid lineage chimerism following nonmyeloablative allogeneic stem cell transplantation. *Exp. Haematol.* **31:** 924–933.
25. Sykes, M., A. Eisenthal & D.H. Sachs. 1988. Mechanism of protection from graft-versus-host disease in murine mixed allogeneic chimeras. Development of a null cell population suppressive of cell-mediated lympholysis responses and derived from the syngeneic bone marrow component. *J. Immunol.* **140:** 2903–2911.
26. Wekerle, T. & M. Sykes. 1999. Mixed hematopoietic chimerism as an approach for the induction of transplantation tolerance. *Transplantation* **68:** 459–467.
27. Diaconescu, R., C.R. Flowers, B. Storer, *et al.* 2004. Morbidity and mortality with nonmyeloablative compared with myeloablative conditioning before hematopoietic cell transplantation from HLA-matched related donors. *Blood* **104:** 1550–1558.
28. McSweeney, P.A., D. Niederwieser, J.A. Shizuru, *et al.* 2001. Hematopoietic cell transplantation in older patients with hematologic malignancies: replacing high-dose cytotoxic therapy with graft-versus-tumor effects. *Blood* **97:** 3390–3400.
29. Slavin, S., A. Nagler, E. Naparstek, *et al.* 1998. Nonmyeloablative stem cell transplantation and cell therapy as an alternative to conventional bone marrow transplantation with lethal cytoreduction for the treatment of malignant and nonmalignant hematologic diseases. *Blood* **91:** 756–763.
30. Krishnamurti L., B. Blazar & J.E. Wagner. 2001. Bone marrow transplantation without myeloablation in sickle cell anemia. *N. Engl. J. Med.* **344:** 68.
31. Horan J.T., J.L. Liesveld, P. Fenton, *et al.* 2005. Hematopoietic stem cell transplantation for multiply transfused patients with sickle cell disease and thalassemia after low-dose total body irradiation, fludarabine, and rabbit anti-thymocyte globulin. *Bone Marrow Transplant.* **35:** 171–177.
32. Hongeng, S., A. Chuansumrit, P. Hathirat, *et al.* 2002. Full chimerism in nonmyeloablative stem cell transplantation in a beta-thalassemia major patient (class 3 Lucarelli). *Bone Marrow Transplant.* **30:** 409–410.
33. Zhu K.E., J. Gu & T. Zhang. 2006. Allogeneic stem cell transplantation from unrelated donor for class 3 β-thalassemia major using reduced-intensity conditioning regimen. *Bone Marrow Transplant.* **37:** 111–112.
34. Locatelli F. 2006. Reduced-intensity regimens in allogeneic hematopoietic stem cell transplantation for hemoglobinopathies. *Hematol. (Am. Soc. Hematol. Educ. Program)* 398–401.
35. Iannone, R., J.F. Casella, E.J. Fuchs, *et al.* 2003. Results of minimally toxic nonmyeloablative transplantation in patients with sickle cell anemia and β-thalassemia. *Biol. Blood Marrow Transplant.* **9:** 519–528.
36. Sodani, P., D. Gaziev, P. Polchi, *et al.* 2004. A new approach for bone marrow transplantation in class 3 thalassemic patients aged less than 17 years. *Blood* **104:** 1201–1203.
37. Casper J., W. Knauf, T. Kiefer, *et al.* 2004. Treosulfan and fludarabine: a new toxicity-reduced conditioning regimen

for allogeneic hematopoietic stem cell transplantation. *Blood* **103:** 725–731.

38. Holowiecki J., S. Giebel, J. Wojnar, *et al.* 2008. Treosulfan and fludarabine low-toxicity conditioning for allogeneic haematopoietic stem cell transplantation in chronic myeloid leukaemia. *Br. J. Haematol.* **142:** 284–292.
39. Ploemacher R.E., K.W. Johnson, E.J.C. Rombouts, *et al.* 2004. Addition of treosulfan to a nonmyeloablative conditioning regimen results in enhanced chimerism and immunologic tolerance in an experimental allogeneic bone marrow transplant model. *Biol. Blood Marrow Transplant.* **10:** 236–245.
40. Bernardo M.E., M. Zecca, E. Piras, *et al.* 2008. Treosulfan-based conditioning regimen for allogeneic haematopoietic stem cell transplantation in patients with thalassaemia major. *Br. J. Haematol.* **143:** 548–551.

Ann. N.Y. Acad. Sci. ISSN 0077-8923

ANNALS OF THE NEW YORK ACADEMY OF SCIENCES
Issue: *Cooley's Anemia: Ninth Symposium*

Progress in hematopoietic stem cell transplantation as allogeneic cellular gene therapy in thalassemia

Antonella Isgrò, Javid Gaziev, Pietro Sodani, and Guido Lucarelli
International Center for Transplantation in Thalassemia and Sickle Cell Anemia, Mediterranean Institute of Hematology, Policlinic of the University of Rome "Tor Vergata," Viale Oxford, Rome, Italy

Addresses for correspondence: Antonella Isgrò, M.D., Ph.D., International Center for Transplantation in Thalassemia and Sickle Cell Anemia, Mediterranean Institute of Hematology, Policlinic of the University of Rome "Tor Vergata," Viale Oxford, 81-00133 Rome, Italy. a.isgro@fondazioneime.org

Allogeneic hemopoietic stem cell transplantation (HSCT) represents one of the best cures for thalassemia. Currently, HSCT for thalassemia consists of allogeneic stem cell gene therapy and still awaits autologous genetically modified stem cell transplantation. HSCT for thalassemia has substantially improved over the last two decades, due in large part to improvements in preventive strategies, the effective control of transplant-related complications, and the development of new preparative regimens. A risk classes-based approach to transplantation in thalassemia has led to disease-free survival probability of 87, 85, and 80% in classes 1, 2, and 3 patients, respectively. Adult thalassemia patients, who are higher risk patients for transplant-related toxicity due to an advanced phase of the disease, have a cure rate of 65% with current treatment protocol. Patients who do not have matched family or unrelated donors could benefit from haploidentical mother-to-child transplantation. Overall, the results of this type of transplantation appear encouraging.

Keywords: thalassemia; HSCT; alternative donors; haploidentical transplant

Introduction

Thalassemia is a genetic disease that requires a hypertransfusion regimen to treat the anemia caused by enhanced red blood cell destruction. However this regimen leads to progressive iron overload and consequent organ deterioration. Regular iron chelation by desferrioxamine treatment slows down this process but the iron overload gradually increases, leading to portal fibrosis that may be enhanced by the concomitant presence of chronic active hepatitis. The only radical cure of thalassemia is to correct the genetic defect by bone marrow transplantation. After transplant, a complete iron overload depletion may be achieved with phlebotomies or 6–12 months of desferrioxamine treatment. Here we describe our experience in the cure of thalassemia by bone marrow transplantation from HLA identical and haploidentical family members.

Bone marrow transplantation

At present, allogeneic hematopoietic cell transplantation (HCT) is the only rational therapeutic modality for the eradication of β-thalassemia major.[1] The purpose of allogeneic HCT for hemoglobinopathies is to correct the basic genetic defect by repleting genes essential for normal hematopoiesis through allogeneic stem cells as vectors following conditioning to overcome the immunological barrier. Therefore allogeneic HCT in these diseases could be considered as allogeneic stem cell gene therapy. It is a form of gene therapy that uses allogeneic stem cells as vectors for genes essential for normal hematopoiesis. Eventually, the vector may well be autologous stem cells transformed by the insertion of normal genes but there is no indication that this approach will be a clinical option in the foreseeable future.

doi: 10.1111/j.1749-6632.2010.05543.x

Preparatory regimens for HCT of patients with diseases other than aplastic anemia must achieve two objectives. One is elimination of the disordered marrow and the other is establishment of a tolerant environment which will permit transplanted marrow to survive and thrive. There is a considerable body of experience with the use of busulfan (BU) and its derivatives in ablating marrow in patients undergoing HCT for the treatment of nonmalignant conditions such as the Wiskott-Aldrich syndrome[2,3] and inborn errors of metabolism.[4] Cyclophosphamide (CY) is an agent that is well established as providing immunosuppression adequate for allogeneic engraftment of patients with aplastic anemia.[5,6] Experience in the use of chemotherapy-only transplant regimens for the treatment of malignancy[7–12] has been pivotal in developing regimens appropriate for the treatment of thalassemia by transplantation.

BU is an alkylating agent with exquisite specificity for the most primitive precursors of the myeloid-erythroid axis. It has been used in low doses for more than 30 years for the treatment of patients with chronic myeloid leukemia, and its toxicity and effectiveness have been well-documented in that setting. Studies in rodents demonstrated that marrow-lethal doses of BU have minor toxicity to the lymphoid system and cause little immunosuppression.[13]

Further, CY has been a component of most conditioning regimens for transplanting patients with hematologic malignancies. Also, CY is most commonly employed for the treatment of lymphoid malignancies and solid tumors, and it has been used as a component of combination chemotherapy for the treatment of acute leukemia. It is not considered a highly effective agent against myeloid malignancies, although single drug studies are not available in this context. The dose-limiting toxicity of CY is to the heart and not to the marrow. Therefore CY alone is not an appropriate conditioning modality for BMT for the treatment of thalassemia because the thalassemic marrow would recover rapidly. On the other hand, BU is an agent which has a good possibility of eradicating a diseased erythron but when used alone is not likely to be sufficiently immunosuppressive to permit sustained allogeneic engraftment. In summary, a combination of BU and CY can eradicate the thalassemia and facilitate sustained allogeneic engraftment.

There are two fundamental treatments in the pretransplant preparation: eradication of the hemopoietic system by administration of a total dose of 14–16 mg/kg of busulfan and suppression of the immune system by administration of a total dose of 200 mg/kg of cyclophosphamide. However there is an overlap of anti-proliferative activity of busulfan on the immune cell system and of cyclophosphamide on the hemopoietic stem cell system. The summed toxicity of these dosages of busulfan and cyclophosphamide reaches the tolerability threshold and therefore cannot be increased.

When the allogeneic graft starts to proliferate in the recipient, an immunological graft-versus-host reaction (graft-versus-host disease) may occur that affects one or more organs to varying degrees, the most frequently affected are the skin, gastrointestinal tract, and liver. GVHD is a serious complication of bone marrow transplantation and can be fatal, therefore the prophylactic administration of cyclosporine (CSA, an immunosuppressive drug), is an important part of the pre- and posttransplant treatment, three or four doses of methotrexate may also be given in addition to CSA in the first 15 days after transplant.

Clinical transplant experience

Analysis of the influence of pretransplant characteristics on the outcome of transplantation was conducted in 161 patients aged less than 17 years who were all treated with exactly the same regimen.[14,15] In multivariate analysis, hepatomegaly more than 2 cm, portal fibrosis, and irregular chelation history were associated with a significantly reduced probability of survival. The quality of chelation was characterized as regular when deferoxamine therapy was initiated no later than 18 months after the first transfusion and administered subcutaneously for 8–10 h continuously for at least 5 days each week. Any deviation from this regimen was defined as irregular chelation. On the basis of these risk factors patients were categorized into three risk classes. Class 1 patients had none of these adverse risk factors, class 3 patients had all three, and class 2 patients had one or two adverse risk factors.

Result of transplant from HLA matched related donors

Class 1 and Class 2 patients

Between May 1985 and December 2003, 498 patients <17 years of age had received HLA-identical transplants using regimens containing BU 14 mg/kg and CY 200 mg/kg. There were 150 class 1 patients, 315 class 2 patients, and 33 class 3 patients. The probabilities of survival, thalassemia-free survival, rejection, and nonrejection mortality for class 1 patients were 90%, 87%, 3%, and 10%, respectively, and for class 2 patients they were 87%, 85%, 3%, and 13%, respectively.

Between October 1985 and August 2007, 515 class 1 and class 2 patients with median age of 7 years (range 1–16 years) were given bone marrow transplantation following conditioning with Bu 3.5 mg/kg/day for four consecutive days and CY 50 mg/kg/day for subsequent 4 days. Since 2003 patients aged less than 4 years were also given Thiotepa 10 mg/kg/day in addition to BU-CY due to a high rejection rate observed in this group of patients (unpublished data). Four hundred and seventy eight of these patients were given transplants at the Hospital of Pesaro[14,16] and 37 patients received BMT at the University Policlinic of Tor Vergata. Graft-versus-host disease prophylaxis consisted of CSA and low-dose methylprednisolone (MP) and since June 2001 CSA, MP and a modified "short course" of methotrexate (MTX).

Class 3 patients

Class 3 younger patients (age <17 years), treated with the same conditioning as class 1 and class 2 patients (BU 14 mg/kg and CY 200 mg/kg), showed a low probability of thalassemia-free survival (53%) and a higher probability of nonrejection transplant related mortality (39%).[17] In an attempt to improve results in class 3 patients, new treatment regimens were devised using BU 14 mg/kg and lower doses of CY (160 or 120 mg/kg). These regimens improved the probability of survival in class 3 younger (age <17 years) patients from 53% to 79%, but were associated with an increase of rejection probability from 7% to 30%, probably due to inadequate immunosuppression and failure to eradicate the massive erythroid hyperplasia characteristic of these patients.[15–17]

In April 1997 a new preparative regimen (Protocol 26) was adopted for class 3 patients <17 years of age, in an attempt to decrease the higher rejection rate through reducing erythroid expansion and increasing immunosuppression over time, to avoid unacceptable drug toxicity during conditioning regimen.[18] Protocol 26 was devised on the assumption that preparation with BU 14 mg/kg and CY 160 mg/kg was inadequate to eradicate thalassemic hematopoiesis in class 3 patients <17 years of age. This protocol involved an intensified preparation with 3 mg/kg of azathioprine and 30 mg/kg hydroxyurea daily from day −45 from the transplant, fludarabine 20 mg/m^2 from day −17 to day −13, followed by the administration of BU 14 mg/kg total dose and CY 160 mg/kg total dose. Graft-versus-host disease prophylaxis consisted of CSA, low-dose MP, and a modified "short course" of MTX. During this time interval patients received a regimen of hypertransfusion to keep the level of hemoglobin >14 g/dL, continuous 24-h infusions of 40 mg/kg of deferoxamine via central venous catheter and growth factors (granulocyte colony-stimulating factor and Globuren) twice weekly to maintain stem cell proliferation in the face of hypertransfusion, thereby facilitating the effect of the hydroxyurea. The probabilities of survival, thalassemia-free survival, rejection and nonrejection mortality in 33 such patients treated with Protocol 26 were 93%, 85%, 8%, and 6%, respectively.[19]

Adult patients

Adult thalassemia patients have more advanced disease with both disease and treatment related organ complications mainly due to prolonged exposure to iron overload. From November 1988 to September 1996, 107 patients older than 16 years received transplants from matched donors. The median age for this population was 20 years (range 17–35 years). Eighteen patients were in class 2 and these received BU 14 mg/kg and CY 200 mg/kg. The other patients were in class 3 and 15 of these received BU 14 mg/kg and CY 120 mg/kg, 13 received BU 16 mg/kg and CY 120 mg/kg, 18 received BU 16 mg/kg and CY 160 mg/kg, and 43 received BU 14 mg/kg and CY 160 mg/kg. The probability of survival, thalassemia-free survival, rejection, and nonrejection mortality for the entire group of these patients were 66%, 62%, 4%, and 37%, respectively.[20,21] For the 18 class 2 adults, the probabilities of survival and of thalassemia-free survival were both 76%.

From April 1997 all adult patients were prepared for transplantation according to Protocol 26 with the only difference that the dose of cyclophosphamide was reduced to 90 mg/kg total dose. The probability of survival, thalassemia-free survival, rejection and nonrejection mortality in 15 high risk group patients were 65%, 65%, 7%, and 28%, respectively.[22]

Transplantation provided what is probably a permanent cure for the marrow defect in nearly all these patients but prolonged follow-up is necessary to determine the long-term outcome. It is reasonable to hope that removal of the continuing cause for extramedullary organ damage will modify disease progression and permit healing of the damaged organs.

The Rome experience

From June 2004 to August 2007, 37 class 1 and class 2 patients with median age of 5 years (range 2–16) and 35 class 3 patients with median age of 10 years (range 5–16) were given BMT from HLA matched related donors in our Center. Class 1 and class 2 patients under 4 years of age were given BU14-CY200 and Thiotepa 10 mg/kg total dose, while patients ≥4 years of age received BU14-CY200 as preparatory regimen. Prophylaxis against GVHD consisted of CSP, low dose of MP and a short course of MTX. Class 3 patients were prepared for BMT according to Protocol 26. Since June 2006, all patients were given targeted dose of intravenous Busilvex instead of oral Busulfan. The probabilities of survival, thalassemia-free survival, rejection and nonrejection mortality of class 1 and class 2 patients aged less than 17 years were 97%, 89%, 8%, and 3%, respectively. The probabilities of survival, thalassemia-free survival, nonrejection mortality, and rejection of class 3 patients were 87%, 80%, 12%, and 10%, respectively. The Rome experience confirmed the results obtained in Pesaro, and showed the reproducibility of the Pesaro experience in other centers.

Result of transplant from haploidentical donors

Approximately 25–30% of patients with thalassemia could have an HLA matched related donor. As HSCT is the only cure for thalassemia, there is need to develop alternative stem cells donations. Our past experience with BMT from alternative donors for 29 patients with β-thalassemia major who received phenotypically matched grafts or haploidentical grafts mismatched for one, two, or three antigens was characterized by higher graft failure (55%), and low thalassemia-free survival (21%).[23] Haploidentical hematopoietic stem cell transplantation from a mismatched family member (HaploHSCT) donor offers an alternative option for patients who lack an human leukocyte antigen (HLA)-matched donor. The main obstacles are represented by graft rejection, delayed immune reconstitution, graft-versus-host disease (GvHD), and higher frequency of opportunistic infections. Haploidentical T-cell depleted HCT from mother to child, assuming that the immunotolerance established during the pregnancy might help to bypass the HLA disparity, is under study at our Center. Preliminary results suggest that haploidentical HSC is a realistic therapeutic option for thalassemic patients without HLA identical donor.

In haploidentical hematopoietic transplantation, donor-versus-recipient NK cell alloreactivity derives from a mismatch between donor NK clones bearing inhibitory Killer Cell Ig-like Receptors (KIRs) for self HLA class I molecules and their HLA class I ligands (KIR ligands) on recipient cells. The mechanism whereby alloreactive NK cells exert their benefits in transplantation has been elucidated. The infusion of alloreactive NK cells (1) ablates recipient T cells which reject the graft and (2) ablates recipient dendritic cells (DCs) which trigger GvHD, thus protecting from GvHD.[24] NK cell alloreactivity also boosts very rapid rebuilding of donor adaptive immunity to infections. Immuno haematological reconstitution was therefore analysed in some patients after HLA-haploidentical transplant.[25] Eight out of 12 patients had sustained engraftment and four had rejected their grafts. Two patients died after full engraftment: one patient died 6 months after transplantation from central nervous system diffuse large B cell lymphoma EBV related and another patient from CMV pneumonia. None developed GVHD. Ten patients are alive, two of them with thalassemia recurrence.

T- and B-cell depletion was carried out with $CD34^+$ coated magnetic microbeads and the CliniMACS device (Miltenyi Biotec©) from peripheral blood and bone marrow of donors (the mothers) and resulted in grafts consisting of stem cells and effector cells (NK cells, monocytes) with the addition of bone marrow mononuclear cells (BMMNCs 3×10^5/kg of the recipient). A total of 12 paediatric patients with β-thalassemia received T and B cell depleted transplants from their haploidentical mothers with a median number of 15×10^6/kg CD34 stem cells. To analyse the mechanisms involved in immunological reconstitution posttransplant, we analysed T cell subsets by flow cytometry, particularly NK sets (CD3-CD56$^+$, CD3-CD16$^+$, and CD56$^+$CD16$^+$ NK cells) at day +20 and +60 posttransplant.

Day +20 posttransplant, the patients had significantly lower CD4$^+$ T cells in comparison to the controls, whereas CD8$^+$ T cells numbers did not statistically differ between patients and controls. NK cells were among the first lymphocytes to repopulate the peripheral blood, and up to 70% of these cells were CD3-CD56$^{+bright}$ cells. Interestingly, a direct correlation has been observed between the percentages of CD56$^+$ CD16$^+$ NK subset and the BM engraftment and in all the patients the origin of the NK subsets was from the mothers. Day +60 posttransplant an increase in the percentages of CD4$^+$ T cells, naïve CD4$^+$ cells, and in thymic naïve Th cells were observed (manuscript in preparation). These data may suggest the importance of NK subsets analyses at the first time of the transplant as an useful parameter for the outcome of the transplant and/or the use of donor's alloreactive NK cells especially in haploidentical recipients (manuscript in preparation).

Conclusion

The only radical cure for homozygous thalassemia is to transplant bone marrow from an HLA identical donor, normal, or heterozygous for thalassemia that is capable of producing and maintaining a normal hemoglobin level in the recipient. All thalassemic patients, together with their parents and siblings, should be HLA typed to this purpose. When an HLA donor is available, we believe that bone marrow transplantation is mandatory in those thalassemic patients in class 1 and in class 2 and in those of class 3 aged less than 17 years. The adult patients should also be offered this possibility of a cure. Patients who do not have matched family or unrelated donors could benefit from haploidentical mother to child transplantation and the results of this type of transplantation are encouraging.

Acknowledgments

The authors are supported by the International Centre for Transplantation in Thalassemia and Sickle Cell Anemia—Mediterranean Institute of Hematology.

Conflicts of interest

The authors declare no conflicts of interest.

References

1. Slavin, S., R. Or, G Cividalli, *et al.* 1988. Bone marrow transplantation in β-thalassemia with prevention of graft-vs.-host disease. In *Birth Defects: Original Article Series. Thalassemia: Pathophysiology and Management*, Vol. 23, Part 5B. Fucharoen S., P.T. Rowley & N.W. Paul, Eds.: 313–316. Alan R Liss. NY, USA.
2. Parkman, R., J. Rappeport, R. Geha, *et al.* 1978. Complete correction of the Wiskott-Aldrich syndrome by allogeneic bone-marrow transplantation. *N. Engl. J. Med.* **298:** 921–927.
3. Kapoor, N., D. Kirkpatrick, J. Oleske, *et al.* 1981. Reconstitution of normal megakaryocytopoiesis and immunologic functions in Wiskott-Aldrich syndrome by marrow transplantation following myeloablation and immunosuppression with busulfan and cyclophosphamide. *Blood* **57:** 692–696.
4. Hobbs, J.R., K. Hugh-Jones, P.J. Shaw, *et al.* 1986. Engraftment rates related to busulphan and cyclophosphamide dosages for displacement bone marrow transplants in fifty children. *Bone Marrow Transplant.* **1:** 201–208.
5. Thomas, E.D., C.D. Buckner, R. Storb, *et al.* 1972. Aplastic anaemia treated by marrow transplantation. *Lancet* **1:** 284–289.
6. Storb, R., R.E. Champlin. 1991. Bone marrow transplantation for severe aplastic anemia. *Bone Marrow Transplant* **8:** 69–72.
7. Santos, G.W., L.L. Sensenbrenner, P.J. Burke, *et al.* 1971. Marrow transplantation in man following cyclophosphamide. *Transplant. Proc.* **3:** 400–404.
8. Tutschka, P.J., G.J. Elfenbein, L.L. Sensenbrenner, *et al.* 1980. Preparative regimens for marrow transplantation in acute leukemia and aplastic anemia. Baltimore experience. *Am. J. Ped. Hematol. Oncol.* **2:** 363–370.
9. Santos, G.W., P.J. Tutschka, R. Brookmeyer, *et al.* 1983. Marrow transplantation for acute nonlymphocytic leukemia after treatment with busulfan and cyclophosphamide. *N. Engl. J. Med.* **309:** 1347–1353.
10. Appelbaum, F.R., R. Storb, R.E. Ramberg, *et al.* 1984. Allogeneic marrow transplantation in the treatment of preleukemia. *Ann. Intern. Med.* **100:** 689–693.
11. Tutschka, P.J., E.A. Copelan, N. Kapoor 1989. Replacing total body irradiation with busulfan as conditioning of patients with leukemia for allogeneic marrow transplantation. *Transplant Proc.* **21:** 2952–2954.
12. Tutschka, P.J., E.A. Copelan, N. Kapoor, *et al.* 1991. Allogeneic bone marrow transplantation for leukemia using chemotherapy as conditioning. Six-year results of a single institution trial. *Transplant Proc.* **23:** 1709–1710.
13. Floersheim, G.L. & L.A. Elson. 1961. Restoration of hematopoiesis following a lethal dose of dimethyl myleran by isologic bone marrow transplantation in mice. Experiments on modification of intolerance to homologous bone marrow by 6-mercaptopurine, amino-chlorambucil and cortisone. *Acta Haematol.* **26:** 233–245.

14. Lucarelli, G., M. Galimberti, P. Polchi, *et al.* 1990. Bone marrow transplantation in patients with thalassemia. *N. Engl. J. Med.* **322:** 417–421.
15. Storb, R., P.L. Weiden, T.C. Graham, *et al.* 1977. Hemopoietic grafts between DLA-identical canine littermates following dimethyl myleran. Evidence for resistance to grafts not associated with DLA and abrogated by antithymocyte serum. *Transplantation* **24:** 349–357.
16. Lucarelli, G., M. Galimberti, P. Polchi, *et al.* 1993. Marrow transplantation in patients with thalassemia responsive to iron chelation therapy. *N. Engl. J. Med.* **329:** 840–844.
17. Lucarelli, G., R. Clift, M. Galimberti, *et al.* 1996. Marrow transplantation for patients with thalassemia: results in Class 3 patients. *Blood* **87:** 2082–2088.
18. Lucarelli, G., M. Andreani & E. Angelucci. 2002. The cure of thalassemia by bone marrow transplantation. *Blood Rev.* **16:** 81–85.
19. Sodani, P., J. Gaziev, P. Polchi, *et al.* 2004. New approach for bone marrow transplantation in patients with class 3 thalassemia aged younger than 17 years. *Blood* **104:** 1201–1203.
20. Lucarelli, G., M. Galimberti, P. Polchi, *et al.* 1992. Bone marrow transplantation in adult thalassemia. *Blood* **80:** 1603–1607.
21. Lucarelli, G., Clift RA, M. Galimberti, *et al.* 1999. Bone marrow transplantation in adult thalassemic patients. *Blood* **93:** 1164–1167.
22. Gaziev, J., P. Sodani, P. Polchi, *et al.* 2005. Bone marrow transplantation in adults with thalassemia. Treatment and long-term follow-up. *Ann. N.Y. Acad. Sci.* **1054:** 196–205.
23. Gaziev, D., M. Galimberti, G. Lucarelli, *et al.* 2000. Bone marrow transplantation from alternative donors for thalassemia: HLA-phenotypically identical relative and HLA nonidentical sibling or parent transplants. *Bone Marrow Transplant.* **25:** 815–821.
24. Ruggeri, L., A. Mancusi, E. Burchielli, *et al.* 2008. NK cell alloreactivity and allogeneic hematopoietic stem cell transplantation. *Blood Cells Mol. Dis.* **40:** 84–90.
25. Isgrò, A., P. Sodani, M. Marziali, *et al.* 2007. Early T cell recovery of thymus-derived naïve T cells and NK cells in paediatrics patients after T-cell depleted HLA-haploidentical stem cell transplantation for thalassemia [abstract]. *Blood* **110:** 336.

Ann. N.Y. Acad. Sci. ISSN 0077-8923

ANNALS OF THE NEW YORK ACADEMY OF SCIENCES
Issue: *Cooley's Anemia: Ninth Symposium*

Emerging insights in the management of hemoglobin E beta thalassemia

Nancy F. Olivieri,[1] Vivekanandan Thayalsuthan,[1] Angela O'Donnell,[2] Anuja Premawardhena,[3] Christopher Rigobon,[1] Giulia Muraca,[1] Christopher Fisher,[4] and David J. Weatherall[2]

[1]Hemoglobinopathy Research Program, Toronto General Hospital, University of Toronto, Toronto, Ontario, Canada. [2]Weatherall Institute of Molecular Medicine, University of Oxford, John Radcliffe Hospital, Headington, Oxford, United Kingdom. [3]Faculty of Medicine, University of Kelaniya, Colombo, Sri Lanka. [4]MRC Molecular Hematology Unit, John Radcliffe Hospital, Headington, Oxford, United Kingdom

Address for correspondence: Nancy F. Olivieri, M.D., F.R.C.P.(C.), Professor, Pediatrics, Medicine and Public Health Sciences, University of Toronto, Canada; University Health Network, 200 Elizabeth Street, Eaton Wing North, 10th Floor, Room 225, Toronto, ON, Canada M5G 2C4. noliv@attglobal.net, nolivi@gmail.com

Globally, hemoglobin (Hb) E β thalassemia accounts for approximately half the severe forms of β thalassemia. Because of its wide clinical diversity and the ability of patients with this condition to adapt unusually well to low hemoglobin levels, the management of Hb E β thalassemia, particularly the decision to instigate regular blood transfusion, is particularly difficult. Here, we present a summary of our work in patients with this condition, which attempts to define clinical, adaptive, and genetic factors of possible value in determining the early management of this condition.

Keywords: hemoglobin; hemoglobin E beta thalassemia; β thalassemia

A recent population analysis suggests that hemoglobin E beta-thalassemia (Hb E β thalassemia) accounts for approximately half of all the cases of severe β thalassemia in the world population.[1] Hb E β thalassemia occurs widely throughout the eastern half of the Indian subcontinent, Bangladesh, Burma, and throughout Southeast Asia.[2] Hb E β thalassemia has a remarkably diverse phenotype, ranging from a transfusion-dependent disorder similar to β thalassemia major, to a condition characterized by relatively normal growth and development with survival into adult life in the absence of red cell transfusions.[2,3] Although the reasons for this clinical heterogeneity are still not fully understood, we and others have demonstrated that this in part reflects the coinheritance of genetic modifiers such as α thalassemia and genetic polymorphisms involved with elevated hemoglobin F production.[4–6] We have identified other genetic modifiers that influence the complications of the disease,[7] together with differences in adaptation to anemia,[8] and the effects of the environment, particularly exposure to malaria.[9]

The remarkable clinical diversity of this condition, which occurs against the background of coinheritance of Hb E with a wide variety of severe β thalassemia mutations,[4] together with its remarkable phenotypic instability during the early years of life,[5,10] presents difficult problems in the early management of this disease. These difficulties are compounded by the fact that it appears that the difference in hemoglobin levels between mild and severely affected patients are remarkably small, in the range of 1–2 g/dL.[5]

Here, we summarize findings obtained in a study of 115 patients with Hb E β thalassemia who had never received regular transfusions during the clinical course of their disease, or in whom regular transfusions had been stopped during the clinical course and in whom there was at least 5 years of followup after regular transfusions had been discontinued. This preliminary analysis attempts to define some clinical and genetic factors, which may assist in deciding whether to initiate regular transfusions, or to stop these when already initiated, in patients with Hb E β thalassemia.

doi: 10.1111/j.1749-6632.2010.05579.x

The study group was composed of patients with Hb E β thalassemia attending the National Thalassaemia Centre, Kurunegala, Sri Lanka, of whom approximately one-third had never been started on regular transfusions, while the remaining patients had been started on regular transfusions, but in whom a decision to stop regular transfusions had been made when the patient was first reviewed between 1996 and 2003. In each patient, it had been decided to stop regular transfusions because it was unclear why each patient had been recommended to begin regular transfusions, noting, in particular, that the pretransfusion hemoglobin concentrations showed little difference from hemoglobin concentrations in patients who had not been supported by regular transfusions. Folate, deferoxamine, and prophylactic penicillin continued to be prescribed as indicated. All these patients were reviewed at least four times a year for a minimum of five years.

The methods for clinical assessment, severity and grading on a scale of 1–5, hematologic and hemoglobin analysis, DNA analysis, serum ferritin and, in some cases, hepatic iron concentrations, and serial assessments of serum erythropoietin concentrations, have been described previously.[4,5,8]

We examined some clinical features, which might distinguish the patients who had never been transfused regularly, from those in whom regular transfusions had been started at some point during their clinical course. Several features suggested that the patients who had not been started on regular transfusions had a milder phenotype. For example, patients never started on regular transfusions were significantly older at diagnosis compared to those in whom regular transfusions had been started. Furthermore, there was a lower rate of splenectomy in the patients who had not been transfused regularly, compared with patients in whom regular transfusions had been initiated and patients in whom regular transfusions had been started had also been splenectomized at an earlier age, compared with those who had never been transfused regularly.

Currently, we are engaged in a detailed analysis of the factors that might underlie the difference in response of the patients in whom regular transfusions were terminated successfully, and those in whom this was unsuccessful and in whom regular transfusions needed to be resumed. Among others, the effect of genetic factors on response to transfusion withdrawal is currently being investigated, particularly with the recent recognition of the variety of different forms of nondeletion α thalassemia in the Sri Lankan population.

It may be possible successfully to stop regular transfusions in a substantial proportion of patients with Hb E thalassemia who have been placed, often for uncertain reasons, on such a regimen. Both genetic factors and the long-term adaptation to anemia may play a part in the successful or unsuccessful withdrawal of transfusions in these patients. We have previously suggested that some of the early phenotypic instability of Hb E thalassemia, including the decline in the rate of splenomegaly with age, might reflect the relatively high erythropoietin response in early life for a particular hemoglobin concentration. This response could certainly be implicated in the increasing spleen size, marrow expansion, and growth disturbances observed in this disorder during infancy and early childhood. Our previous findings that response to a given hemoglobin concentration declines throughout late childhood suggests the possibility arises that as patients with Hemoglobin E thalassemia age, it may be possible to stop transfusions in many.[8,10]

The management of Hb E β thalassemia is going to place an enormous burden on the limited health services of many of the poorer countries in Asia, particularly as they enter the epidemiological transition whereby, due to improved public health and social conditions, more affected children are surviving in early life. Undoubtedly, there are many children at the severe end of the spectrum of this disorder, who will require lifelong transfusions on a regular basis, along with a significant proportion of patients who may grow and develop relatively normally without ever being begun on such a regimen. Further work may help to define which patients of this type do require regular transfusions and who do not. Clearly, many such patients may be receiving unnecessary chronic transfusions because of its phenotypic variability during early life, and the difficulty of defining its future course.

It is possible that many patients might be spared the proliferative complications of the high erythropoietin response for a particular hemoglobin concentration in early life through the initiation of regular transfusions, which can then be stopped at or during early puberty. Given the vast numbers of patients with this disease in Asia, this approach would lead to an enormous sparing of health resources. Further work is required to try to determine the factors, which might predict the successful cessation of transfusion in patients with Hb E β thalassemia.

Conflicts of interest

The authors declare no conflicts of interest.

References

1. Modell, B. & M. Darlison. 2008. Global epidemiology of haemoglobin disorders and derived service indicators. *Bull. World Health Organ.* **86:** 480–487.
2. Weatherall, D.J. & J.B. Clegg. 2001. *The Thalassaemia Syndromes* (4th ed.). Oxford: Blackwell Science.
3. Penman, B.S., O.G. Pybus, D.J. Weatherall & S. Gupta. 2009. Epistatic interactions between genetic disorders of hemoglobin can explain why the sickle-cell gene is uncommon in the Mediterranean. *Proc. Natl Acad. Sci. USA* **106:** 21242–21246.
4. Fisher, C.A., A. Premawardhena, S. de Silva, *et al.* 2003. The molecular basis for the thalassaemias in Sri Lanka. *Br. J. Haematol.* **121:** 662–671.
5. Premawardhena, A., C.A. Fisher, N.F. Olivieri, *et al.* 2005. Haemoglobin E β thalassaemia in Sri Lanka. *Lancet* **366:** 1467–1470.
6. Sripichai, O., T. Munkongdee, C. Kumkhaek, *et al.* 2008. Coinheritance of the different copy numbers of alpha-globin gene modifies severity of beta-thalassemia/Hb E disease. *Ann. Hematol.* **87:** 375–379.
7. Premawardhena, A., C.A. Fisher, F. Fathiu, *et al.* 2001. Genetic determinants of jaundice and gallstones in haemoglobin E beta thalassaemia. *Lancet* **357:** 1945–1946.
8. O'Donnell, A., A. Premawardhena, M. Arambepola, *et al.* 2007. Age-related changes in adaptation to severe anemia in childhood in developing countries. *Proc. Natl Acad. Sci. USA* **104:** 9440–9444.
9. O'Donnell, A., A. Premawardhena, M. Arambepola, *et al.* 2009. Interaction of malaria with a common form of severe thalassemia in an Asian population. *Proc. Natl Acad. Sci. USA* **106:** 18716–18721.
10. Olivieri, N.F., G.M. Muraca, A. O'Donnell, *et al.* 2008. Studies in haemoglobin E beta-thalassaemia. *Br. J. Haematol.* **141:** 388–397.

Ann. N.Y. Acad. Sci. ISSN 0077-8923

ANNALS OF THE NEW YORK ACADEMY OF SCIENCES
Issue: *Cooley's Anemia: Ninth Symposium*

Fetal globin gene inducers: novel agents and new potential

Susan P. Perrine,[1,3] Serguei A. Castaneda,[1] David H.K. Chui,[2] Douglas V. Faller,[1] Ronald J. Berenson,[3] Noppadol Siritanaratku,[4] and Suthat Fucharoen[4]

[1]Cancer Center and Hemoglobinopathy-Thalassemia Research Unit, Department of Medicine, Pediatrics, Pharmacology and Experimental Therapeutics, Boston University School of Medicine, Boston, Massachusetts. [2]Center of Excellence in Sickle Cell Disease, Department of Medicine, Pathology and Laboratory Medicine, Boston University School of Medicine, Boston, Massachusetts. [3]HemaQuest Pharmaceuticals, Boston, Massachusetts and Seattle, Washington. [4]Thalassemia Research Centre, Mahidol University, Nakhonpathon, Thailand. [5]Siriraj Hospital, Bangkok, Thailand

Address for correspondence: Susan P. Perrine, Hemoglobinopathy Thalassemia Research Unit, Boston University School of Medicine, 72 East Concord Street, L-909, Boston, MA 02118. sperrine@bu.edu

Inducing expression of endogenous fetal globin (γ-globin) gene expression to 60–70% of alpha globin synthesis produces β-thalassemia trait globin synthetic ratios and can reduce anemia to a mild level. Several classes of therapeutics have induced γ-globin expression in beta-thalassemia patients and subsequently raised total hemoglobin levels, demonstrating proof-of-concept of the approach. Butyrate treatment eliminated transfusion requirements in formerly transfusion-dependent patients with treatment for as long as seven years. However, prior generation inducers were not readily applicable for widespread use. Currently, a novel oral dual-action therapeutic, sodium 2,2-dimethylbutyrate, is in clinical trials, an oral decitabine formulation is under development, and agents with complementary mechanisms of action can be applied in combined regimens. Identification of three major genetic trait loci which modulate clinical severity provides avenues for developing tailored regimens. These refinements offer renewed potential to apply fetal globin induction as a treatment approach in patient-friendly regimens that can be used worldwide.

Keywords: thalassemia; short chain fatty acids; erythropoiesis; fetal globin, quantitative trait loci

Introduction

β-thalassemia syndromes are the most common monogenic disorders worldwide, characterized by molecular mutations of the β-globin chain of adult hemoglobin (HbA; $\alpha_2\beta_2$), with resulting defective or deficient β-globin chains and an excess of unmatched α-globin chains.[1–8] The excess α-globin damages the red blood cell membrane and causes apoptosis of developing erythroblasts and intramedullary hemolysis.[1–8] In patients with coinheritance of β-thalassemia and hereditary persistence of fetal hemoglobin (HbF; $\alpha_2\gamma_2$) mutations, high-level expression of fetal globin (γ-globin) ameliorates the clinical severity of thalassemia, particularly the degree of anemia.[1] Many patients with higher γ-globin levels than their counterparts with the same mutations often do not require regular transfusions, or do not require transfusions on a regular basis as early in life as do others with lower γ-globin levels. These observations, and clinical trials of fetal globin inducers, have clearly established that patients with β-thalassemia benefit from persistence of, or pharmacologic induction of, γ-globin.[1–20] Inducing γ-globin expression by even small increments is an established therapeutic approach that is most likely to be feasible to apply worldwide, as the γ-globin genes are universally present and normally integrated in hematopoietic stem cells.[1,2]

Lessons from prior trials and factors for tailored regimens

Proof-of-principle has been demonstrated in clinical trials in which pharmacological reactivation of γ-globin expression has reduced anemia and eliminated transfusion requirements in patients with thalassemia. Fetal globin reinduction was

doi: 10.1111/j.1749-6632.2010.05593.x

accomplished with chemotherapeutic agents, particularly 5-azacytidine, and 5-aza-2-deoxy-cytidine (decitabine),[14–20] and with short-chain fatty acids (SCFAs), such as arginine butyrate (AB) and sodium phenylbutyrate.[2,9,10,12,13,21] SCFAs would be preferable for a long-term therapy compared to chemotherapeutics, which typically are cytotoxic and have carcinogenicity risks long-term. However, while SCFAs have not been found to be mutagenic, many prototype SCFAs also have limitations, including rapid metabolism and requirements for high doses, and those which are also global HDAC inhibitors cause inhibition of erythropoiesis.[2] Erythropoiesis stimulating agents are limiting for long term application, also due to parenteral administration and high costs.[22–25] However, these three classes of therapeutics have already rendered some thalassemia patients transfusion independent in small trials. Agents which are more tolerable would allow for broader application, particularly where thalassemia is common globally and transfusions carry particularly high risks of infections.[2]

In the SCFA clinical trials, several observations were highly informative regarding magnitude of responses and patterns of thalassemia mutations, which appear to respond differently. Several γ-globin inducers have produced significant hematologic responses with increases in total hemoglobin of 2–5 g/dL or more above baseline, and although the clinical trials have been small, patients with diverse thalassemia syndromes have had significant responses, including transfusion-independence.[2,9–19] Clinical trials of 5-azacytidine, phenylbutyrate, arginine butyrate, and EPO preparations have all demonstrated responses of this magnitude in thalassemia patients. Collins and colleagues found that sodium phenylbutyrate could increase total Hgb by 2 g/dL above baseline, and that responses occurred more frequently in patients with EPO levels >130 mU/mL.[9] Increases in total Hgb levels of 1–5 g/dL above baseline were achieved when these agents were administered for at least 3–6 months.[9,10,26] This is remarkable, because thalassemic cells survive for only a few days,[4–8] compared to the normal red cell survival of 120 days.

Of the chemotherapeutic agents, hydroxyurea (HU) treatment has increased total Hgb by 0.6–1.0 g/dL in HbE/β-thalassemia patients, and although not as great an effect in magnitude, was still significant.[2,16,17] Hajjar and Pearson reported

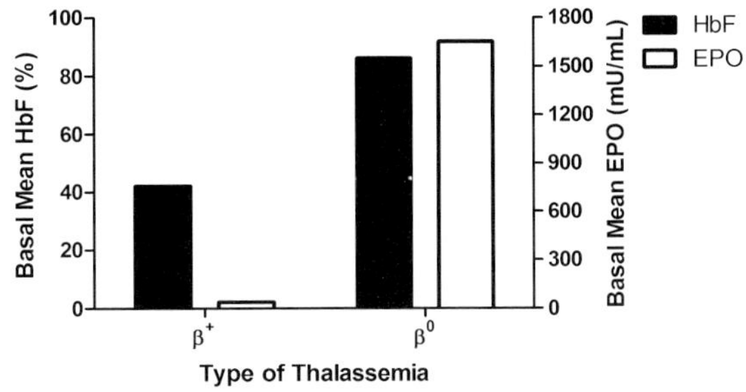

Figure 1. Basal levels of fetal hemoglobin (HbF) and endogenous erythropoietin (EPO) in patients with β^+- and β°-thalassemia. Values represent the mean baseline levels in the two groups enrolled in a trial of arginine butyrate + erythropoietin.

that γ-globin increased rapidly with HU treatment, with a 6-week treatment time-frame required for a peak response, but was followed by a decline in total Hgb, suggesting cellular growth inhibition.[15] 5-Azacytidine administration has increased total Hgb levels by an average of 2.5 g/dL (range 1–4 g/dL), even in end-stage patients with life-threatening severe anemia.[1,2,18,19]

Of the SCFAs and histone deacetylase (HDAC) inhibitors, arginine butyrate (AB), administered first intensively and then intermittently, increased total Hgb levels by 1–5 g/dL (mean 2.9 g/dL) when administered frequently for at least three months, as shown in Figure 2.[10] AB treatment has made four patients transfusion independent for several years with home therapy, given initially for 5 days/week for 4 weeks, followed by intermittent or pulse therapy for 4 nights every other week, to optimize γ-globin induction and simultaneously avoid the antiproliferative effects common to HDAC inhibitors. AB has been safe in long-term use, with no butyrate-related adverse events in more than 16 patient-years of home administration provided by parents. A representative profile of rises in total hemoglobin levels in a formerly transfusion-dependent patient is shown in Figure 2(C). Isobutyramide has also increased fetal globin within 28 days of treatment and has reduced transfusion requirements.[12,13]

EPO preparations have increased Hgb levels by 1–3 g/dL above baseline in thalassemia intermedia patients, with highest responses in children, and have decreased transfusion requirements in thalassemia major.[1,2,22–25] The studies generally found that HbF did not increase, so that thalassemic red blood cell production increased with EPO. All of these trials have already shown proof-of-principle of the utility of therapeutic induction of γ-globin ± enhancement of erythropoiesis in β-thalassemia patients.

Studies with HbF inducers with differing mechanisms of action

For a long-term therapeutic strategy, γ-globin inducers with high potency or improved pharmacokinetic profiles are desirable, so that smaller, more tolerable doses than those required for SPB or AB, and combination of agents with complementary actions, can be administered, as required in most medical conditions. Agents with differing mechanisms of action, such as agents with global epigenetic actions and targeted activity, could be combined sequentially (Table S1). Chemotherapeutic agents are not suitable for simultaneously dosed combinations, as this would result in additive cytotoxicity and greater degrees of erythroid cell apoptosis. Combinations of butyrate and 5-azacytidine in the baboon were shown by Stamatoyannopoulos and colleagues to produce a synergistic threefold increase in γ-globin expression, above the significant levels induced by each drug alone.[2] Higher responses than those achieved with single agents alone, with both additive and synergistic effects, have been found in cell culture studies and in animal models using hydroxyurea, decitabine, or MS-275 with a novel SCFAD which is not a global HDAC inhibitor, sodium 2,2 dimethylbutyrate.[27]

Clinical trials of AB ± EPO have shown that β^+-thalassemia patients often require EPO in addition to a SCFA to achieve substantial increase in total Hgb levels. Hgb can be increased on average by 3 g/dL above baseline with AB ± EPO.[2] We studied AB and EPO in combination and found that a subset of β^+-thalassemia patients had relatively low HbF (<30%) and low baseline EPO levels (<130 mU/mL), as shown in Figure 1. The β^+-thalassemia group responded to the therapeutic combination with higher rises in total hemoglobin to a greater degree than they did with either agent administered alone.[2] Examples of HbF and total Hgb responses in representative β-thalassemia patients with higher versus lower baseline EPO levels to treatment with arginine butyrate (AB) ± EPO are shown in Figure 2A,B. Patients with baseline EPO levels <80 mU/mL required AB and EPO in combination to elicit a high hematologic response (a rise in total hemoglobin of 3 g/dL above baseline); neither agent alone was as effective as the two agents together.

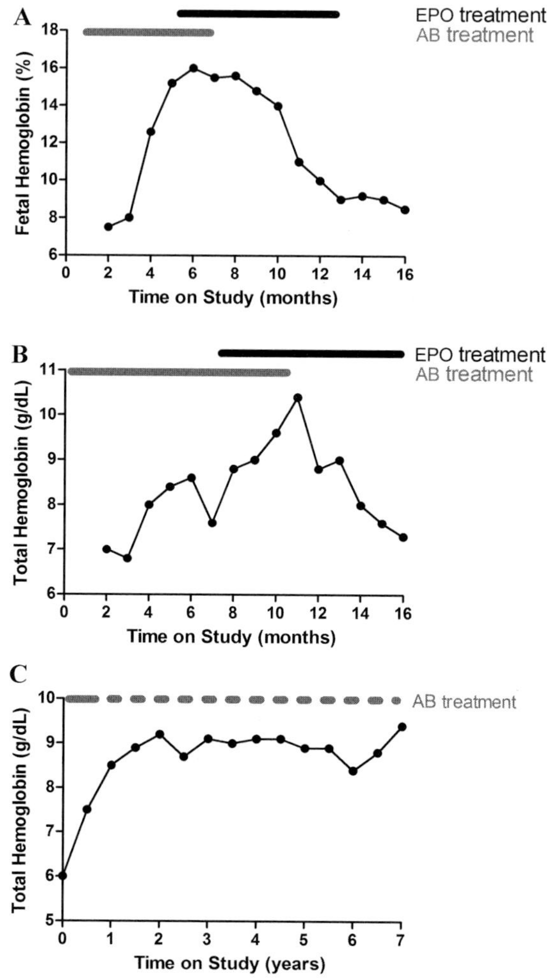

Figure 2. (A) Representative responses in fetal hemoglobin and (B) total hemoglobin to arginine butyrate (AB) ± erythropoietin (EPO) in a patient with β^+-thalassemia. The combination of the two therapeutics produced the highest rise in total hemoglobin and required both agents; while only butyrate treatment produced an increase in fetal globin, (C) AB treatment rendered a formerly transfusion-dependent $\beta^{0/+}$-thalassemia patient transfusion independent for seven years. An initial frequent dose regimen (solid line) and a maintenance pulse regimen, administered 4 nights, twice per month (shown by the dotted line) was used. Addition of EPO to the butyrate regimen did not produce any added therapeutic benefit in this type of thalassemia patient.

When butyrate was discontinued and EPO administered alone, HbF and total Hgb gradually declined back to baseline. AB and EPO in combination were therefore more effective than either agent alone in β^+-thalassemia. In contrast, patients with at least one β°-thalassemia mutation and baseline EPO levels >130 mU/mL have responded to the arginine

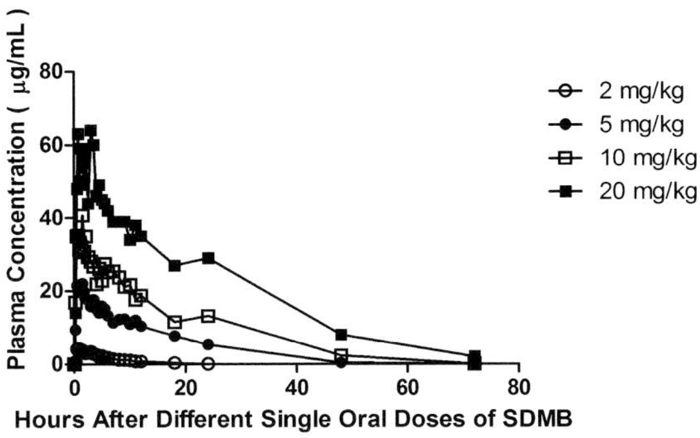

Figure 3. Pharmacokinetic profiles of sodium 2,2-dimethyl butyrate (SDMB) in healthy human volunteers. Mean drug levels are shown after administration in single oral doses at 2 mg/kg (○), 5 mg/kg (●), 10 mg/kg (□), and 20 mg/kg (■). The drug was detectable in the plasma after single oral doses with a $t_{1/2}$ of 9–11 h.

butyrate alone, increasing total Hgb levels by 2–4 g/dL, without any further rise in total Hgb when EPO was added, as shown in Figure 2C, in a formerly transfusion-dependent patient who became transfusion independent with home therapy, with arginine butyrate administered 4 nights, twice per month, for 7 years. These clinical findings indicated that combinations of agents with complementary, yet distinct, molecular mechanisms of actions can produce significantly higher responses than single agents. Based on these collective observations, our group hypothesized that prolonging the survival of erythroid precursor cells as EPO does, for a sufficient interval may allow a γ-globin inducer to then reduce the proapoptotic α:β globin chain imbalance. Identifying a therapeutic with these dual actions became a therapeutic goal.

A novel oral fetal globin inducer: sodium 2,2-dimethylbutyrate

Based on the beneficial therapeutic effects of sodium phenylbutyrate, arginine butyrate, and isobutyramide, an orally active SCFAD, which requires more tolerable doses, would be of benefit for long-term treatment in beta-thalassemia. An oral butyrate derivative, sodium 2,2-dimethylbutyrate (SDMB), has entered clinical trials. This therapeutic stimulates γ-globin production in erythroid cell cultures, anemic baboons, and transgenic mice.[28] The agent also enhances thalassemic erythroid cell survival through Bcl-family prosurvival proteins.[29] SDMB has an excellent safety profile in long-term animal studies in two species and tested negative in mutagenicity testing. In normal volunteers, the therapeutic was found to have a half-life of 9–11 h at tolerable doses from 2 to 20 mg/kg/dose, allowing for once per day dosing (shown in Fig. 3).[30] These actions, and the pharmacologic profile, defines SDMB as an excellent candidate for single-use therapy and for combined modality therapy in thalassemia, as it can be used with therapeutics which are cytotoxic or suppress erythropoiesis, such as the global HDAC inhibitors, decitabine, or hydroxyurea. SDMB is now undergoing initial evaluation in short-term studies in β-thalassemia intermedia patients in dose-escalation trials. With beneficial dual actions on fetal globin induction and in prolonging erythroid cell survival, the agent offers potential for providing a potential mainstay or maintenance therapeutic,[28,29,31] to which the cytotoxic agents might be intermittently added or "pulsed."

The influence of quantitative trait loci on basal and induced levels of HbF

HbF and proportions of F-cells can vary by 10-fold in different normal subjects and in patients with the same molecular mutations; it has been difficult to predict whether clinical courses will become thalassemia intermedia or major with the same globin mutations. The influence of specific genetic modifiers, including single nucleotide polymorphisms (SNPs) and quantitative trait loci (QTL), which alter basal HbF levels in both normal and hemoglobinopathy subjects and ameliorate clinical severity has been recognized for many years, but is now considered to be influenced by the presence of genetic modifiers, such as a T-allele present at promoter nucleotide (nt) –158 5′ upstream of the HBG ($^{G}\gamma$-globin gene) on chromosome 11p15 (rs7482144), associated with elevated HbF levels particularly during stress erythropoiesis.[32,33] More recently, this and two other QTL have been found to account for nearly 50% of the variation in basal HbF/F-cell levels.[32–38] Genome-wide SNP association studies by Thein and colleagues yielded the unexpected finding that *BCL11A* is a major QTL for HbF and F-cell production in normal individuals and in patients with β-thalassemia, which subsequently was confirmed in sickle cell disease; *BCLIIA* was found to have profound effects in preventing the fetal to adult globin switch when absent.[32–38] Thein and colleagues also showed that the *HBS1L-MYB* intergenic polymorphism (*HMIP*) on chromosome

Table 1. Genetic modifiers of fetal globin gene expression

Quantitative trait locus	Activity
BCLIIA	Repressor of γ-globin
−158 C→T $^{G}\gamma$ promoter	Increases $^{G}\gamma$-globin
6p22.3–23.2, *myb*	Decreases F-cell proportions
Xp22	Increases F-cells proportions
PDE 7B	Reduces γ-globin
MAPK5	Increases γ-globin through distant upstream site
PEX7	Binds factor that binds a negative regulator
TOX	Not determined

6q23 exerts significant negative effects.[32,35,36] Other groups have confirmed that *BCL11A* on chromosome 2p16 is a major HbF QTL in populations both with or without β-hemoglobinopathies. Further, Chui and colleagues reported that *BCL11A* is a transcriptional repressor of *HBG* ($^{G}\gamma$-globin) proximal promoter activity, which is abolished by butyrate *in vitro*.[37] (Modifiers of fetal globin expression are listed in Table 1). *BCL11A* binds to the GGCCGG motif in nucleotide −56 to −51 on the gamma globin proximal promoter, a region in which our group previously identified alterations in protein binding in the nucleated erythroid cells of patients who responded to butyrate therapy, including disappearance of a putative repressor from the region.[21,26] Those, and our more recent findings demonstrated that with butyrate and a newer agent, RB7, identified through molecular modeling, displacement of a repressor complex (potentially *BCL11A*) occurs in the promoter, leading to histone acetylation and γ-globin transcription, highly targeted effects.[21,26,39,40]

Differences in QTLs occur commonly. In a recent analysis of random sickle cell and thalassemia patients enrolled in clinical trials, more than 50% of the sickle cell subjects were found to have a high basal HbF genotype at the *BCL11A* locus and 70% of Thai HbE-beta-thalassemia patients had a high HbF genotype including the XmnI polymorphism and a *BCL11A* QTL. Three QTLs in the Thai population which produce low or high F genotypes in genome wide screening studies have been found to profoundly alter thalassemia severity, producing an average 1 g/dL difference in total hemoglobin levels with the same globin mutations.[34] It is entirely possible that the presence or absence of genetic modifiers (QTL) will also affect inducibility of responses to different HbF-inducing therapeutic agents. Determination of whether the presence of QTL polymorphisms are associated with differential responses to epigenetic modifiers, such as HDAC inhibitors or demethylating agents, or with targeted SCFA derivatives (SCFADs) which are *not* global HDAC inhibitors, will allow design of clinical trial protocols tailored for a greater likelihood of success in patients with different QTLs.

Summary

Proof-of-concept of fetal globin induction as an approach to improve globin chain balance and reduce the anemia in β-thalassemia has been established with three different therapeutic classes of γ-globin inducers. Chemotherapeutic agents and global HDAC inhibitors, which inhibit cellular proliferation probably should be used intermittently at most in beta-thalassemia, as cell growth arrest can aggravate apoptosis. A novel oral HbF inducer, SDMB, which is not cytotoxic, can be used in combination regimens with the epigenetic and cytotoxic agents. An oral formulation of decitabine is being developed, and higher potency oral inducers have been identified. Targeting clinical trials now for specific agents directed to low F versus high F QTL may identify regimens predictive of responses to different agents. These new options for HbF induction should benefit many thalassemia patients globally, particularly many who chronically live with very low hemoglobin levels (<7 g/dL) without transfusions.

Acknowledgments

This work was supported by grants from the National Institutes of Health, DK-52962, HL-61208, and FS-R 002170 (S. Perrine), MOI R00533, and HL-007501–28 (S. A. Castaneda).

Conflicts of interest

Drs. S. Perrine and R.J. Berenson have salary support and equity interest in HemaQuest Pharmaceuticals. Dr. D.V. Faller has equity interest in HemaQuest Pharmaceuticals.

Supporting Information

Additional Supporting Information may be found in the online version of this article:

Table S1. HbF-inducing gents with complementary mechanisms of action

Please note: Wiley-Blackwell are not responsible for the content or functionality of any supporting materials supplied by the authors. Any queries (other than missing material) should be directed to the corresponding author for the article.

References

1. Steinberg, M.H. & G.P. Rodgers. 2001. Pharmacologic modulation of fetal hemoglobin. *Med. (Baltimore)* **80:** 328–344.
2. Perrine, S.P. 2008. Fetal globin stimulant therapies in the beta-hemoglobinopathies: principles and current potential. *Pediatr. Ann.* **37:** 339–346.
3. Gallo, E., P. Massaro, R. Miniero, *et al.* 1979. The importance of the genetic picture and globin synthesis in determining the clinical and haematological features of thalassaemia intermedia. *Br. J. Haematol.* **41:** 211–221.
4. Schrier, S.L. 1997. Pathobiology of thalassemic erythrocytes. *Curr Opin. Hematol.* **4:** 75–78.
5. Stamatoyannopoulos, G. 2005. Control of globin gene expression during development and erythroid differentiation. *Exp. Hematol.* **33:** 259–271.
6. Centis, F., L. Tabellini, G. Lucarelli, *et al.* 2000. The importance of erythroid expansion in determining the extent of apoptosis in erythroid precursors in patients with beta-thalassemia major. *Blood* **96:** 3624–3629.
7. Mathias, L.A., T.C. Fisher, L. Zeng, *et al.* 2000. Ineffective erythropoiesis in beta-thalassemia major is due to apoptosis at the polychromatophilic normoblast stage. *Exp. Hematol.* **28:** 1343–1353.
8. Pootrakul, P., P. Sirankapracha, S. Hemsorach, *et al.* 2000. A correlation of erythrokinetics, ineffective erythropoiesis, and erythroid precursor apoptosis in Thai patients with thalassemia. *Blood* **96:** 2606–2612.
9. Collins, A.F., H.A. Pearson, P. Giardina, *et al.* 1995. Oral sodium phenylbutyrate therapy in homozygous beta thalassemia: a clinical trial. *Blood* **85:** 43–49.
10. Perrine, S.P., G.D. Ginder, D.V. Faller, *et al.* 1993. A short-term trial of butyrate to stimulate fetal-globin-gene expression in the beta-globin disorders. *N. Engl. J. Med.* **328:** 81–86.
11. Cao, H., G. Stamatoyannopoulos & M. Jung. 2004. Induction of human gamma globin gene expression by histone deacetylase inhibitors. *Blood* **103:** 701–709.
12. Domenica Cappellini, M., G. Graziadei, L. Ciceri, *et al.* 2000. Oral isobutyramide therapy in patients with thalassemia intermedia: results of a phase II open study. *Blood Cells Mol. Dis.* **26:** 105–111.
13. Reich, S., C. Buhrer, G. Henze, *et al.* 2000. Oral isobutyramide reduces transfusion requirements in some patients with homozygous beta-thalassemia. *Blood* **96:** 3357–3363.
14. Dunbar, C., W. Travis, Y.W. Kan, *et al.* 1989. 5-Azacytidine treatment in a beta (0)-thalassaemic patient unable to be transfused due to multiple alloantibodies. *Br. J. Haematol.* **72:** 467–468.
15. Hajjar, F.M. & H.A. Pearson. 1994. Pharmacologic treatment of thalassemia intermedia with hydroxyurea. *J. Pediatr.* **125:** 490–492.
16. Singer, S.T., F.A. Kuypers, N.F. Olivieri, *et al.* 2005. Fetal haemoglobin augmentation in E/beta(0) thalassaemia: clinical and haematological outcome. *Br. J. Haematol.* **131:** 378–388.
17. Fucharoen, S., N. Siritanaratkul, P. Winichagoon, *et al.* 1996. Hydroxyurea increases hemoglobin F levels and improves the effectiveness of erythropoiesis in beta-thalassemia/hemoglobin E disease. *Blood* **87:** 887–892.
18. Lowrey, C.H. & A.W. Nienhuis. 1993. Brief report: treatment with azacitidine of patients with end-stage beta-thalassemia. *N. Engl. J. Med.* **329:** 845–848.
19. Ley, T.J., J. DeSimone, N.P. Anagnou, *et al.* 1982. 5-azacytidine selectively increases gamma-globin synthesis in a patient with beta+ thalassemia. *N. Engl. J. Med.* **307:** 1469–1475.
20. Saunthararajah, Y., C.A. Hillery, D. Lavelle, *et al.* 2003. Effects of 5-aza-2′-deoxycytidine on fetal hemoglobin levels, red cell adhesion, and hematopoietic differentiation in patients with sickle cell disease. *Blood* **102:** 3865–3870.
21. Perrine, S.P., R. Mankidy, M.S. Boosalis, *et al.* 2009. Erythroid Kruppel-like factor (EKLF) is recruited to the gamma-globin gene promoter as a co-activator and is required for gamma-globin gene induction by short-chain fatty acid derivatives. *Eur. J. Haematol.* **82:** 466–476.
22. Bourantas, K., G. Economou & J. Georgiou. 1997. Administration of high doses of recombinant human erythropoietin to patients with beta-thalassemia intermedia: a preliminary trial. *Eur. J. Haematol.* **58:** 22–25.
23. Nisli, G., K. Kavakli, C. Vergin, *et al.* 1996. Recombinant human erythropoietin trial in thalassemia intermedia. *J. Trop. Pediatr.* **42:** 330–334.
24. Rachmilewitz, E.A. & M. Aker. 1998. The role of recombinant human erythropoietin in the treatment of thalassemia. *Ann. N.Y. Acad. Sci.* **850:** 129–138.
25. Galanello, R., S. Barella, M.P. Turco, *et al.* 1994. Serum erythropoietin and erythropoiesis in high- and low-fetal hemoglobin beta-thalassemia intermedia patients. *Blood* **83:** 561–565.
26. Ikuta T, Kan YW, Swerdlow PS, *et al.* 1998 Alterations in protein-DNA interactions in the γ globin gene promoter in response to butyrate therapy. *Blood* **92:** 2924–2933.
27. Perrine, S., D.V. Faller, L. Shen, *et al.* 2009. HQK-1001 has additive HbF-inducing activity in combination with hydroxyurea and decitabine [abstract]. *Blood* **114:** 977.
28. Pace, B.S., G.L. White, G.J. Dover, *et al.* 2002. Short chain fatty acid derivatives induce fetal globin expression and erythropoiesis in vivo. *Blood* **100:** 4640–4648.
29. Castaneda, S., M.S. Boosalis, D. Emery, *et al.* 2005. Enhancement of growth and survival and alterations in Bcl-family proteins in beta-thalassemic erythroid progenitors by novel short-chain fatty acid derivatives. *Blood Cells Mol. Dis.* **35:** 217–226.
30. Perrine, S., W.C. Welch, J. Keefer, *et al.* 2008. Phase 1 clinical testing of HQK-1001, a novel oral fetal globin gene inducer [abstract]. *Blood* **112:** 130.

31. Boosalis, M.S., R. Bandyopadhyay, E.H. Bresnick, *et al.* 2001. Short-chain fatty acid derivatives stimulate cell proliferation and induce STAT-5 activation. *Blood* **97:** 3259–3267.
32. Thein, S.L., S. Menzel, M. Lathrop, *et al.* 2009. Control of fetal hemoglobin: new insights emerging from genomics and clinical implications. *Hum. Mol. Genet.* **18:** R216–R223.
33. Labie, D., J. Pagnier, C. Lapoumeroulie, *et al.* 1985. Common haplotype dependency of high G gamma-globin gene expression and high Hb F levels in beta-thalassemia and sickle cell anemia patients. *Proc. Natl. Acad. Sci. USA* **82:** 2111–2114.
34. Nuinoon, M., W. Makarasara, T. Mushiroda, *et al.* 2010. A genome-wide association identified the common genetic variants influence disease severity in beta°-thalassemia/hemoglobin E. *Hum. Genet.* **127:** 303–314.
35. Jiang, J., S. Best, S. Menzel, *et al.* 2006. cMYB is involved in the regulation of fetal hemoglobin production in adults. *Blood* **108:** 1077–1083.
36. Garner, C., J. Mitchell, T. Hatzis, *et al.* 1998. Haplotype mapping of a major quantitative-trait locus for fetal hemoglobin production, on chromosome 6q23. *Am. J. Hum. Genet.* **62:** 1468–1474.
37. Chen, Z., H.Y. Luo, M.H. Steinberg, *et al.* 2009. BCL11A represses HBG transcription in K562 cells. *Blood Cells Mol. Dis.* **42:** 144–149.
38. Sankaran, V.G., J. Xu, T. Ragoczy, *et al.* 2009. Developmental and species-divergent globin switching are driven by BCL11A. *Nature* **460:** 1093–1097.
39. Bohacek, R., M.S. Boosalis, C. McMartin, *et al.* 2006. Identification of novel small-molecule inducers of fetal hemoglobin using pharmacophore and 'PSEUDO' receptor models. *Chem. Biol. Drug. Des.* **67:** 318–328.
40. Mankidy, R., D.V. Faller, R. Mabaera, *et al.* 2006. Short-chain fatty acids induce gamma-globin gene expression by displacement of a HDAC3-NCoR repressor complex. *Blood* **108:** 3179–3186.

Ann. N.Y. Acad. Sci. ISSN 0077-8923

ANNALS OF THE NEW YORK ACADEMY OF SCIENCES
Issue: *Cooley's Anemia: Ninth Symposium*

Detection of the cardiovascular complications of thalassemia by echocardiography

John Malcolm Walker and Sunil Nair
Hatter Cardiovascular Institute, University College Hospital, London, United Kingdom

Address for correspondence: Dr. John Malcolm Walker, M.D., F.R.C.P., Clinical Director Hatter Cardiovascular Institute, University College Hospital, 67 Chenies Mews, London WC1E 6HX, United Kingdom. malcolm.walker@uclh.nhs.uk

The thalassemia syndromes are associated with cardiovascular complications, which differ with the varying phenotypes encountered. The well-recognized paradigm of heart failure induced by myocardial iron overload, in thalassemia major (TM), has now been joined by pulmonary arterial hypertension (mostly seen in thalassemia intermedia) among other more subtle disorders of the cardiovascular system, including endothelial dysfunction. Cardiovascular magnetic resonance (T2*) has allowed cardiac iron load to be quantified noninvasively, and the routine measurement of T2* has been associated with a marked improvement in the outlook for patients with TM, in particular. Echocardiography remains an indispensable tool in the cardiovascular assessment of patients, it provides many insights into cardiovascular function, and its use allows improved management of patients. It is particularly suited to assess diastolic function, diagnose intracardiac masses (usually thrombus), and assess right ventricular function and pulmonary pressure.

Keywords: thalassemia syndromes; echocardiography; ventricular dysfunction; iron overload; pulmonary hypertension

Introduction

Treatment of thalassemia major (TM) consists of regular blood transfusions and iron chelation therapy, which can delay cardiac complications and improve longevity. Even when severe the cardiomyopathy, which may be accounted for by accumulation of iron within myocytes,[1] may be reversed by treatment with iron chelators.[2,3] The development of the T2* parameter using cardiac magnetic resonance (cMR) scanning has provided a robust tool for assessing tissue levels of iron and has contributed to the recently observed reduction in deaths from cardiac iron overload.[4] Despite the fundamental importance of cMR scanning and T2* assessment of tissue iron content, the scans are relatively expensive and not available universally. Transthoracic echocardiography (TTE) is widely available at relatively low cost, but conventional TTE parameters have been unhelpful in estimating risk from iron overload in TM.[5] Once abnormalities in left ventricular (LV) systolic function become detectable significant iron deposition has occurred and survival is reduced.[3] Abnormalities of diastolic function may occur earlier[6,7] and dynamic studies may highlight abnormalities of function not apparent at rest. Newer techniques for assessing ventricular function by echocardiography include tissue Doppler imaging that may detect abnormalities despite normal global LV function in iron overload.[8] The syndrome of thalassemia intermedia (TI) poses different cardiovascular challenges, but not iron cardiac overload in most cases.[9,10] These patients, who characteristically have sufficient residual hemoglobin production to survive without regular blood transfusion, have significant risk of pulmonary hypertension;[11] the chronic anemia is associated with increased chamber size and probable long-term changes in ventricular function that remain poorly characterized. The clinical management of thalassemia patients is complex due to the variable phenotype, the chronicity, and multisystem nature of the condition but also complications

doi: 10.1111/j.1749-6632.2010.05643.x

arising from some of the treatments required, for instance, the use of implanted central vein access lines and ports. These features mandate knowledge of the tissue specific iron load, assessed by cMR and regular cardiovascular examinations and imaging to pick up complications, a role well suited to TTE.

Iron and the heart

The human body has no mechanism for excreting excess iron, which is stored as crystalline iron oxide within ferritin and hemosiderin. At normal body iron levels, plasma iron is bound to transferrin, preventing catalytic activity, and free radical production.[12] In thalassemia the combination of increased gastrointestinal iron absorption and iron from red cell breakdown in the reticuloendothelial system saturates this iron binding capacity and this results in the emergence of nontransferrin bound iron (NTBI).[13] NTBI is more toxic than bound iron and promotes hydroxyl free radical formation[14] resulting in damage to membrane lipids and proteins. NTBI is taken up more readily by cardiac myocytes than transferrin bound iron.[15]

In the heart, free intracellular iron results in impaired Na-K-ATPase activity,[15] increased lysosomal fragility[16] and impaired mitochondrial respiratory chain activity,[17] and leads to heart failure. Iron deposition in the heart follows a characteristic pattern,[1] with the LV wall containing the most iron[18]; the tissue distribution of iron is nonuniform, with the epicardial layer containing the most iron, the endocardium containing a moderate amount and the intermediate layer containing the least amount of iron. The degree of cardiac dysfunction depends on the quantity of iron deposited in individual myocardial fibers and the number of fibers affected. The relatively mild degree of fibrosis in most autopsy studies of iron overload suggests that even when advanced, the cardiomyopathy could be reversible.[19]

Historically, risk of cardiac siderosis was assessed indirectly by association with consistently high ferritin levels >2,500 and high liver iron measures from liver biopsy >15 gm/100 gm dry weight.[20] We now know that although some assessment of risk can be extrapolated from these measures of iron exposure they are both imprecise surrogate estimates for cardiac iron load. In fact, cardiac MRI studies have elegantly demonstrated that at any particular time in an individual patient there may exist discordance between iron load in the heart and liver.[21]

Conventional transthoracic echocardiography

For many countries the mainstay of assessing cardiac involvement in thalassemia has been by TTE. This technique is widely available at relatively low cost and has the advantage of being obtainable at the bedside. TTE uses high frequency ultrasound waves to obtain real time moving images of the heart. From the images obtained the chamber sizes, contractility, and valve function can be studied and quantified. As a technique it does have limitations, including subjectivity in interpretation, user dependency, and being subject to poor acoustic windows (e.g., in obese patients, those with significant lung disease or chest wall deformities; rare occurrences in thalassemia), which may limit image acquisition and quality. Conventional echocardiograpic markers of LV function, such as the left ventricular ejection fraction (LV EF) have traditionally been used as a surrogate marker to predict the degree of cardiac iron loading. On the whole they have been unhelpful in this role, as the absence of a reduced EF does not exclude significant iron overload and a risk of sudden cardiac decompensation (Fig. 1). M mode techniques for evaluating LV systolic function have remained normal,[22] and have failed to identify thalassemia patients with iron overload from normal controls. Once abnormalities in LV systolic function become detectable significant iron deposition has occurred and survival is reduced, suggesting this is a late stage in the disease process.[23,24] Measures of diastolic function, or ventricular relaxation, may occur earlier[25,26] and detailed analysis of digitized M mode tracings has detected abnormalities in contraction and relaxation in children with thalassemia.[27] Other echo techniques involving dynamic studies have highlighted abnormalities of function not apparent at rest.[28]

Normal ranges may be difficult to define in the thalassemia population. Anemia is associated with a compensatory increase in cardiac output, so that normal values taken from nonanemic, nonthalassemia populations are not applicable to this group, where normality of cardiac function is associated with high LV EF of >60% (compared to quoted normal ranges in standard age matched populations of >50%). Thus reports of "normal" ventricular

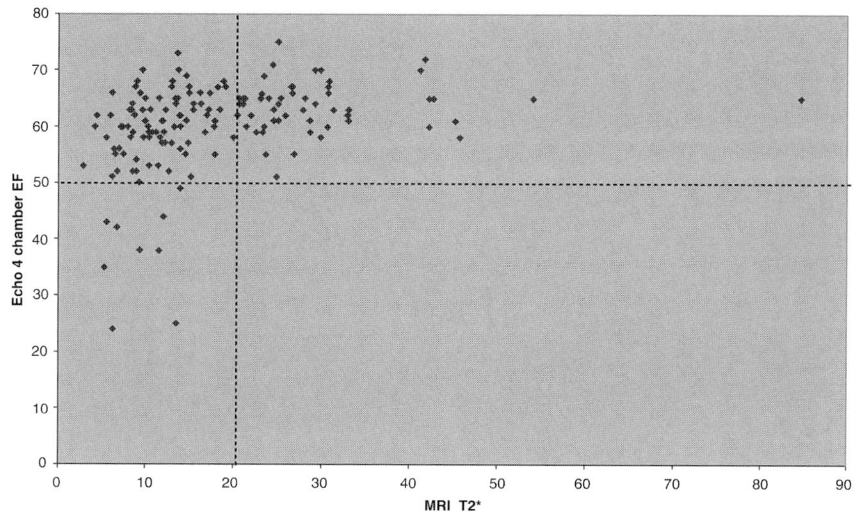

Figure 1. A plot of left ventricular ejection fraction measured by echocardiography (Teichholz method) against cardiac T2* obtained from a cMR scan obtained at the same clinic visit for a group of thalassemia major patients undergoing clinical screening. A cardiac T2* under 20 ms denotes significant myocardial iron overload, with a value of <10 ms being severe iron overload. It can be seen that there are a significant number of individuals with T2* <20 ms and even some with a T2* <10 ms where the EF is within conventional normal limits of >50%. No patient with a T2* > 20 ms has an EF <50%, and this populations average EF for the noniron overloaded group (T2* > 20 ms) appears to be >60% (unpublished observations).

function provided by ultrasound laboratories without a significant experience in this condition may falsely reassure the unwary clinician/ hematologist. Therefore, although the conventional measure of LV function, the ejection fraction (EF) undoubtedly identifies at risk individuals when abnormal, it may remain normal despite high iron content within the heart (Fig. 1). There is at least 10% interstudy and interoperator variation in the measurement of EF, making it a poor choice as a single descriptor of overall cardiac function. Despite these limitations, serial measurements in individuals can identify those at risk if the EF is noted to be consistently falling; conversely an improving EF is a good prognostic indicator and can track falling myocardial iron content shown by a rising T2* (Fig. 2).

Tissue doppler imaging

Newer techniques for assessing ventricular function include tissue Doppler imaging (TDI). TDI involves obtaining regional information regarding wall motion and velocity.[29,30] Tissue Doppler techniques include TDI velocity measurements, strain, strain rate and longitudinal deformation, or tissue tracking (TT). Over the past decade there have been numerous studies published addressing the feasibility and potential clinical applications of TDI and its derived techniques of strain and strain rate.[31] Despite promising publications the clinical uptake of these methods has been slow, especially so in thalassemia, although some preliminary studies are now being published.

TDI allows the analysis of velocities with high amplitude and low frequency, which originate from the myocardial tissue. TDI images are obtained by gain adjustment and elimination of the high pass filter, they require modifications of the software and hardware of the ultrasound platform.

Tissue Doppler derived velocities can be obtained by using pulsed Doppler, with a sample volume placed at various points on an apical four-chamber view of the heart, or by color-coded Doppler (Fig. 3). Both methods give the same mechanical information but differences exist in the peak values obtained. Pulsed Doppler techniques measure peak velocity approximately 20–30% higher than the mean velocity obtained with color Doppler. This difference must be considered when estimating LV filling pressure using the ratio of early diastolic velocities measured from the Doppler mitral flow profile (E) and from the mitral annular velocity obtained by TDI (E′ or Ea).[32] One of the main reasons for skepticism toward TDI lies in its physical principles. Doppler is the ideal method for examining

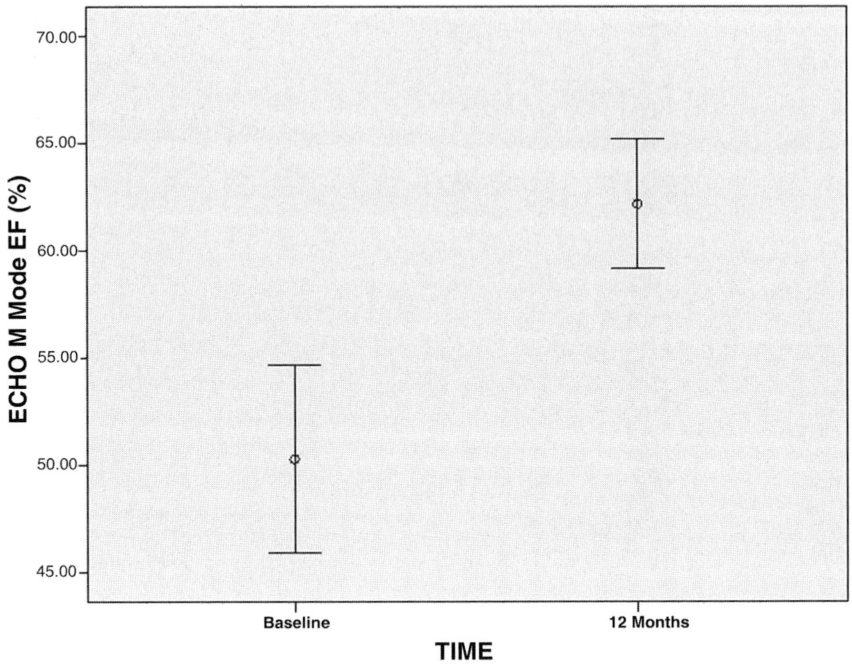

Figure 2. A group of patients with severe iron overload (T2* < 8 ms) underwent intensification of chelation, by the introduction of combination treatment with deferioxamine plus oral deferiprone. At the first visit there is a mean EF 50%, which improves after 12 months of intensive chelation to a mean >60%; this was associated with an improvement in cMR T2*. The LV EF can be used to track changes in patient iron burden across time and across treatment changes.

intracardiac and vascular flow that obeys the laws of fluid dynamics. Myocardial motion is different, occurring in multiple planes and directions. It is influenced by motion of other organs and structures within the thoracic cage and follows complex mechanical phenomena for which there exists no reference method.[33] Nevertheless, normal values for tissue Doppler derived velocities have been established.[34] A peak mitral annular velocity of >5.4 cm/s averaged from six annular sites predicts an EF > 50%.[35] In a general population study, reduced TDI velocities were associated with increased mortality, rates suggesting that these new techniques were able to identify early, subtle changes in cardiac performance before the onset of clinically evident disease,[36] a situation of potential great importance in the thalassemic population.

A previous study by our group[8] in 52 thalassemia patients found that color-coded TDI annular velocities of the mitral and tricuspid valves detected abnormalities, despite normal LV EF in a high proportion of patients with iron overload. This suggested that TDI may be able to identify abnormalities in asymptomatic patients with iron overload (Fig. 4). A similar observation has been made in thalassemic children,[37] but others have failed to confirm an advantage of TDI over conventional Doppler indices.[38] Resolution of the place of TDI parameters in the assessment of thalassemic patients will therefore depend on larger studies.

The limitations of TDI in respect of tethering from collateral segments can be overcome by strain imaging. Strain is a measure of tissue deformation and is defined as the change in length normalized to the original length. If the segment gets shorter in length then the strain is value is a negative number, conversely, if the segment gets longer then the strain is a positive number.

Strain imaging introduced the concept of myocardial deformation as a marker of contractility intrinsic to the myocardium. Strain rate is the speed at which this change occurs. Strain rate and strain are similar to shortening velocity and shortening fraction respectively. By TDI strain rate is the difference in velocity between two points along the myocardial wall (velocity gradient) normalized to the distance between the two points. Strain rate measures the rate at which two points move toward

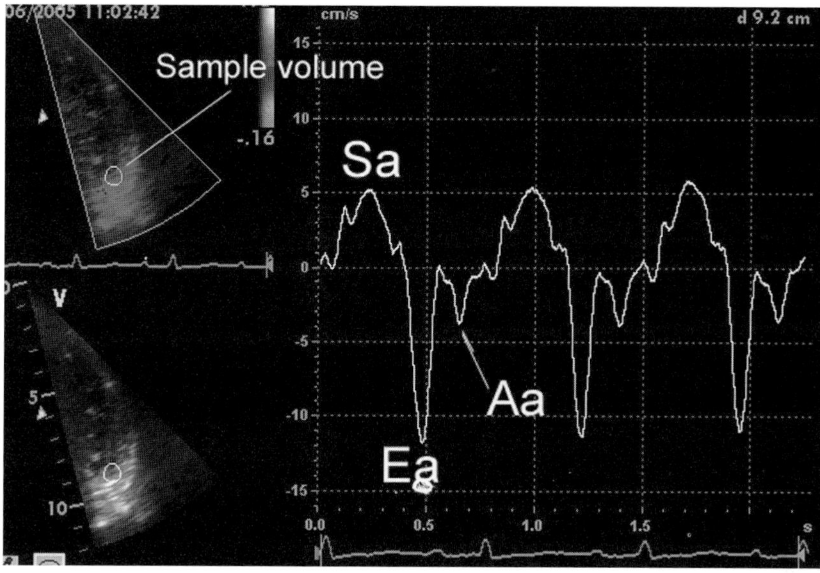

Figure 3. A color-coded TDI signal from the lateral mitral annulus border. The sample volume is labeled. The image was obtained at a frame rate > 150 fps, and the velocity peaks are labeled: Sa, the peak systolic velocity; Ea, the peak early diastolic velocity; and Aa, the peak late diastolic velocity.

or away from each other. Integration of strain rate yields strain, the normalized change in length between two points. But strain is not without its limitations. As it is derived from TDI, limitations in terms of angle dependency apply. In addition, the signal is subjected to noise problems especially in the apical views. This affects the profile of the spectral curve and can make interpretation difficult and reproducibility very challenging. Strain rate and strain are theoretically less susceptible to translational motion and tethering artifacts and thus may be superior to tissue velocity in depicting regional or global myocardial function. In general peak systolic strain comes closest to measuring local contractile function. It is relatively volume independent and less pressure dependent than strain. Despite these theoretical advantages and promising experience in the preclinical detection of myocardial dysfunction in other cardiomyopathies, systematic studies of these parameters have not been published yet in the thalassemic population. TDI has the potential for providing rapidly obtained, bedside assessment of diastolic function,[39] more easily than with many other parameters, such as pulmonary vein flow analysis and for the determination of right ventricular function both in systole and diastole. These parameters deserve to be analyzed prospectively in suitably large cohorts of thalassemia patients to achieve clinical credibility and more widespread adoption.

General echocardiographic assessment

The echocardiogram is above all an accessible widely available imaging tool, which should be used in the cardiovascular assessment of all thalassemic patients on a regular basis. It complements the information obtained by cMR imaging and even simple measurements of ventricular dimensions in systole and diastole obtained by m-mode imaging in the parasternal long axis with even the most basic of ultrasound equipment, can be used to track the progress of individual patients across time. Atrial dimensions can alert physicians to the likely future risk of the development of arrhythmia, particularly atrial fibrillation, which is now commonly encountered in the aging population of thalassemic patients, even in the absence of current significant iron overload (>40% incidence of AF in TM patients >40 years; personal observations). Echocardiography may reveal mobile masses within the heart, usually thrombus within atria, or occasionally within the right ventricle (RV), associated with the current or previous use of long-term indwelling central venous lines. These may not be detected by MR, owing to

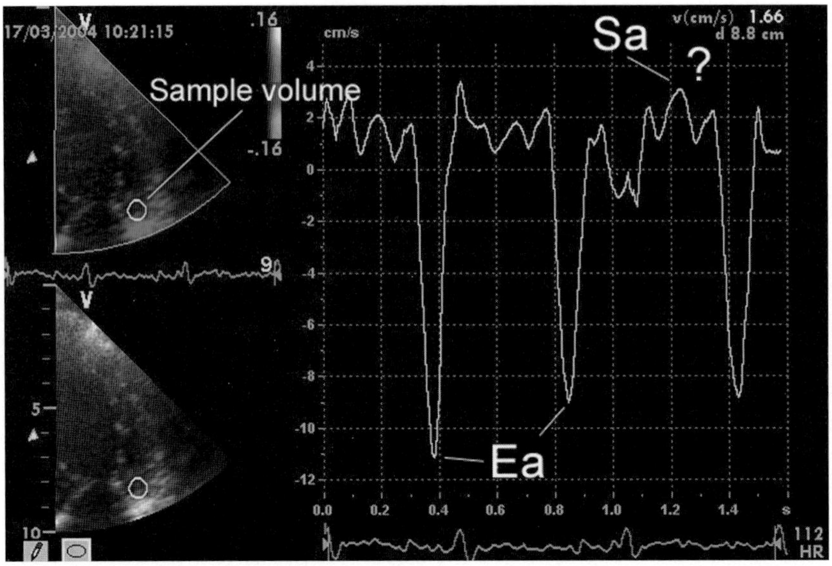

Figure 4. A color-coded TDI signal obtained from the same patient 15 months prior to the image in Figure 3. Note the virtual absence of a peak systolic velocity wave form and preservation of the diastolic velocity curve (peak Ea), which is unitary in the absence of atrial systole (patient in AF). This recording was obtained when the patient had severe myocardial iron overload, with a cMR T2* <6 ms and overt biventricular failure. The change in TDI velocity profile toward a normal appearance in Figure 3 followed intensive chelation therapy with a combination of desferoxamine plus deferiprone.

the averaging techniques required to construct images.

Most importantly, the emerging risk associated with pulmonary hypertension, particularly in thalassemia intermedia, in the absence of myocardial iron overload, or LV disease, is best documented noninvasively by conventional Doppler interrogation of the tricuspid valve. The velocity of the tricuspid regurgitant jet (TR jet) accurately reflects the pressure drop between RV and right atrium and thus of pulmonary arterial pressure (Pressure in mmHg $= 4 \times$ velocity in m/s).[40] Conventional definitions suggest a TR velocity >2.5 m/s is abnormal and > 3.0 m/s significant pulmonary hypertension. Some cautions need to be understood. Many patients with thalassemia are anemic at the time of assessment and, owing to the cardiovascular compensatory mechanisms, have a hyperdynamic circulation, so that increased velocities may reflect healthy physiological responses and not pathological changes in the pulmonary circulation. These issues require to be resolved for this population. Nevertheless regular screening for elevated TR velocities is now necessary as, despite the caveats mentioned above, clinical experience suggests once pulmonary hypertension is established, prognosis is poor. Approaches using more intensive management of the anemia in TI, or the introduction of specific medication to reduce pulmonary pressures (e.g., sildenafil), are currently under investigation.

Conclusions

It appears that TDI techniques can usefully supplement the conventional LV EF to characterize ventricular function in TM and follow changes brought about by treatment. It remains to be proven that the TDI velocities are superior to classical measurements of global ventricular function, exemplified by the ejection fraction (EF). However, the TDI annular velocity measurements (Sa, Ea, and Aa) are rapidly obtained and are less reliant on image quality than EF. For the quantification of diastolic function the use of early (Ea) and, particularly late (Aa) TDI velocities appear promising and are certainly less cumbersome than many echo parameters classically used to assess diastolic dysfunction. It will require a cohort of patients to derive reliable normal values for these parameters and to establish if they are less susceptible to operator and interindividual variability than classical measurements of function. The RV is particularly susceptible to impaired function associated with iron overload. The tricuspid annular velocity signal from the TDI (RV Sa, Ea, and Aa) may prove to be a very useful bedside tool to assess the RV, which has been notoriously difficult to study using conventional echo techniques.

In summary, the echo still has the capacity to help clinicians manage patients and monitor the effects of changes in therapy, but it does not have the capacity to estimate the myocardial tissue iron content. With the advent of simplified, rapid MR scans at a much reduced cost, able to provide a rapid assessment of cardiac T2* without analysis of ventricular function, at the same time as liver iron assessment, opens the prospect of wider application of the T2* but would mandate the careful collection of anatomical and functional data by echocardiography using standardized protocols that should include conventional measurements and the tissue Doppler annular velocities introduced above, with a special emphasis on right ventricular function and assessments of pulmonary hypertension by TR jet velocity.

Conflicts of interest

Dr. Nair was in receipt of a British Heart Foundation Fellowship award during the period of this study and has received support from Novartis in attending educational symposia. Dr. Walker has received support for attending educational meetings from Novartis and ApoPharma.

References

1. Buja, L.M. & W.C. Roberts. 1971. Iron in the heart. Etiology and clinical significance. *Am. J. Med.* **51:** 209–221.
2. Weatherall, D.J. 1997. The thalassaemias. *BMJ* **314:** 1675–1678.
3. Olivieri, N.F. 1999. The beta-thalassemias. *N. Engl. J. Med.* **341:** 99–109.
4. Modell, B., M. Khan, M. Darlison, *et al.* 2008. Improved survival of thalassaemia major in the UK and relation to T2* cardiovascular magnetic resonance. *J. Cardiovasc. Magn. Reson.* **10:** 42.
5. Schafer, A.I., R.G. Cheron, R. Dluhy, *et al.* 1981. Clinical consequences of acquired transfusional iron overload in adults. *N. Engl. J. Med.* **304:** 319–324.
6. Brittenham, G.M., P.M. Griffith, A.W. Nienhuis, *et al.* 1994. Efficacy of deferoxamine in preventing complications of iron overload in patients with thalassemia major. *N. Engl. J. Med.* **331:** 567–573.
7. Olivieri, N.F., D.G. Nathan, J.H. MacMillan, *et al.* 1994. Survival in medically treated patients with homozygous beta-thalassemia. *N. Engl. J. Med.* **331:** 574–578.
8. Vogel, M., L.J. Anderson, S. Holden, *et al.* 2003. Tissue Doppler echocardiography in patients with thalassaemia detects early myocardial dysfunction related to myocardial iron overload. *Eur. Heart J.* **24:** 113–119.
9. Taher, A.T., K.M Musallam, M. Karimi, *et al.* 2010. Overview on practices in thalassemia intermedia management aiming for lowering complication rates across a region of endemicity: the OPTIMAL CARE study. *Blood* **115:** 1886–1892.
10. Cappellini, M.D., K.M. Musallam & A.T. Taher. 2009. Insight onto the pathophysiology and clinical complications of thalassemia intermedia. *Hemoglobin* **33**(Suppl 1): S145-S159.
11. Aessopos, A., M. Tsironi, A. Andreopoulos & D. Farmakis. 2009. Heart disease in thalassemia intermedia. *Hemoglobin* **33**(Suppl 1): S170-S176.
12. Hershko, C. & T.E. Peto. 1987. Non-transferrin plasma iron. *Br. J. Haematol.* **66:** 149–151.
13. Hershko, C., G. Graham, G.W. Bates & E.A. Rachmilewitz. 1978. Non-specific serum iron in thalassaemia: an abnormal serum iron fraction of potential toxicity. *Br. J. Haematol.* **40:** 255–263.
14. Gutteridge, J.M., D.A. Rowley, E. Griffiths & B. Halliwell. 1985. Low-molecular-weight iron complexes and oxygen radical reactions in idiopathic haemochromatosis. *Clin. Sci. (Lond)* **68:** 463–467.
15. Link, G., A. Pinson & C. Hershko. 1994. Ability of the orally effective iron chelators dimethyl- and diethyl-hydroxypyrid-4-one and of deferoxamine to restore sarcolemmal thiolic enzyme activity in iron-loaded heart cells. *Blood* **83:** 2692–2697.
16. Link, G., A. Pinson & C. Hershko. 1993. Iron loading of cultured cardiac myocytes modifies sarcolemmal structure and increases lysosomal fragility. *J. Lab. Clin. Med.* **121:** 127–134.
17. Link, G., R. Tirosh, A. Pinson & C. Hershko. 1996. Role of iron in the potentiation of anthracycline cardiotoxicity: identification of heart cell mitochondria as a major site of iron-anthracycline interaction. *J. Lab. Clin. Med.* **127:** 272–278.
18. Schellhammer, P.F., M.A. Engle & J.W. Hagstrom. 1967. Histochemical studies of the myocardium and conduction system in acquired iron-storage disease. *Circulation* **35:** 631–637.
19. Levin, E.B. & A. Golum. 1953. The heart in hemochromatosis. *Am. Heart. J.* **45:** 277–288.
20. Telfer, P.T., E. Prestcott, S. Holden, *et al.* 2000. Hepatic iron concentration combined with long-term monitoring of serum ferritin to predict complications of iron overload in thalassaemia major. *Br. J. Haematol.* **110:** 971–977.
21. Anderson, L.J., B. Wonke, E. Prescott, *et al.* 2002. Comparison of effects of oral deferiprone and subcutaneous desferrioxamine on myocardial iron concentrations and ventricular function in beta-thalassaemia. *Lancet* **360:** 516–520.
22. Hoffbrand, A.V. 2001. Diagnosing myocardial iron overload. *Eur. Heart J.* **22:** 2140–2141.
23. Brili, S.V., A.I. Tzonou, S.S. Castelanos, *et al.* 1997. The effect of iron overload in the hearts of patients with beta-thalassemia. *Clin. Cardiol.* **20:** 541–546.
24. Olson, L.J., W.P. Baldus & A.J. Tajik. 1987. Echocardiographic features of idiopathic hemochromatosis. *Am. J. Cardiol.* **60:** 885–889.

25. Kremastinos, D.T., D.P. Tsiapras, G.A. Tsetsos, *et al.* 1993. Left ventricular diastolic Doppler characteristics in beta-thalassemia major. *Circulation* **88:** 1127–1135.
26. Nienhuis, A.W., P. Griffith, H. Strawczynski, *et al.* 1980. Evaluation of cardiac function in patients with thalassemia major. *Ann. N. Y. Acad. Sci.* **344:** 384–396.
27. Valdes-Cruz, L.M., C. Reinecke, M. Rutkowski, *et al.* 1982. Preclinical abnormal segmental cardiac manifestations of thalassemia major in children on transfusion-chelation therapy: echographic alterations of left ventricular posterior wall contraction and relaxation patterns. *Am. Heart J.* **103:** 505–511.
28. Mariotti, E., A. Agostini, E. Angelucci, *et al.* 1993. Cardiac study by dobutamine stress echocardiography in thalassemic patients. *Bone Marrow Transplant.* **12**(Suppl 1): 14–15.
29. Miyatake, K., M. Yamagishi, N. Tanaka, *et al.* 1995. New method for evaluating left ventricular wall motion by color-coded tissue Doppler imaging: in vitro and in vivo studies. *J. Am. Coll. Cardiol.* **25:** 717–724.
30. Fleming, A.D., W.N. McDicken, G.R. Sutherland & P.R. Hoskins. 1994. Assessment of colour Doppler tissue imaging using test-phantoms. *Ultrasound Med. Biol.* **20:** 937–951.
31. Abraham, T.P., V.L. Dimaano & H.Y. Liang. 2007. Role of tissue Doppler and strain echocardiography in current clinical practice. *Circulation* **116:** 2597–2609.
32. McCulloch, M., W.A. Zoghbi, R. Davis, *et al.* 2006. Color tissue Doppler myocardial velocities consistently underestimate spectral tissue Doppler velocities: impact on calculation peak transmitral pulsed Doppler velocity/early diastolic tissue Doppler velocity (E/Ea). *J. Am. Soc. Echocardiogr.* **19:** 744–748.
33. Thomas, G. 2004. Tissue Doppler echocardiography—a case of right tool, wrong use. *Cardiovasc. Ultrasound* **2:** 12.
34. Palka, P., A. Lange, A.D. Fleming, *et al.* 1996. Age-related transmural peak mean velocities and peak velocity gradients by Doppler myocardial imaging in normal subjects. *Eur. Heart J.* **17**:940–950.
35. Gulati, V.K., Katz, W.E., Follansbee, W.P. & Gorcsan, J. 1996. Mitral annular descent velocity by tissue Doppler echocardiography as an index of global left ventricular function. *Am. J. Cardiol.* **77:** 979–984.
36. Mogelvang, R., P. Sogaard, S.A. Pedersen, *et al.* 2009. Cardiac dysfunction assessed by echocardiographic tissue Doppler imaging is an independent predictor of mortality in the general population. *Circulation* **119:** 2679–2685.
37. Uçar, T., T. Ileri, S. Atalay, *et al.* 2009. Early detection of myocardial dysfunction in children with beta-thalassaemia major. *Int. J. Cardiovasc. Imaging* **25:** 379–386.
38. de Gregorio, C., B. Piraino, G. Morabito, *et al.* 2009. On the use of conventional and tissue Doppler echocardiography in patients with beta-Thalassemia major and myocardial iron-overload: preliminary data by a single centre study. *Int. J. Cardiol.* Advance online publication. doi:10.1016/j.ijcard.2009.06.013.
39. Gurunath P. Parale, S. Pawar Swapnil & S. Tapare Vinay. 2009. Assessment of LV diastolic function in patients with β-thalassemia major with special reference to E/Eann ratio. *J. Pediatr. Hematol. Oncol.* **31:** 69–73.
40. Sallach, S.M., R.M. Peshock & S. Reimold. 2007. Noninvasive cardiac imaging in pulmonary hypertension. *Cardiol. Rev.* **15:** 97–101.

Ann. N.Y. Acad. Sci. ISSN 0077-8923

ANNALS OF THE NEW YORK ACADEMY OF SCIENCES
Issue: *Cooley's Anemia: Ninth Symposium*

Cardiovascular MRI in thalassemia major

John C. Wood and Leila Noetzli
Divisions of Pediatric Cardiology and Radiology, Children's Hospital Los Angeles, Los Angeles, California

Address for correspondence: John C. Wood, M.D., Ph.D., Divisions of Pediatric Cardiology and Radiology, Children's Hospital Los Angeles, MS#34, 4650 Sunset Blvd, Los Angeles, CA 90027-0034. jwood@chla.usc.edu

MRI assessment of myocardial iron and function has revolutionized the treatment of thalassemia major patients. While knowledge of somatic iron stores is vital for iron chelation management, it does not adequately monitor cardiac risk. MRI monitoring of cardiac T2* allows preclinical recognition of myocardial iron, stratifies prospective cardiac risk, and tracks response to modifications in iron chelation therapy. MRI assessment of cardiac function complements T2* measurements by offering highly accurate and reproducible assessments of ventricular function. This manuscript describes the historical context of cardiac toxicity in thalassemia major, the introduction of cardiac T2* methods in the early 2000s, and the impact of these techniques on patient care as well as our fundamental understanding of iron cardiomyopathy. Technical details regarding T2* image acquisition and postprocessing are also discussed. As barriers to widespread implementation are being overcome, cardiac T2* is rapidly transitioning from a clinical research tool to the standard of care.

Keywords: thalassemia; iron; MRI; heart

Historical background

Prior to the introduction of deferoxamine in the early 1970s, patients with thalassemia major universally succumbed to iron cardiomyopathy in the second decade of life.[1] Cardiac symptoms were a relatively late finding, often preceding death by only 6–12 months. Availability of effective iron chelation has marked prolonged life expectancy and quality of life.[2] Nonetheless, cardiac toxicity remains the leading cause of death in thalassemia, primarily because it is clinically silent until it has reached advanced stages. Traditionally, markers of somatic iron stores, such as liver iron and serum ferritin, were used as surrogates for cardiac iron risk. In general, survival was improved in patients who maintain lower overall iron stores.[2–4] Although liver iron and serum ferritin were and continue to be vital for guiding iron chelation therapy, they incompletely convey cardiac risk. Some patients developed cardiac symptoms despite apparently adequate control of overall iron burden.[5,6] In such patients, myocarditis was postulated as the causative agent as there is considerable overlap in the clinical presentation of myocarditis and iron cardiomyopathy.[7]

Initial T2* studies

The introduction of cardiac MRI in the early 2000s completely changed our fundamental understanding and management of iron cardiomyopathy. Anderson et al published a seminal paper in 2001 describing the relationship between cardiac T2* and left ventricular ejection fraction in 104 patients with thalassemia major (Fig. 1).[8] T2* is a fundamental MRI relaxation time that shortens in the presence of iron. Cardiac T2* in normal volunteers is greater than 25 msec[9] but a cutoff of 20 msec is typically used in clinical practice to improve specificity. Ejection fraction is simply the percent of blood expelled from the ventricle with each beat. The manuscript had six core findings: (1) all patients with a T2* greater than 20 msec (no detectable cardiac iron) had normal cardiac function. The negative predictive value of cardiac T2* was high; (2) thalassemia patients lacking cardiac iron (T2* $>$ 20 msec) exhibited higher ejection fractions than population norms. Westwood and colleagues later confirmed these findings in a larger sample; the differences likely reflect lower cardiac afterload and greater cardiac

doi: 10.1111/j.1749-6632.2010.05571.x

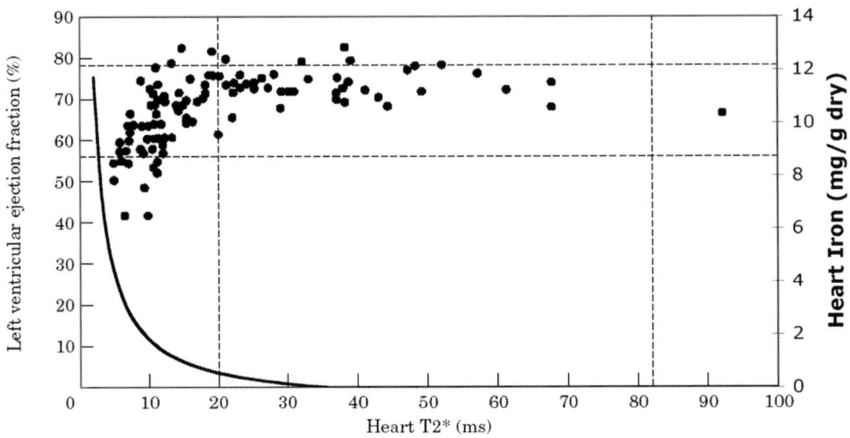

Figure 1. Plot of ejection fraction (left axis) versus heart T2* in milliseconds. T2* greater than 20 msec represents patients with no detectable cardiac iron. Horizontal dotted lines represents predicted population norms for ejection fraction in non thalassemia subjects. Solid line represents calibration curve for cardiac iron (right axis) as a function of cardiac T2*. Predicted cardiac iron for patients having a T2* of 2–10 msec is 1.8–10 mg/g dry weight, consistent with published autopsy studies. Figure reprinted from *Circulation*, with permission.

preload associated with chronic anemia;[10] (3) as T2* decreased below 20 msec, there was a proportional decline in cardiac ejection fraction indicating an association between increased cardiac iron and cardiac dysfunction; (4) many patients with detectable cardiac iron exhibited normal cardiac function, suggesting that T2* was identifying preclinical iron deposition; (5) iron cleared more rapidly from the liver than from the heart in response to intensive chelation. The same authors later demonstrated that the effective half life of cardiac iron clearance was 13.5 months compared with 1.4 months for liver iron reduction, in response to continuous deferoxamine therapy[11]; and (6) finally, cardiac T2* was uncorrelated with liver iron concentration and serum ferritin.

MRI controversy

The final observation was particularly challenging for many in the thalassemia community because it appeared to contradict established disease models and treatment paradigms. Some challenged the relationship between cardiac T2* and iron as well as transferability of the technique.[12,13] Since that time, however, the reciprocal relationship between cardiac T2* and iron has been validated in animals and in autopsy specimens.[14,15] *In vivo* validation is lacking for cardiac iron given the unacceptable risk of cardiac biopsy for research purposes, but several studies have validated *in vivo* liver T2* measurements.[8,16,17] In fact, if one simply applies the liver T2* calibration to heart, accounting for differences in tissue water concentration, the predicted cardiac iron concentrations agree favorably with autopsy specimens (Fig. 1).[14] The predicted cardiac iron concentration for T2* values less than 10 msec rise sharply, mirroring the change in observed ejection fractions, and are in the potentially lethal range.

The disparity between cardiac and liver iron levels can best be explained by differences in mechanisms and kinetics of cardiac and hepatic iron uptake/clearance. Serial assessment of liver and cardiac iron demonstrate that cardiac iron changes lag corresponding changes in liver iron concentration.[6] The liver is the dominant storage organ for excess iron and readily acquires excess transferrin and nontransferrin bound iron; it also mobilizes iron rapidly and efficiently in times of demand or in response to iron chelation. In contrast, the heart has robust mechanisms to prevent excessive transferrin-mediated uptake. Pathologic myocardial iron overload occurs when iron binding capacity is saturated and labile free iron species begin to circulate. Even then, cardiac iron uptake is delayed compared to many other extrahepatic organs, including the pancreas.[9,18,19] Thus many young patients can exhibit severe hepatic iron loading with no evidence of cardiac iron loading. Nonetheless, severely elevated hepatic iron levels are associated with prospective risk of cardiac iron uptake. Once the heart begins to accumulate iron, it can do so rapidly. Cardiac iron can also accumulate even in the presence of negative liver iron balance or at extremely low liver iron concentrations (<5 mg/g dry weight).[6] Cardiac iron balance appears to depend upon the hours per week of chelation coverage more than the grams per week of drug administered. This observation probably accounts for the critical dependence of chelation compliance on survival.[4,20]

A second point of contention for the initial T2* studies was the heterogeneity in ventricular function observed for any given T2* value. Many patients with severe cardiac iron loading were completely asymptomatic. One key explanation was that MRI methods are primarily sensitive to the safely stored hemosiderin iron fraction, not free iron species associated with ventricular dysfunction.[21] Toxic free iron is magnetically silent at physiologic concentrations. Free iron entering the heart is initially buffered by myocardial ferritin to prevent oxidative damage. Excess ferritin is digested in lysosomes to form insoluble hemosiderin. Tissue ferritin fraction is relatively magnetically weak compared with aggregated ferritin complexes and hemosiderin degradation products. Hence, patients could have severely elevated siderosomal iron stores (low T2*) with relatively low labile iron pools (normal function). However, labile iron pools will generally increase proportionally to the amount of stored iron (1/T2*), creating the statistical link between abnormal T2* and cardiomyopathy.

Closing the loop

This mechanistic explanation raised another important question: How should a patient with a low T2* and normal function be treated? Prior work suggests that waiting for ventricular function to decline is risky because patients will die if they cannot or will not comply with years of intensified chelation therapy.[22] Cross-sectional results imply that low T2* conveys prospective risk of developing cardiac failure but it was not until this year that this hypothesis was confirmed.[23] Kirk and colleagues demonstrated that the prospective risk of symptomatic heart failure over a 1 year period was 50% for a T2* < 6 msec, 30% for T2* between 6 and 8 msec, and 14% for T2* between 8 and 10 msec.[23] Thus, T2* has been confirmed as a powerful predictor of clinical cardiac risk, with the longitudinal risk closely mirroring projections from cross-sectional studies.

Technical aspects of T2* imaging

The cardiac T2* technique is relatively robust. Differences exist in image acquisition and post processing. For acquisition, one can either use a technique that collects multiple echoes during a single breath-hold or one that collects a single echo time per breath-hold. Both give comparable numbers.[24] Transferability among different centers has been demonstrated for both approaches as well.[25,26] The choice of minimum echo time is important because it determines the smallest T2* that can be measured. A minimum echo time at or below 2 msec is preferable; this is readily accomplished on most modern scanners. The longest echo time should be between 17–20 msec, balancing adequate characterization of the signal decay while not becoming too vulnerable to cardiac motion. The number of echoes collected is relatively unimportant as long as it is greater than 5. Most centers use 8–12.

A second acquisition option is to suppress signal from the left and right ventricle through a MRI-trick known as a blood suppression pulse. This produces a so-called "black blood" T2* image; standard T2* techniques produce a "white-blood" image. Black blood techniques enhance boundary definition and reduce T2* contributions from blood motion artifacts. This technique is particularly helpful in improving reproducibility when no myocardial iron is present, but white-blood and black-blood techniques yield similar T2* numbers at high iron concentrations.[27]

Some centers have chosen to use T2 rather than T2* methods to characterize tissue iron.[28–31] T2 techniques are more robust to susceptibility artifacts from the lung, liver, and cardiac veins which is potentially quite helpful for 3 Tesla magnets.[32] Good reproducibility and intermachine transferability have been demonstrated for machines from the same manufacturer.[31] However, cardiac T2 techniques are not as readily available as T2* sequences and have greater intermachine differences in implementation that could influence the calibration. Cardiac T2 methods are also more vulnerable to motion artifacts introduced from breathing. Thus cardiac T2 methods remain primarily a research tool except for a few sites which have been using them for many years.

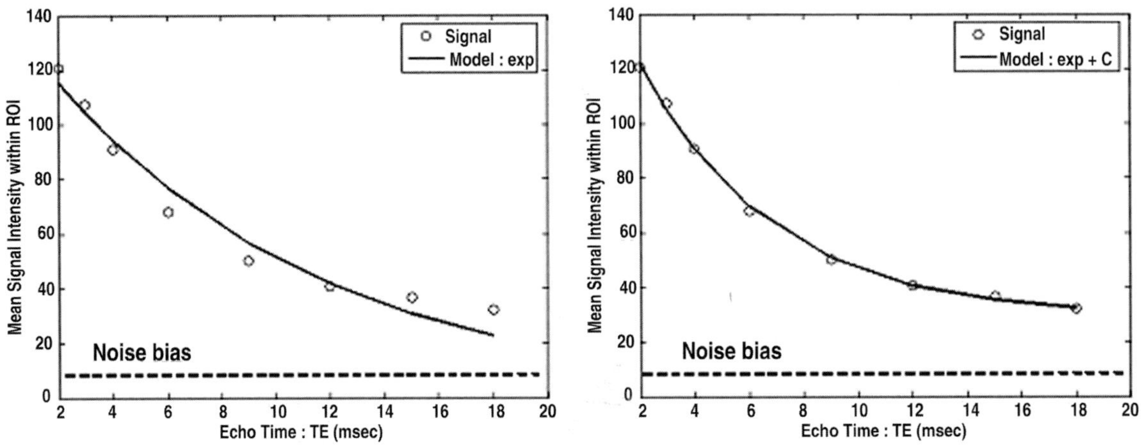

Figure 2. Signal decay curve from a representative patient with severe cardiac iron (T2* ~ 5 msec). The dotted horizontal line represents the estimated constant offset produced from rectified noise. A simple monoexponential decay curve (left panel) cannot fit the data well because there is contribution from low-iron containing tissues at longer echo times. The right hand panel demonstrates improvement if the model includes a constant term to account for bias from noise, low-iron containing tissues, or instrumentation offsets. Figure reprinted from *Journal of Magnetic Resonance Imaging*, with permission.

Postprocessing of T2* images

In addition to differences introduced during image acquisition, image processing can also be a source of error. In principle, the concept is straightforward. T2* images darken exponentially with echo time; this can be fit easily by simple mathematical models, including Excel spreadsheets. The difficulty arises in patients having severe cardiac iron overload, because the tissue has both iron-rich muscle fibers and iron-poor vascular spaces (capillaries, arterioles, venules constitute ~10% of the volume in the heart). Signal from the heavily iron loaded muscle will decay quickly, while contributions from the myocardial blood volume will not. Thus no single exponential describes the image darkening. An example is shown in Figure 2. Simple exponential fit in this situation overestimates true T2 decay. There are at least three solutions to this problem. Some investigators advocate truncating the exponential fit when the signal approaches background level.[33,34] This approach is simple and fairly robust. Clarke and colleagues try to fit the signal decay to two exponential functions, one which decays rapidly (iron-rich) and one which decays slowly (iron-poor).[35] The primary difficulty with this approach is mathematical instability because of the need to estimate four parameters instead of two. Our approach has been a compromise, approximating the slow decay component by a constant offset.[36] All three approaches will work, if proper constraints are placed on the fitting parameters. The Royal Brompton group has published comparisons suggesting that the truncated two-component model is superior,[33,34] contrary to our findings.[36] However, the optimal model probably depends on many detailed and machine/pulse sequence dependent factors, including how MRI scanners reconstruct the images from phased-array imaging coils. From a practioner's perspective, either approach will yield clinically valid results. Small biases exist between the methods but are widest at T2* values below 5 msec where treatment should be maximized regardless of the absolute value.

A more practical consideration is how to obtain software to perform the analysis. CMR Tools markets a thalassemia tool kit that is easy to use and FDA approved. Unfortunately, the licensing fee may be prohibitive for some centers. Some of the major MRI vendors have software on their offline workstations that is suitable for T2* analysis. It also is not free, but some sites may have obtained the software anyway for other, higher volume applications. Since the programming involved to calculate T2* is straightforward, some sites have simply contracted local physicists or engineers to write MATLAB or IDL programs for display and T2* measurement. As a cost-free solution to the problem, some sites have even simply used their image archive (PACS) systems, such as OSIRIX, to calculate region of interest (ROI) values for the different echo times; ROI values

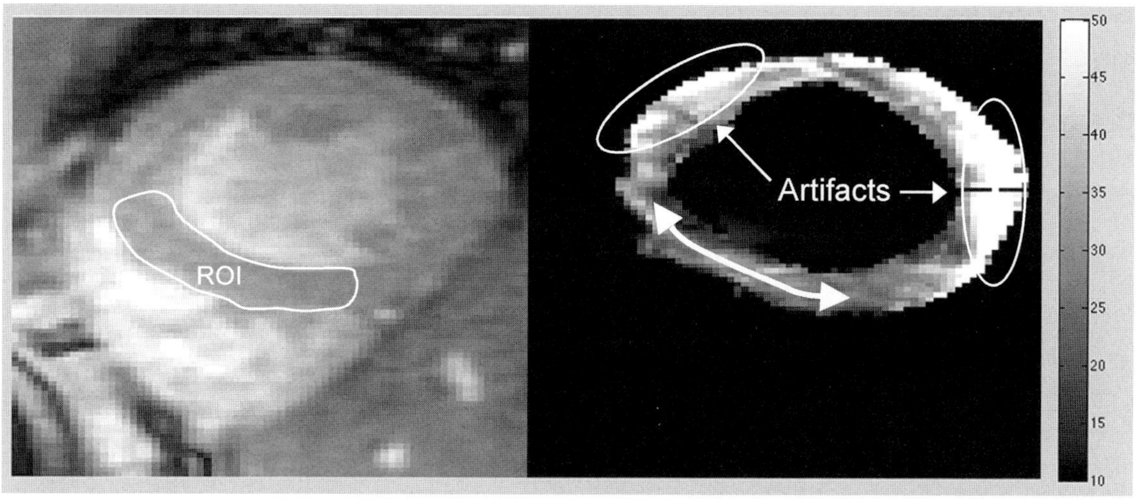

Figure 3. (Left) Short axis gradient echo image from a patient with sickle cell disease and no cardiac iron. (Right) Corresponding R2*, or 1/T2*, map of the left ventricle; R2* is proportional to iron. Two large susceptibility artifacts are indicated. R2* values in these regions is more than 50 Hz (or equivalently T2* < 20), representing "false-positive" iron detection in these regions. Large curved arrow in left and right images represents region of interest selection avoiding these "hot spots."

can subsequently be easily displayed and fit to an exponential function in Microsoft Excel. Nonetheless, this approach is somewhat tedious and most high-volume sites opt for a more automated technique.

With standardized acquisition and postprocessing software, interexam and intersite variability are low. One key factor is the standardization of the ROI determination. Myocardial iron is heterogeneously distributed and there are systematic susceptibility artifacts that should be avoided near the great cardiac veins. Figure 3 demonstrates a R2* (1/T2*) map from a SCD patient lacking cardiac iron. The local T2* near the great veins is 10 msec (which would suggest high iron concentration) but the rest of the myocardium has a normal T2*; this represents a well-described susceptibility artifact from deoxygenated blood in the epicardial cardiac veins. We, and others, have documented this circumferential variation in cardiac T2*.[37,38] To minimize contribution from this artifact, we advocate full thickness interventricular septal tracing that does not entirely extend to the right ventricular insertion points. In fact, the R2* maps often delineate where the ROI should be terminated. Ramazzotti and colleagues promote a different approach, using both segmental and global T2* information from three slices to generate a robust metric of overall myocardial iron concentration.[39,40] This approach has merit but is more labor intensive. Further work is necessary to determine trade-offs between effort and efficacy.

Conclusion

In summary, cardiac T2* assessment is rapidly becoming the standard of care for chronically transfused patients. Imaging principles for tissue iron measurements have been validated computationally, *in vitro*, *in situ*, and *in vivo*. From a practical perspective, cardiac T2* is reproducible and accurately stratifies prospective risk of cardiac decompensation. Cardiac T2* measurements have also provided insights into relative interorgan differences in iron loading/unloading kinetics. Cost remains the single largest barrier to widespread use, particularly in regions of high disease prevalence.

Acknowledgments

This work is supported by an investigator-initiated research grant from Novartis, USA, General Clinical Research Center at CHLA/USC (NIH #RR00043-43), NHLBI (1 RO1 HL075592-01A1), and the Center for Disease Control (Thalassemia Center Grant U27/CCU922106).

Disclosure statement

Drs. Wood and Coates have research funding from Novartis for basic and clinical research studies.

Conflicts of Interest

The authors declare no conflicts of interest.

References

1. Ehlers, K.H., A.R. Levin, A.L. Markenson, *et al.* 1980. Longitudinal study of cardiac function in thalassemia major. *Ann. N.Y. Acad. Sci.* **344:** 397–404.
2. Borgna-Pignatti, C., S. Rugolotto, P. De Stefano, *et al.* 2004. Survival and complications in patients with thalassemia major treated with transfusion and deferoxamine. *Haematologica* **89:** 1187–1193.
3. Olivieri, N.F., D.G. Nathan, J.H. MacMillan, *et al.* 1994. Survival in medically treated patients with homozygous beta-thalassemia. *N. Engl. J. Med.* **331:** 574–578.
4. Brittenham, G.M., P.M. Griffith, A.W. Nienhuis, *et al.* 1994. Efficacy of deferoxamine in preventing complications of iron overload in patients with thalassemia major. *N. Engl. J. Med.* **331:** 567–573.
5. Anderson, L.J., M.A. Westwood, E. Prescott, *et al.* 2006. Development of thalassaemic iron overload cardiomyopathy despite low liver iron levels and meticulous compliance to desferrioxamine. *Acta Haematol.* **115:** 106–108.
6. Noetzli, L.J., S.M. Carson, A.S. Nord, *et al.* 2008. Longitudinal analysis of heart and liver iron in thalassemia major. *Blood* **112:** 2973–2978.
7. Kremastinos, D.T., G. Tiniakos, G.N. Theodorakis, *et al.* 1995. Myocarditis in beta-thalassemia major: a cause of heart failure. *Circulation* **91:** 66–71.
8. Anderson, L.J., S. Holden, B. Davis, *et al.* 2001. Cardiovascular T2-star (T2*) magnetic resonance for the early diagnosis of myocardial iron overload. *Eur. Heart J.* **22:** 2171–2179.
9. Wood, J.C., J.M. Tyszka, N. Ghugre, *et al.* 2004. Myocardial iron loading in transfusion-dependent thalassemia and sickle-cell disease. *Blood* **103:** 1934–1936.
10. Westwood, M.A., L.J. Anderson, A.M. Maceira, *et al.* 2007. Normalized left ventricular volumes and function in thalassemia major patients with normal myocardial iron. *J. Magn. Reson. Imaging* **25:** 1147–1151.
11. Anderson, L.J., M.A. Westwood, S. Holden, *et al.* 2004. Myocardial iron clearance during reversal of siderotic cardiomyopathy with intravenous desferrioxamine: a prospective study using T2* cardiovascular magnetic resonance. *Br. J. Haematol.* **127:** 348–355.
12. Fischer, R., & R. Engelhardt. 2003. Deferiprone versus desferrioxamine in thalassaemia, and T2* validation and utility. *Lancet* **361:** 182–183; author reply 183–184.
13. St Pierre, T.G. 2003. Deferiprone versus desferrioxamine in thalassaemia, and T2* validation and utility. *Lancet* **361:** 182; author reply 183–184.
14. Wood, J.C., M. Otto-Duessel, M. Aguilar, *et al.* 2005. Cardiac iron determines cardiac T2*, T2, and T1 in the gerbil model of iron cardiomyopathy. *Circulation* **112:** 535–543.
15. Ghugre, N., C. Enriquez & J.C. Wood. 2005. Myocardial R2 and R2* vary linearly with cardiac iron in human heart. In *Paper presented at the International Society of Magnetic Resonance in Medicine*, Miami Beach, FL.
16. Wood, J.C., C. Enriquez, N. Ghugre, *et al.* 2005. MRI R2 and R2* mapping accurately estimates hepatic iron concentration in transfusion-dependent thalassemia and sickle cell disease patients. *Blood* **106:** 1460–1465.
17. Hankins, J.S., McCarville, M.B., Loeffler, R.B., *et al.* 2009. R2* magnetic resonance imaging of the liver in patients with iron overload. *Blood* **113:** 4853–4855.
18. Noetzli, L.J., J. Papudesi, T.D. Coates & J.C. Wood. 2009. Pancreatic iron loading predicts cardiac iron loading in thalassemia major. *Blood* **114:** 4021–4026.
19. Wood, J.C., R. Origa, A. Agus, *et al.* 2008. Onset of cardiac iron loading in pediatric patients with thalassemia major. *Haematologica* **93:** 917–920.
20. Gabutti, V. & C. Borgna-Pignatti. 1994. Clinical manifestations and therapy of transfusional haemosiderosis. *Baillieres Clin. Haematol.* **7:** 919–940.
21. Wood, J.C., J. Fassler & T. Meade. 2004. Mimicking liver iron overload using liposomal ferritin preparations. *Mag Res Med.* **51:** 607–611.
22. Davis, B.A., C. O'Sullivan, P.H. Jarritt & J.B. Porter. 2004. Value of sequential monitoring of left ventricular ejection fraction in the management of thalassemia major. *Blood* **104:** 263–269.
23. Kirk, P., M. Roughton, J.B. Porter, *et al.* 2009. Cardiac T2* magnetic resonance for prediction of cardiac complications in thalassemia major. *Circulation* **120:** 1961–1968.
24. Westwood, M., L.J. Anderson, D.N. Firmin, *et al.* 2003. A single breath-hold multiecho T2* cardiovascular magnetic resonance technique for diagnosis of myocardial iron overload. *J. Magn. Reson. Imaging.* **18:** 33–39.
25. Westwood, M.A., D.N. Firmin, M. Gildo, *et al.* 2005. Intercentre reproducibility of magnetic resonance T2* measurements of myocardial iron in thalassaemia. *Int. J. Cardiovasc. Imaging* **21:** 531–538.
26. Tanner, M.A., T. He, M.A. Westwood, *et al.* 2006. Multicenter validation of the transferability of the magnetic resonance T2* technique for the quantification of tissue iron. *Haematologica* **91:** 1388–1391.
27. He, T., P.D. Gatehouse, P. Kirk, *et al.* 2007. Black-blood T2* technique for myocardial iron measurement in thalassemia. *J. Magn. Reson. Imaging* **25:** 1205–1209.
28. Mavrogeni, S.I., T. Maris, A. Gouliamos, *et al.* 1998. Myocardial iron deposition in beta-thalassemia studied by magnetic resonance imaging. *Int. J. Card. Imaging* **14:** 117–122.
29. Voskaridou, E., M. Douskou, E. Terpos, *et al.* 2004. Magnetic resonance imaging in the evaluation of iron overload in patients with beta thalassaemia and sickle cell disease. *Br. J. Haematol.* **126:** 736–742.
30. Papakonstantinou, O., E. Alexopoulou, N. Economopoulos, *et al.* 2009. Assessment of iron distribution between liver, spleen, pancreas, bone marrow, and myocardium by means of R2 relaxometry with MRI in patients with beta-thalassemia major. *J. Magn. Reson. Imaging* **29:** 853–859.
31. He, T., P. Kirk, D.N. Firmin, *et al.* 2008. Multi-center transferability of a breath-hold T2 technique for myocardial iron assessment. *J. Cardiovasc. Magn. Reson.* **10:** 11.
32. Guo, H., W.Y. Au, J.S. Cheung, *et al.* 2009. Myocardial T2 quantitation in patients with iron overload at 3 Tesla. *J. Magn. Reson. Imaging* **30:** 394–400.
33. He, T., P.D. Gatehouse, P. Kirk, *et al.* 2008. Myocardial T(*)2 measurement in iron-overloaded thalassemia: an ex

vivo study to investigate optimal methods of quantification. *Magn. Reson. Med.* **60:** 350–356.
34. He, T., P.D. Gatehouse, G.C. Smith, *et al.* 2008. Myocardial T2* measurements in iron-overloaded thalassemia: an *in vivo* study to investigate optimal methods of quantification. *Magn. Reson. Med.* **60:** 1082–1089.
35. Clark, P.R., W. Chua-anusorn & T.G. St Pierre. 2003. Bi-exponential proton transverse relaxation rate (R2) image analysis using RF field intensity-weighted spin density projection: potential for R2 measurement of iron-loaded liver. *Magn. Reson. Imaging* **21:** 519–530.
36. Ghugre, N., C. Enriquez, T.D. Coates, *et al.* 2005. Improved R2* Measurements in Myocardial Iron Overload. *J. Cardiovasc. Magn. Reson.* **7:** 32–33.
37. Ghugre, N.R., C.M. Enriquez, T.D. Coates, *et al.* 2006. Improved R2* measurements in myocardial iron overload. *J. Magn. Reson. Imaging* **23:** 9–16.
38. Pepe, A., V. Positano, M.F. Santarelli, *et al.* 2006. Multislice multiecho T2* cardiovascular magnetic resonance for detection of the heterogeneous distribution of myocardial iron overload. *J. Magn. Reson. Imaging* **23:** 662–668.
39. Ramazzotti, A., A. Pepe, V. Positano, *et al.* 2009. Multicenter validation of the magnetic resonance T2* technique for segmental and global quantification of myocardial iron. *J. Magn. Reson. Imaging* **30:** 62–68.
40. Ramazzotti, A., A. Pepe, V. Positano, *et al.* 2008. Standardized T2* map of a normal human heart to correct T2* segmental artefacts; myocardial iron overload and fibrosis in thalassemia intermedia versus thalassemia major patients and electrocardiogram changes in thalassemia major patients. *Hemoglobin* **32:** 97–107.

Ann. N.Y. Acad. Sci. ISSN 0077-8923

ANNALS OF THE NEW YORK ACADEMY OF SCIENCES
Issue: *Cooley's Anemia: Ninth Symposium*

Complexity of alpha thalassemia: growing health problem with new approaches to screening, diagnosis, and therapy

Elliott Vichinsky
Children's Hospital & Research Center Oakland, Oakland, Califorina

Address for correspondence: Elliott Vichinsky, MD, Children's Hospital & Research Center Oakland, 747 52nd Street, Oakland, CA 94609. evichinsky@mail.cho.org

Alpha thalassemia, the most common genetic disorder of hemoglobin synthesis, affects up to 5% of the world's population. It represents a group of conditions with reduced or absent synthesis of one to all four of α globin genes. Deletional or nondeletional mutations occur on chromosome 16. Its severity ranges from asymptomatic to fatal *in utero*. Hemoglobin H disease, a mutation of three α globin genes, is more severe than previously recognized. Anemia, hypersplenism, hemosiderosis, growth failure, and osteoporosis are commonly noted as the patient ages. Alpha thalassemia major, a usually fatal *in utero* disease, is now recognized to have a complex molecular and phenotypic expression with increasing births being reported. Surviving newborns without intrauterine transfusion often have congenital anomalies and neurocognitive injury. Serious maternal complications often accompany pregnancy. Doppler ultrasonography with intrauterine transfusion ameliorates these complications. The high incidence in many populations mandates population screening and prenatal diagnosis of at-risk couples. Universal newborn screening has been adopted in several regions with DNA confirmatory testing. These advances have resulted in ethical dilemmas for the family and the provider.

Keywords: alpha thalassemia; thalassemia; hemoglobin H; hydrops; Bart's

Overview

Alpha thalassemia, affecting 5% of the world's population, is probably the most common of all single gene disorders. It refers to a group of hereditary anemias caused by absent or decreased production of the α chain of hemoglobin. Its severity is quite variable and ranges from asymptomatic carriers to a fatal *in utero* disease. Early in gestation, embryonic hemoglobins (Gower1, Gower2, and Portland), which do not contain α globin chains, are the predominant hemoglobins. They are rapidly replaced by fetal and then adult hemoglobin, which contain α globin chains. Therefore, α thalassemia mutations become phenotypically evident by 12 weeks of gestation.

The α gene cluster is located on chromosome 16, which includes α gene 1 and α gene 2. Upstream on the chromosome are the embryonic genes and a major regulatory element, HS-40, that controls the α globin gene activity.[1]

When both α genes on a single chromosome are inactive, the designation α° thalassemia is used. When there is some production of α globin chains, α^+ thalassemia is designated. Alpha thalassemia is divided into deletional and nondeletional types.[1] (Tables 1 and 2[1]) There are at least 40 different deletions. The size of the deletion is important and affects the clinical phenotype. Common α thalassemia deletions which spare the embryonic gene allow for the production of functional embryonic hemoglobin early in gestation. In contrast, the large deletions lack the benefit of embryonic hemoglobin. These large deletions are particularly severe. The nondeletional mutations have a more severe phenotype than most of the deletional mutations. The most common nondeletional α thalassemia mutation is Hemoglobin Constant Spring (Hb CS); this

doi: 10.1111/j.1749-6632.2010.05572.x

Table 1. Classification of deletional α thalassemia, modified from Bain *et al.*[1]

Type of deletion	Phenotype	Number of examples recognized	Examples
Deletion involving one or both α genes			
Deletion of all or part of one α gene	α^+ thalassemia	7	$-\alpha^{4.2}$, $-\alpha^{3.71}$, $-\alpha^{3.711}$, $-\alpha^{3.5}$, $\alpha(\alpha)^{5.3a}$, $-\alpha^{2.7}$
Deletion of all or part of both α genes, but without deletion of HS-40	α^0 thalassemia	20	$\_^{SEA}$, $\_^{THAI}$, $\_^{MED}$, $\_^{FIL}$, $\_^{BRIT}$, $\_^{SPAN}$, $-(\alpha)^{20.5a}$, $-(\alpha)^{5.2a}$
Deletion of both α genes and of HS-40 (100–250 kb)	α^0 thalassemia	8, without other phenotypic abnormality	$\_^{DUTCHII}$
Extensive loss of 16p13.3 (1–2 Mb) including both α genes and HS-40[b]	α^0 thalassemia	17, with mental retardation and dysmorphism	$\_^{BO}$
Deletion of α1 gene and 18–20 kb downstream of α1 gene	α^0 thalassemia	1	$(\alpha)^{-ZFa}$
Deletion leaving α genes intact			
Deletion of upstream major regulatory element (HS-40) without deletion of α genes	α^0 or very severe α^+ thalassemia	12	$(\alpha\alpha)^{RAc}$, $(\alpha\alpha)^{TATc}$, $(\alpha\alpha)^{MMc}$, $(\alpha\alpha)^{IJc}$

[a](α) Indicates that the gene is present but nonfunctional.
[b]Loss of 16p13.3 may be the result of deletion, inversion plus deletion, formation of a ring chromosome 16 that lacks the α gene cluster, or un-balanced inheritance of a derivative (16) lacking 16p13.3 from a parent who had a balanced translocation, e.g., *t*(1;16), *t*(5;16), or *t*(16;20).
[c](αα) Indicates that both α genes are present but nonfunctional.

mutation of the stop codon results in 31 amino acids being added to the α chain. Mutations of a terminal codon to a coding sequence often lead to an elongated α chain that is unstable and produced at a very limited rate.

Historically, the phenotype of α thalassemia mutations was directly related to the number of α globin genes affected. One gene deletion resulted in a silent carrier; 2-gene deletions: α-thalassemia trait; 3-gene deletions: Hemoglobin H (Hb H), and 4-gene deletions: hydrops fetalis. However, the genotype and phenotype of α thalassemia syndrome is now recognized to be more complex and variable. The phenotype varies depending not only on the number of alpha genes affected, but the type of α thalassemia mutation. Large deletions, nondeletional mutations, alterations in the regulatory region, and unstable mutations all increase the severity of the phenotype.

Epidemiology

Alpha thalassemia is particularly common in China and Southeast Asia, with up to 40% of the regional population being carriers.[1–5] One of the most frequent α- thalassemia mutations is the $–^{SEA}$ deletion, which deletes both α globin genes but spares the embryonic gene. Homozygosity for this deletion ($–^{SEA}$) is the most common cause of hydrops fetalis.[2,5] The

Table 2. Classification of nondeletional α thalassemia[1]

Type of mutation	Phenotype	Number of examples recognized	Examples
RNA splice site mutation α1 or α2 gene	α+ thalassemia	3(α2 donor site, α2/α1 acceptor site)	α2IVS1(-5nt) donor splice site Mediterranean/Middle East
RNA polyadenylation signal mutations	α+- α0 thalassemia (i.e., severe α+) or α+	4 (α2 gene account for the severe phenotype)	α2AATAAA→AATAAG (αPA6A→ Gα, αTSaudiα)
Impaired RNA translation consequent on initiation codon	α+ thalassemia, α+- α0 or, when mutation occurs w/deletional	5 (2 in α2 gene, 1 in α1 gene, 2 in single α2 gene)	α2ATG→ACG, GTG or A-G; -α3.7 ATG→GTG (mutation with deletional gives α0 phenotype)
Impaired RNA translation consequent on a frame shift or nonsense mutation	α+ or α0 thalassemia	5 (4 frame shift plus 1 nonsense)	Codon 30/31 (-4nt) frame shift and α2 CD116 GAG→TAG nonsense mutation
Impaired RNA translation consequent on a termination codon mutation	α+ thalassemia	5 (all α2 gene)	Hb Constant Spring TAA→CAA (αCSα), Hb Icaria TAA→AAA (αICα), Hb Koya Dora TAA→TCA
Production of highly unstable α chain as a result of point mutation or a small deletion	α+ thalassemia	At least 18: 14 point mutations, 4 small deletions	Hb Agrinio (αAgrα), Hb Petah Tikvah (αPT), Hb Quong Sze (αQSα), Hb Suan Dok (αSDα)
Lack of transactivating factor encoded by *ATRX* gene	α+ thalassemia		ATR-X syndrome

sparing of the embryonic gene allows enough functional embryonic hemoglobin (hemoglobin Portland 1 and hemoglobin Portland 2) to allow gestation to continue and the phenotype of hydrops fetalis to develop. In contrast, other common α-thalassemia mutations ($–^{FIL}$, $–^{THAI}$) also lack the entire embryonic α globin cluster, and therefore do not produce the functional embryonic Hemoglobin Portland. These embryos may terminate unnoticed early in gestation.[2] Over 5% of individuals in the Philippines are carriers for the $–^{SEA}$ or $–^{FIL}$ mutation. Hydrops fetalis, while most common in Southeast Asia, is found worldwide among many ethnic groups; $–^{MED}$ is a common α° thalassemia mutation in Mediterranean regions, particularly Greece and Cyprus. It has resulted in hydrops fetalis. Nondeletional α thalassemia is found throughout the world. Up to 8% of Southeast Asians are carriers of Hb CS. In the Middle East, Hemoglobin α^{TSaudi} α is a common α-thalassemia nondeletional mutation. It is a mutation of the polyadenylation signal sequence of the α2 gene, resulting in decreased expression of structurally normal alpha chains. Hemoglobin Koya Dora, another structural nondeletional mutation, is found in India. Other structural mutations, such as hemoglobin Quong Sze found in Southeast Asia, are highly unstable and result in defects in the hem pocket.[1,3,6,7]

Hemoglobin H

Hemoglobin H (Hb H) disease is caused by the inactivation of three α-globin genes either by deletional or nondeletional mutations. Deletional Hb H is the most common type. While milder than the nondeletional Hb H, it is not a benign disorder.[8–11] The recognition of its clinical morbidity, increasing prevalence, and benefit of early detection has resulted in universal Hb H newborn screening programs to be developed. In California, demographic changes have resulted in Hb H being commonly diagnosed in the newborn. Over 500 cases have recently been diagnosed between 1998 and 2006 (Table 3[12]).

Significant hemolytic anemia can occur during fever, infections, and pregnancy that may necessitate the need for blood transfusions. Infection with parvovirus B19 can lead to severe aplastic crises. In addition, this condition can lead to growth retardation during childhood, and iron overload in adults regardless of previous transfusion history, leading to hepatic, cardiac, and endocrine dysfunction.[9,11] As these patients age, one-third will eventually develop cholelithiasis and the risk of iron-induced cardiomyopathy will increase. In deletional Hb H, the average hemoglobin is 9.6 with an MCV of 63 fL. In contrast, nondeletional Hb H, such as Hb H Constant Spring, the average hemoglobin is 7.6 with an MCV of 73 fL.[8,9,13,14]

Approximately 15% of Hb H disease is due to a nondeletional mutations. The deficit in α globin expression is more severe in the nondeletional Hb H disease and the hemoglobin mutation is more unstable. The oxidative damage and membrane dysfunction observed results in rigid overhydrated cells with a shortened red cell survival. The loss of phospholipid asymmetry with phosphatidylserine exposure increases the morbidity of this disease and the risk of thrombosis. Recent studies demonstrate Hb HCS patients have significant ineffective erythropoiesis. The hemolytic anemia and ineffective erythropoiesis results in the patient having a more severe clinical and laboratory course (Fig. 1[14]).

Hemoglobin H Constant Spring (Hb HCS) is the most common nondeletional Hb H, with up to one third of these patients being transfusion dependent.[14–16] The clinical severity of nondeletional Hb H may be variable but is often moderately severe. The majority of patients have a beneficial response to splenectomy. However, the high rate of thrombosis following splenectomy in these patients often requires chronic anticoagulation therapy. At least 25% of Hb HCS requires chronic transfusions with chelation therapy. Medical problems including growth delay, osteoporosis, and iron overload are greater in Hb HCS than deletional Hb H.

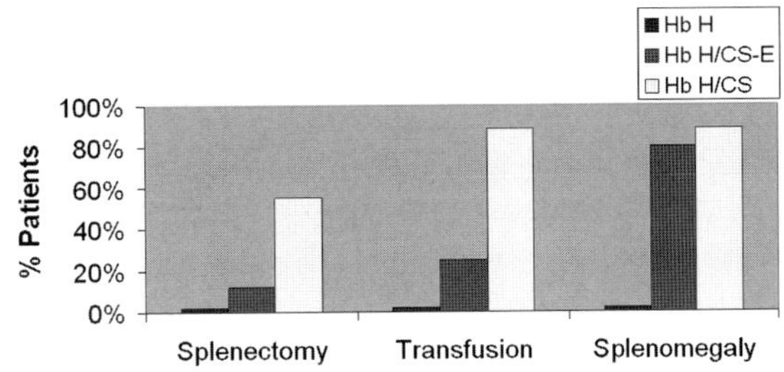

Figure 1. Comparison of the rate of splenectomy, transfusion, and splenomegaly history in three types of Hb H disease – Hb H (three gene deletion), Hb HCS, Hb H with Constant Spring ($\alpha^\circ\,\alpha^{CS}$), Hb H/CS-E (Hb HCS + heterozygote for Hb E).

Hydrops fetalis

The incidence of Hydrops fetalis appears to be increasing.[2,12,17–19] Advances in perinatal care and recognition of surviving homozygous thalassemia newborns has precipitated studies of long-term survivors with this disorder. In southern China, the prevalence of homozygous α thalassemia[2,5,20,21] births is 0.23%. Nonimmune hydrops fetalis is most often caused by α thalassemia in these regions.[5,22] In addition to China and Southeast Asia, Bart's hydrops fetalis is now being recognized in Greece, Turkey, Cyprus, India, Sardinia, United States, and other parts of the world.[1–3,5,22]

In the first 8 weeks of gestation, functional embryonic hemoglobin is responsible for oxygen delivery. These embryonic hemoglobins (hemoglobin Gower 1, hemoglobin Gower 2, and Hemoglobin Portland) are replaced early in gestation. By 8 weeks of gestation, a switch to fetal hemoglobin production (Hemoglobin F $\alpha 2/\gamma 2$) occurs. Since α globin chains are absent, hemoglobin F cannot be synthesized and hemoglobin Bart's becomes the dominant hemoglobin. Hemoglobin Bart's is a γ tetromere, which is unable to deliver oxygen to tissues because of its very high oxygen affinity. This results in a progressive severe anemia.[23] Mid-trimester intrauterine hemoglobin analysis demonstrates an average hemoglobin (g/dL) of 6.4 in homozygous Bart's[23]

Table 3. Thalassemia newborn screening in California

Diagnosis/Genotype	No. identified	Incidence (per 100,000)
Alpha thalassemia syndromes	502	11.1
Hb H disease	406	9.0
Hb H with Hb E trait	35	0.8
Hb H with Hb EE	16	0.4
Hb H-Constant Spring	25	0.6
Hb H with other variants	8	0.2
Hb H with SS	7	0.2
Hydrops fetalis (SEA)	8	0.2
Beta thalassemia syndromes	79	1.8
Hb β°	19	0.4
Hb Eβ	34	0.8
Hb Cβ	21	0.5
Hb Dβ°	5	0.1
Other mutations	862	19.1
Hb EE	514	11.4
Hb CC, HPFH	44	1.0
Heterozygote variants	304	6.7

This anemia underestimates the severity of hypoxia because Hemoglobin Bart's has no hem/hem interaction or Bohr effect and binds oxygen irreversibly tight. There is severe ineffective erythropoiesis with marked extramedullary hematopoiesis.[2] These factors result in massive organomegaly, severe albuminemia, and heart failure. This leads to gross body edema, growth failure, and intrauterine demise.

Most cases of α thalassemia major, or hydrops fetalis, are consistent with the above description. However there is a marked variability in the intrauterine clinical course of these mutations. Many of the pregnancies, especially those with large α thalassemia deletions involving the embryonic gene, terminate unnoticed or early in gestation. Others continue throughout pregnancy and are born as stillbirths or critically ill. Some do not become hydropic and are born spontaneously.[23–25]

The environmental and genetic factors responsible for the diverse intrauterine course of hydrops fetalis are not all known. The specific α globin mutations are a major factor in the severity of the disease.[1,2,26–28] Deletional, nondeletional, hyperunstable, and compound α globin mutations affect red cell survival. Severe hemoglobin H mutations can result in hydrops fetalis even when the hemoglobin Bart's levels are as low as 40%. Hydrops fetalis from three-gene deletions include Hb H, $-^{MED}/\alpha^{\mathrm{TSaudi}}\alpha$, and Hb H α-serine to proline/ α^{FIL}.[1,2,10,27–30] In addition, hydrops fetalis has been reported from homozygous Hb HCS and other unexpected alpha thalassemia combinations.[1,29,31,32] Nonthalassemia factors may affect the occurrence and severity of hydrops.[33] Hydrops fetalis caused by homozygous α thalassemia, in combination with Rh antigen alloimmunization, has been observed. In some cases, the immune hemolytic anemia may worsen a hemoglobin H disorder to have the phenotype of α-hydrops. Some of these rare hydrops fetalis cases with co-morbid variables become mild after the neonatal period.

Associated fetal anomalies

Developmental abnormalities are commonly seen in hydrops fetalis. At least 17% of newborns have one congenital anomaly.[1–3,34,35] It is likely that fetal hypoxia disturbs organogenesis and fetal development. Most of these anomalies are mild and often affect the genitourinary system.[35,36] In particular, hypospadias has been reported. Musculoskeletal defects, such as limb malformations, occur in 8% of fetuses.[1,2,34,35] Skeletal malformations may be common because normal limb development occurs around 6 weeks of gestation. Many other anomalies have been reported including microcephaly, hydrocephaly, hypoplasia of lungs, anomalous genitalia, and cardiac defects.[1,34,36] Central nervous anomalies are uncommon. A fetus with a malformation consisting of a neuronal migrational defect has been reported.[34] A serious developmental problem is hypoxia-induced central nervous system injury particularly observed in the surviving hydrops fetalis children who are not transfused *in utero*.

Maternal complications

Serious maternal complications may occur during the pregnancy. In fact, in women with a hydropic fetus who are not receiving adequate medical care, the maternal mortality rate could approach 50%.[2,36] Sixty-one percent of women with an affected fetus develop hypertension, 30% develop severe preeclampsia, and 11% develop antepartum hemorrhage.[36,37] Other serious complications that may occur include renal failure, premature labor, congestive heart failure, abruptio placenta, and oligohydramios.[1,2,17,37] Overall, these are high-risk pregnancies and almost always associated with some obstetrical complication.

Prevention and screening

Prevention of hydrops fetalis by education, counseling, and screening the at-risk population is the most effective therapy. The approach to screening and counseling is dependent upon community resources. Commonly, microcytosis using an MCV < 82 fL and/or hypochromia (MCH <27 pg) is often used as a population screening technique.[2–4,17,21] Anemia is unreliable and is often not present in adults with two α globin gene deletions. Once iron deficiency is ruled out or corrected, microcytosis should be further evaluated in the individual and his or her partner in order to determine their risk for hydrops. Hemoglobin electrophoresis and quantitative hemoglobin A2 levels are often used to diagnose β thalassemia carriers. In the past, diagnosis of α thalassemia was made if the electrophoresis and hemoglobin A2 levels were normal. However, this is unreliable and will result in missed index cases.[1] Many individuals are carriers of both α thalassemia and β thalassemia, and an elevated hemoglobin A2 level may mask a couple at risk.[2,20] Molecular diagnosis for α globin mutations is essential for at-risk couples. Newer screening techniques using multiplex gap-PCR with deletional and nondeletional H mutations has made screening more efficient and rapid.[38] When parents have α thalassemia trait, DNA analysis on the fetus is required. Fetal tissue obtained by chorionic villus sampling early in the first trimester is indicated. Prenatal diagnosis for hydrops fetalis can also be conducted using fetal blood obtained by cordocentesis, or amniocentesis.

Prenatal ultrasonography and intrauterine fetal blood sampling

Anemia increases fetal blood velocities by increasing cardiac output and decreasing blood viscosity.[7,17,39–43] Ultrasound measurements can reliably detect fetal anemia. Doppler ultrasonography of the middle cerebral arteries report 88% sensitivity and 87% specificity for the prediction of fetal anemia.[42] In addition to increased velocity, other ultrasound abnormalities develop in homozygous α thalassemia before hydrops fetalis occurs. Placentomegaly, cardiothoracic ratio abnormalities, and increased placental thickness can be detected as early as 12–14 weeks and predict the development of ascites and hepatomegaly of hydrops fetalis.[6,7,39,41]

Screening of the middle cerebral artery is recommended because it is easily visualized and correlates well to tissue hypoxia and anemia. Middle cerebral artery measurements can be initiated weekly as early as 16 weeks of gestation. The results can be plotted on a normal, validated curve. However, the actual values are most commonly converted to multiples of the median to account for changes in gestational age.[40,41] While the peak middle cerebral artery Doppler measurement is highly reliable for anemia, its validity decreases following intrauterine transfusion.[43] Therefore, serial empiric monitoring of the fetal hemoglobin after the first transfusion is generally necessary. Although direct measurement of fetal hemoglobin is associated with risks (such as bleeding or fetal bradycardia), the overall procedure-related pregnancy loss is approximately 1%.[44]

Intrauterine transfusion therapy

Most fetuses with homozygous α thalassemia are not treated. The majority of cases go undetected. This has resulted in fetal loss and serious maternal complications, especially if the mother is not being monitored. Despite the lack of prenatal treatment, fetal survival is increasingly being recognized. Respiratory distress and severe anemia associated with marked hepatosplenomegaly have been noted in almost all of the births that did not receive intrauterine therapy. Those not transfused died shortly after birth. Long-term surviving patients had major neurologic deficits.[2,24,45] In contrast, the outcome of approximately 20 patients receiving intrauterine therapy was markedly better;[35,45–49] long-term neurologic function of those patients transfused *in utero* appears good. Intrauterine transfusion therapy appears promising in minimizing the morbidity and mortality of homozygous α thalassemia. However, most of these patients will require lifetime transfusion therapy and chelation. Recent advances in stem cell transplantation have resulted in some patients being cured. Successful cases of related, unrelated, and mismatched stem cell transplantation for alpha thalassemia major have been reported.[48,49]

Conclusion

In summary, homozygous α thalassemia and hydrops fetalis is a complex, usually fatal disease that is devastating to the entire family. There is diversity in the genotype and phenotype expression of this syndrome that presents challenges in at-risk couple counseling and population screening. Presently, counseling and testing of at-risk populations is inadequate. More cases are being diagnosed unexpectedly. Advances in diagnosis and treatment have raised ethical dilemmas for the patient and provider.

Acknowledgments

I would like to thank Erica Riray and Shanda Robertson for providing assistance with editing and manuscript preparation.

Conflicts of Interest

The author declares no conflicts of interest.

References

1. Bain, B.J. 2006. *Haemoglobinopathy Diagnosis.* 2nd ed. Blackwell Pub. Malden, Mass.
2. Chui, D.H. & J.S. Waye. 1998. Hydrops fetalis caused by alpha-thalassemia: an emerging health care problem. *Blood* **91:** 2213–2222.
3. Gibbons, R., D.R. Higgs, N.F. Olivieri & W.G. Wood 2001. The alpha thalassaemias and their interaction with structural hemoglobin variants. In *The Thalassaemia Syndromes.* D.J. Weatherall & J.B. Clegg, Eds.: 4th ed., 484. Blackwell Science. Oxford, England.
4. Lau, Y.L., L.C. Chan, Y.Y. Chan, *et al.* 1997. Prevalence and genotypes of alpha- and beta-thalassemia carriers in Hong Kong—implications for population screening. *New Engl. J. Med.* **336:** 1298–1301.
5. Yang, Y. & D.Z. Li. 2009. A survey of pregnancies with Hb Bart's disease in Mainland China. *Hemoglobin* **33:** 132–136.
6. Hofstaetter, C., M. Hansmann, S.H. Eik-Nes, *et al.* 2006. A cardiovascular profile score in the surveillance of fetal hydrops. *J. Matern. Fetal Neonatal Med.* **19:** 407–413.
7. Leung, W.C., D. Oepkes, G. Seaward & G. Ryan. 2002. Serial sonographic findings of four fetuses with homozygous alpha-thalassemia-1 from 21 weeks onwards. Ultrasound Obstet. Gynecol. **19:** 56–59.
8. Chen, F.E., C. Ooi, S.Y. Ha, *et al.* 2000. Genetic and clinical features of hemoglobin H disease in Chinese patients. *N. Engl. J. Med.* **343:** 544–550.
9. Chui, D.H., S. Fucharoen & V. Chan. 2003. Hemoglobin H disease: not necessarily a benign disorder. *Blood* **101:** 791–800.
10. Lorey, F., P. Charoenkwan, H.E. Witkowska, *et al.* 2001. Hb H hydrops foetalis syndrome: a case report and review of literature. *Br. J. Haematol.* **115:** 72–78.
11. Origa, R., M.C. Sollaino, N. Giagu, *et al.* 2007. Clinical and molecular analysis of haemoglobin H disease in Sardinia: haematological, obstetric and cardiac aspects in patients with different genotypes. *Br. J. Haematol.* **136:** 326–332.
12. Michlitsch, J., M. Azimi, C. Hoppe, *et al.* 2009. Newborn screening for hemoglobinopathies in California. *Pediatr. Blood Cancer* **52:** 486–490.
13. Weatherall, D.J. 2001. Phenotype-genotype relationships in monogenic disease: lessons from the thalassaemias. *Nat. Rev. Genet.* **2:** 245–255.
14. Styles, L.A., D.H. Foote, K.M. Kleman, *et al.* 1997. Hemoglobin H-constant spring disease: an under recognized, severe form of a tahlassemia. *Int. J. Ped. Hematol/Oncol.* **4:** 69–74.
15. Vichinsky, E.P. 2005. Changing patterns of thalassemia worldwide. *Ann. N. Y. Acad. Sci.* **1054:** 18–24.
16. Singer, S.T., H.Y. Kim, N.F. Olivieri, *et al.* 2009. Hemoglobin H-constant spring in North America: an alpha thalassemia with frequent complications. *Am. J. Hematol.* **84:** 759–761.
17. Leung, W.C., K.Y. Leung, E.T. Lau, *et al.* 2008.Alpha-thalassaemia. *Semin. Fetal Neonatal Med.* **13:** 215–222.
18. Lorey, F., G. Cunningham, E.P. Vichinsky, *et al.* 2001. Universal newborn screening for Hb H disease in California. *Genetic Testing* **5:** 93–100.
19. Weatherall, D.J. 2008. Hemoglobinopathies worldwide: present and future. *Curr. Mol. Med.* **8:** 592–599.
20. Li, D., C. Liao, J. Li, *et al.* 2006. Detection of alpha-thalassemia in beta-thalassemia carriers and prevention of Hb Bart's hydrops fetalis through prenatal screening. *Haematologica* **91:** 649–651.
21. Liao, C., Q. Li, J. Wei, *et al.* 2007. Prenatal control of Hb Bart's disease in southern China. *Hemoglobin* **31:** 471–475.
22. Suwanrath-Kengpol, C., O. Kor-anantakul, T. Suntharasaj & R. Leetanaporn. 2005. Etiology and outcome of nonimmune hydrops fetalis in southern Thailand. *Gynecol. Obstet. Invest.* **59:** 134–137.
23. Srisupundit, K., W. Piyamongkol & T. Tongsong. 2008. Comparison of red blood cell hematology among normal, alpha-thalassemia-1 trait, and hemoglobin Bart's fetuses at mid-pregnancy. *Am. J. Hematol.* **83:** 908–910.
24. Lee, S.Y., C.B. Chow, C.K. Li & M.C. Chiu. 2007. Outcome of intensive care of homozygous alpha-thalassaemia without prior intra-uterine therapy. *J. Paediatr. Child Health* **43:** 546–550.
25. Monaco, S.E., M. Davis, A.C. Huang, *et al.* 2005. Alpha-thalassemia major presenting in a term neonate without hydrops. *Pediatr. Dev. Pathol.* **8:** 706–709.
26. Chan, V., T.K. Chan, S.T. Liang, *et al.* 1985. Hydrops fetalis due to an unusual form of Hb H disease. *Blood* **66:** 224–228.
27. Chan, V., V.W. Chan, M. Tang, *et al.* 1997. Molecular defects in Hb H hydrops fetalis. *Br. J. Haematol.* **96:** 224–228.
28. Ko, T.M., F.J. Hsieh, P.M. Hsu & T.Y. Lee. 1991. Molecular characterization of severe alpha-thalassemias causing hydrops fetalis in Taiwan. *Am. J. Med. Genet.* **39:** 317–320.
29. Siriratmanawong, N., C. Pinmuang-Ngam, G. Fucharoen & S. Fucharoen. 2007. Prenatal diagnosis of Hb Bart's hydrops fetalis caused by a genetic compound heterozygosity for two different alpha-thalassemia determinants. *Fetal Diagn. Ther.* **22:** 264–268.
30. Viprakasit, V., S. Green, S. Height, *et al.* 2002. Hb H hydrops fetalis syndrome associated with the interaction of two common determinants of alpha thalassaemia (–MED/(alpha)TSaudi(alpha)). *Br. J. Haematol.* **117:** 759–762.

31. Ne, W., K. Harano, T. Harano, *et al.* 2008. Hb Constant Spring [alpha 142, Term–>Gln (TAA>CAA in alpha2)] in the alpha-thalassemia of anemic patients in Myanmar. *Hemoglobin* **32:** 454–461.
32. Charoenkwan, P., S. Sirichotiyakul, P. Chanprapaph, *et al.* 2006. Anemia and hydrops in a fetus with homozygous hemoglobin constant spring. *J. Pediatr. Hematol. Oncol.* **28:** 827–830.
33. Joshi, D.D., H.J. Nickerson & M.J. McManus. 2004. Hydrops fetalis caused by homozygous alpha-thalassemia and Rh antigen alloimmunization: report of a survivor and literature review. *Clin. Med. Res.* **2:** 228–232.
34. Adam, M.P., J. Chueh, Y.Y. El-Sayed, *et al.* 2005. Vascular-type disruptive defects in fetuses with homozygous alpha-thalassemia: report of two cases and review of the literature. *Prenat. Diagn.* **25:** 1088–1096.
35. Singer, S.T., L. Styles, J. Bojanowski, *et al.* 2000. Changing outcome of homozygous alpha-thalassemia: cautious optimism. *J. Pediatr. Hematol. Oncol.* **22:** 539–542.
36. Dame, C., N. Albers, C. Hasan, *et al.* 1999. Homozygous alpha-thalassaemia and hypospadias–common aetiology or incidental association? Long-term survival of Hb Bart's hydrops syndrome leads to new aspects for counselling of alpha-thalassaemic traits. *Eur. J. Pediatr.* **158:** 217–220.
37. Liang, S.T., V.C. Wong, W.W. So, *et al.* 1985. Homozygous alpha-thalassaemia: clinical presentation, diagnosis and management. A review of 46 cases. *Br. J. Obstet. Gynaecol.* **92:** 680–684.
38. Kidd, J.L., M. Azimi, B. Lubin, *et al.* 2009. Application of an expanded multiplex genotyping assay for the simultaneous detection of Hemoglobin Constant Spring and common deletional alpha-thalassemia mutations. *Int. J. Lab Hematol.* [Epub ahead of print].
39. Lam, Y.H. & M.H. Tang. 2002. Middle cerebral artery Doppler study in fetuses with homozygous alpha-thalassaemia-1 at 12–13 weeks of gestation. *Prenat. Diagn.* **22:** 56–58.
40. Mari, G., R.L. Deter, R.L. Carpenter, *et al.* 2000. Noninvasive diagnosis by Doppler ultrasonography of fetal anemia due to maternal red-cell alloimmunization. Collaborative Group for Doppler Assessment of the Blood Velocity in Anemic Fetuses. *New Engl. J. Med.* **342:** 9–14.
41. Moise, K.J., Jr. 2008. The usefulness of middle cerebral artery Doppler assessment in the treatment of the fetus at risk for anemia. *Am. J. Obstet. Gynecol.* **198:** 161 e1–e4.
42. Oepkes, D., P.G. Seaward, F.P. Vandenbussche, *et al.* 2006. Doppler ultrasonography versus amniocentesis to predict fetal anemia. *New Engl. J. Med.* **355:** 156–164.
43. Zimmermann, R., P. Durig, R.J. Carpenter, Jr., G. Mari. 2002. Longitudinal measurement of peak systolic velocity in the fetal middle cerebral artery for monitoring pregnancies complicated by red cell alloimmunisation: a prospective multicentre trial with intention-to-treat. *Bjog* **109:** 746–752.
44. Daffos F, M. Capella-Pavlovsky, F. Forestier. 1985. Fetal blood sampling during pregnancy with use of a needle guided by ultrasound: a study of 606 consecutive cases. *Am. J. Obstet. Gynecol.* **153:** 655–660.
45. Lucke, T., S. Pfister & M. Durken. 2005. Neurodevelopmental outcome and haematological course of a long-time survivor with homozygous alpha-thalassaemia: case report and review of the literature. *Acta Paediatr.* **94:** 1330–1333.
46. Carr, S., L. Rubin, D. Dixon, *et al.* 1995. Intrauterine therapy for homozygous alpha-thalassemia. *Obstet. Gynecol.* **85:** 876–879.
47. Weisz, B., O. Rosenbaum, B. Chayen, *et al.* 2009. Outcome of severely anaemic fetuses treated by intrauterine transfusions. *Arch.Dis. Child.* **94:** F201–F204.
48. Yi, J.S., C.L. Moertel & K.S. Baker. 2009. Homozygous alpha-thalassemia treated with intrauterine transfusions and unrelated donor hematopoietic cell transplantation. *J. Pediatr.* **154:** 766–768.
49. Zhou, X., S.Y. Ha, G.C. Chan, *et al.* 2001. Successful mismatched sibling cord blood transplant in Hb Bart's disease. *Bone Marrow Transplant.* **28:** 105–107.

Ann. N.Y. Acad. Sci. ISSN 0077-8923

ANNALS OF THE NEW YORK ACADEMY OF SCIENCES
Issue: *Cooley's Anemia: Ninth Symposium*

Nutritional deficiencies in patients with thalassemia

Ellen B. Fung

Department of Hematology/Oncology, Children's Hospital and Research Center at Oakland, Oakland, California

Address for correspondence: Ellen B. Fung, Ph.D., R.D., Department of Hematology/Oncology, Children's Hospital and Research Center, Oakland, HEDCO Health Science Building, 5700 Martin Luther King Jr. Way, Oakland, CA 94609. efung@mail.cho.org

Optimal nutritional status is imperative for growth, development, immune function, and bone health. Patients with thalassemia are known to have poor growth, altered puberty, and immune function as well as reduced bone mineral acquisition. The etiology of these comorbidites is typically ascribed to the toxic effects of transfusion-related iron-overload. Recently, our group and others have observed marked nutritional deficiencies in key fat and water-soluble vitamins as well as important essential minerals. Depressed circulating levels of nutrients have been observed despite seemingly adequate dietary intake. This disconnect between intake and circulating levels suggests that patients with thalassemia may have increased needs for certain nutrients due to either poor nutrient absorption, elevated losses, or increased nutrient turnover. Randomized controlled clinical trials are needed to test the efficacy of nutritional therapies toward improving the overall health in thalassemia, as well as decreasing long-term comorbidities such as reduced bone mass.

Keywords: nutrition; thalassemia; zinc; vitamin D; iron, dietary intake

Nutritional red flags: growth deficits and pubertal delay

Optimal nutritional status is imperative for achieving the genetic potential for growth and pubertal development in children, and poor growth and delayed puberty is considered a red flag to any pediatrician leading to exploration of possible nutrient specific or global nutritional deficiencies.[1] In the adult patient, altered nutritional status may adversely affect immune function, oxidative stress, bone health, and/or may limit the effectiveness of some medications.[2]

Growth failure is common in patients with thalassemia. Various reports suggest the incidence of growth deficits ranges from 25% to 75% depending on thalassemia syndrome and severity of disease.[3–5] Height Z-score tends to decrease with age, commonly associated with pubertal deficits.[3,5] However, growth failure is multifactorial in thalassemia, related to chronic anemia, chelation toxicity, and iron-associated endocrinopathies such as hypogonadism, hypothyroidism, and growth hormone deficiency. Ethnicity may also be considered when making generalized comparisons of growth to reference populations; however, ethnic disparity alone does not explain the extent of the deficits observed. Little attention has historically been given to the role nutrition may play to growth failure in thalassemia.

A few reports from investigators outside the United States suggest that suboptimal nutritional status plays a role in growth failure and pubertal development. Fikry and colleagues observed a positive correlation between serum zinc level and linear growth in 46 young Egyptian patients with thalassemia.[6] Filosa and colleagues reported that delays in pubertal development were related to poor overall nutritional status in young Italian males with thalassemia.[7] Others have shown in small groups of toddlers with thalassemia that nutrition support for one month improves markers of immune function and growth.[8,9] Soliman and colleagues went one step further and conducted a randomized nutrition intervention in 30 prepubertal children with transfusion-dependent thalassemia.[10] Of interest, when compared to age and gender matched controls, the children with thalassmia had similar dietary intake at baseline despite marked growth and

doi: 10.1111/j.1749-6632.2010.05578.x

body fat deficits. After increasing caloric intake by 30–50% over an 8-week period, they observed significant improvements in weight, fat stores, albumin and insulin-like growth factor 1 (IGF-1) levels compared to the nonsupplemented Thal group. The improvement in IGF-1 following nutritional therapy supports the notion that a component of the growth failure in Thal is related to nutritional deficiency. Unfortunately, the majority of the published work in this area has summarized observations or interventions in relatively small numbers of subjects primarily conducted outside of North America in low profile journals, therefore has received little attention.

Nutrient intake, requirements, and expenditure

Nutritional adequacy is predicated on a balance between intake and requirements. One explanation for the reduced growth rates in thalassemia despite seemingly adequate caloric intake could be increased caloric expenditure. This is quite possible given the existence of hyperactive bone marrow and increased cardiac output due to chronic anemia. In 1995, Vaisman and colleagues evaluated seven adult patients with thalassemia before and 3 days after red blood cell transfusion.[11] Hemoglobin concentration was negatively associated with energy expenditure. They observed energy expenditure to be 12% higher than expected, which decreased to near normal levels following transfusion, presumably due to a reduction in protein turnover and reduced cardiac output.

In addition to the potential increased requirement for total calories, others have shown that the requirements for specific nutrients may be increased in patients with thalassemia. The clearest example of this is with regard to folate metabolism. Folate, an essential nutrient required for normal erthropoietic activity, has been shown recently to be readily catabolized by ferritin.[12] Thus, in patients with thalassemia with hyperactive erythropoiesis, confounded by iron overload, folate requirements are increased and deficiencies are commonly reported.[13] Increased markers of oxidative stress have been reported in Thal by many investigators most frequently associated with iron overload.[14] This topic will be explored in more detail in the paper presented by Lal and colleagues.[15] Insufficient antioxidant intake has been associated with oxidative stress. In the early 1990s, a group in Thailand was able to reduce circulating glutathione peroxidase in young patients with thalassemia through supplementation with 200 mg of vitamin E for 4–8 weeks.[16] Iron overload may also perturb essential trace element status. There is the potential for sequestration of zinc and copper in the liver of iron-overloaded subjects due to the upregulation of metallothionien by high iron concentrations. Depressed circulating zinc and copper levels[17] have been reported, although there is a paucity of data on hepatic concentration of minerals other than iron in transfusion-dependent patients with thalassemia.

Recently, Claster and colleagues reported the circulating levels of a variety of essential nutrients in a convenience sample of 24 chronically transfused patients with thalassemia (age range: 1.5–31.4 years, ferritin 2089 ± 1920 ng/mL).[18] They found surprisingly low levels of both water soluble and fat soluble vitamins (Table 1). For a few nutrients, over half of the patients sampled had low levels; these included vitamins A, C, D, and selenium. In fact only a few nutrients did not appear to be reduced, which included serum copper, vitamin B-12, and γ-tocopherol, the supplemental form of vitamin E. Circulating levels of many nutrients tended to decrease with increasing age, that is younger subjects tended to have higher circulating nutrient levels compared to older subjects. Although this level of nutritional deficiency has been shown in other studies to be associated with poor health outcomes, the small sample size and cross-sectional study design in this study by Claster and colleagues precluded a cause and effect type analysis.

As summarized thus far, patients with thalassemia may be at increased risk for nutritional deficiencies due to elevated nutrient requirements. However, nutrient balance is related not only to requirement and output, but input: patients with thalassemia may also have inadequate intake or absorption of nutrients. Our group assessed typical dietary intake in 38 patients with thalassemia (21 female, 17.1 ± 5.4 years, mean ± *SD*; 28 transfusion dependent) and compared them to 36 age, gender, and ethnically similar controls (20 females, 17.8 ± 6.2 years). Each subject completed a 160-question Block©2005, food frequency questionnaire. Questionnaires were analyzed and nutrient inadequacy defined as less than two-thirds the current age and gender specific U.S. Dietary Reference Intake value. Overall kcal, and protein, fat, and cholesterol intake were

Table 1. **Circulating nutrient levels in patients with thalassemia**

Nutrient	Normal range	Value	% Abnormal
Fat soluble vitamins			
Vitamin A (μg/dL)	38–98	34.6 ± 12.2	52.4%
Vitamin D (ng/mL)	20–100	17.1 ± 8.5	50.0%
α-Tocopherol (mg/dL)	5.7–19.9	7.5 ± 7.5	29.2%
γ-Tocopherol (mg/dL)	<4.3	3.0 ± 5.0	4.2%
Water soluble vitamins			
Thiamin (μg/L)	2.4–11.7	4.1 ± 4.0	37.5%
Vitamin B-6 (ng/mL)	3.3–26	7.0 ± 5.9	34.8%
Vitamin B-12 (pg/mL)	200–1100	528 ± 152	0%
Folate (ng/mL)	>8	11.8 ± 7.7	37.5%
Trace elements			
Copper (μg/dL)	59–118	85.1 ± 15.5	0%
Selenium (μg/dL)	110–160	99.5 ± 20.7	75.0%
Zinc (μg/dL)	65–124	83.0 ± 15.6	8.3%

Adapted from Claster *et al.* (2009).[18]
Mean ± *SD*.
Vitamin D: 25-hydroxy vitamin D.

similar between Thal and control subjects, (kcal: 107 ± 41%, Thal vs. 105 ± 38%, Control, NS; macro nutrient data not shown). The percentage of subjects with inadequate specific nutrient intakes are shown in Figure 1. Across the board, more Thal subjects had inadequate nutrient intake. Vitamin D, folate, calcium, and magnesium were significantly lower in Thal compared to controls ($P = 0.02$). These nutrients are of particular concern as they are critical for optimal bone mineralization and low bone mass is a particularly common comorbidity in thalassemia.[19] The number of dairy servings consumed per day were consistent with the specific nutrient intakes. That is, subjects with thalassemia consumed significantly lower servings of dairy compared to the health controls (1.3 vs. 2.0 servings per day, $P = 0.02$).

From these data it is clear that patients with thalassemia have frequently reported depressed circulating nutrient levels, the potential for increased requirements of specific nutrients and some indication that dietary intake is inadequate. Few studies have explored overall dietary intake in large samples of contemporary patients with thalassemia. The Thalassemia Clinical Research Network recently completed a cross-sectional analysis of dietary intake in nearly 200 patients with a variety of thalassemia syndromes.[20] It is anticipated this group will publish further information on dietary intake and body composition in this large cohort of patients with thalassemia within the year.

Specific micronutrients

Vitamin D: skeletal and extra skeletal effects

Vitamin D deficiency has received much attention in the scientific literature recently.[21] Numerous studies have reported on a variety of chronic disease states are apparently at risk for inadequacy or deficiency. Thalassemia is one of the chronic disease states identified that is at particular risk. Last year we reported that only 18% of a contemporary sample of 361 patients with thalassemia residing in North America had sufficient levels of 25-OH vitamin D (defined as >30 ng/mL).[3] Others have reported similar levels of inadequacy.[18,22,23]

Vitamin D is unique in that it is the only essential nutrient for which we are also able to synthesize in the body. It has been estimated that up to 80% of the vitamin D requirement is synthesized in the skin, whereas the remainder is obtained from dietary sources. There are many factors to consider when it comes to the cutaneous synthesis of vitamin D: geographic latitude, season, altitude, cloud cover, air quality, time of day, as well as an individual's clothing, skin pigmentation, and sun screen use. For

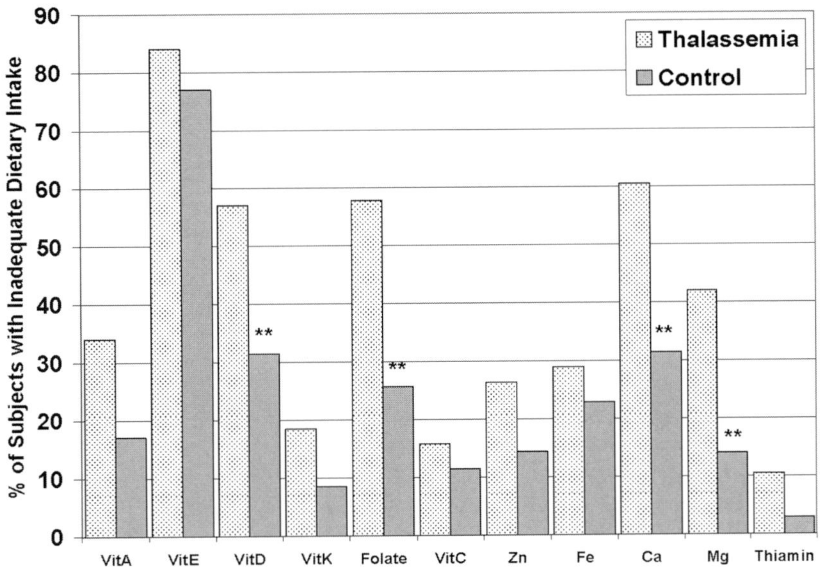

Figure 1. Percentage of subjects with thalassemia ($n = 38$) compared to healthy age and ethnically similar controls ($n = 36$) with inadequate dietary intake of essential nutrients, defined as intake less than two-thirds the recommendation for healthy people. **Denote significant difference between Thal and Controls of $P < 0.02$.

those cities that lie north of 42° latitude, sunlight is too weak to synthesize vitamin D from late October to early March,[24] and for those cities that lie north of 40° latitude, sunlight is too weak to synthesize vitamin D during January and February. Therefore, vitamin D status should be monitored more carefully in those patients with thalassemia who reside in Northern latitudes, are naturally dark skinned, who customarily shroud themselves, or who have limited exposure to sunlight during mid-day hours when the sun is at its highest in the sky, 10:00 am to 2:00 pm. Although dietary intake is not the primary contributor to vitamin D status, it must still be considered as a possible risk factor for deficiency. There are few natural sources of vitamin D in the diet, primarily fatty fish and cod liver oil. As a result, in many countries vitamin D is fortified in the food supply. In the United States, fluid milk is fortified to 100 IU vitamin D per 8 ounces. Therefore, patients with thalassemia who are lactose intolerant or who avoid milk for other reasons may be at greater risk for vitamin D deficiency.

Vitamin D also has unique hormonal functions; its active form, 1,25-OH vitamin D has been shown to have multiple roles in the body not only related to bone health and fracture reduction but also cardiovascular health, immune function, blood pressure, and cancer prevention. A report released this past year thoroughly reviewed the literature that relates to vitamin D and functional outcomes in the U.S. population.[25] In this exhaustive report, a consistent relationship between vitamin D and cardiovascular health was not observed. However, individuals with thalassemia may be at greater risk for vitamin D deficiency and therefore have a greater response to supplementation.

Wood and colleagues found a weak though significant correlation between 25-OH vitamin D levels and left ventricular ejection fraction in patients with thalassemia who were not on vitamin D supplementation, $r^2 = 0.35$.[26] In this small study, all four subjects who had ejection fractions that were considered dysfunctional (LVEF <57%) also had deficient levels of vitamin D. They also observed a correlation between the ratio of 25 to 1,25 hydroxy vitamin D and R2, a level of iron concentration within the heart by magnetic resonance imaging. More recently, Dimitriadou and colleagues reported that PTH was higher in β-thalassemia major patients with increased myocardial iron compared to those with normal levels ($P = 0.017$).[27] Patients with thalassemia and reduced levels of vitamin D have been shown to have a 10-fold greater risk of low bone mass after controlling for age, weight Z-score, and hypogonadism.[19] In addition, those patients with thalassemia who have the vitamin D receptor Bsml polymorphism, may be further risk for osteoporosis.[28]

With so many subjects at risk for vitamin D insufficiency, how can the medical team tackle this pandemic? Vitamin D is a fat-soluble vitamin, as such, it is stored in the tissues and can be provided in high doses in low frequency. The current guidelines from the National Kidney Foundation for replacement suggest a 50,000 IU supplement be provided every other week for 8 weeks for subjects with 25-OH vitamin D levels less than 15 ng/mL or 50,000 IU every 4 weeks for those with levels <30 ng/mL. At Children's Hospital Oakland, we have observed that many patients continue to have 25-OH vitamin D levels below the optimal range of 30 ng/mL despite a prescribed dose of 1000 IU per day, or 7000 IU per week. Given this, we modified the current guideline to coincide with the thalassemia transfusion regimen. Thirteen patients with transfusion-dependent thalassemia and vitamin D levels ≤20 ng/mL were given 50,000 IU of ergocalciferol (D2) orally at time of transfusion for six to eight transfusion cycles or 18–24 weeks. This dosage translates to approximately 1700–2300 IU per day depending upon the frequency of transfusion. We found 25-OH vitamin D increased from baseline in all but one patient, but only reached a level of sufficiency in one patient (defined as >30 ng/mL, Fig. 2). Therefore, this pilot program was successful at improving adherence to the vitamin D supplementation regimen; however, this dosage for patients with low vitamin D levels may be insufficient to boost their levels within a six-month period. Soliman and colleagues suggest a higher dose (100,000 IU/kg with a max of 600,000 IU) or greater frequency (e.g., weekly), may be required to increase circulating levels in many subjects.[23] Vitamin D replacement has been successful in other chronic disease states using similar high-dose, low-frequency supplementation regimens.[29,30]

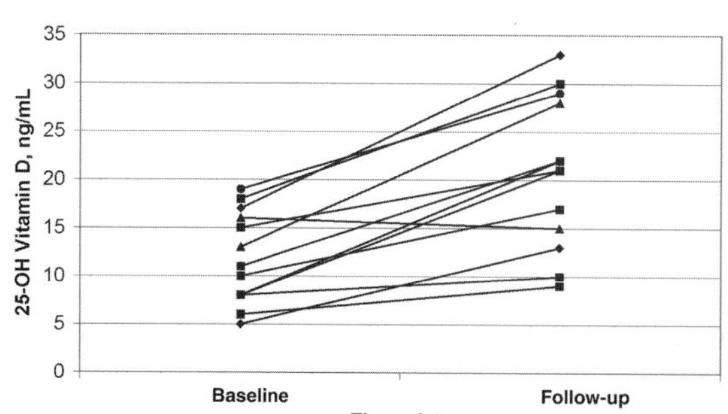

Figure 2. Response of serum 25-OH vitamin D levels before and after high dose ergocalciferol supplementation in patients with thalassemia.

Zinc deficiency: growth, immune function, and bone health

Zinc is an essential trace mineral required for cell division, differentiation, and gene expression. It is critical to the function of over 300 enzymes, as such it is important to a myriad of bodily functions including development and maintenance of the immune system, bone health, vitamin A metabolism, and actions of thyroid, insulin, testosterone, and growth hormone.

Zinc is a particularly important mineral to transfused patients with thalassemia because it is similar enough in size and charge to iron, therefore it has the potential to be chelated along with iron in those patients treated for iron overload.

Zinc deficiency has been documented in both transfused and nontransfused patients with thalassemia.[17,31] A 2003 report from Iran found that 80% of adolescent patients with beta thalassemia exhibited poor zinc status defined by depressed plasma zinc.[32] Depletion of circulating zinc may be due in part to the presence of proximal tubular damage[33] and hyperzincuria, as urinary zinc is elevated 4-fold in patients with thalassemia compared to controls.[34] Increases in urinary zinc may be related to the presence or absence of diabetes, a comorbidity also associated with increased zinc losses.[35] Alternatively, chelators used to treat iron overload may also place these patients at risk for zinc deficiency.[35,36] Arcasoy and colleagues conducted a zinc supplementation study in 32 young regularly transfused, nonchelated patients with thalassemia (1–18 years).[37] Twenty-one patients received between 22 and 90 mg Zn/day over a period of 1–7 years, the remaining patients received only their usual transfusion regimen. Although only 50% of the sample were considered growth delayed at study initiation, they observed an increase in height velocity in the zinc compared to the nonsupplemented group ($P < 0.01$). This result suggests patients within their clinic were experiencing a zinc-limiting growth failure.

Abnormalities of zinc metabolism may also play a role in the pathology of osteoporosis in patients with thalassemia. In 2004, Bekheirnia and colleagues observed that female patients with thalassemia and severe zinc deficiency had lower lumbar BMD Z-scores in comparison to the other females (-3.26 vs. -2.54).[32] Serum zinc was 16.4 μg/dL lower in females with low femoral bone mass compared to those with normal bone mass. More recently, this same group observed a similar relationship between depressed serum zinc and low bone mass in both males and females with thalassemia.[38] Similar to the previous report, low bone mass was common in the 203 adolescent patients studied (50% had Z-score <-2.5 in the spine), and low bone mass was strongly associated with low serum zinc. Our group has recently completed a randomized placebo controlled trial of zinc supplementation on bone health in patients with thalassemia (Clinical Trials.gov #NCT00480415). The results from this trial are pending.

Within the last few years, others have explored the relationship between zinc deficiency and diabetes in patients with thalassemia. Dehshal and colleagues measured serum zinc, insulin, and glucose in 70 patients with thalassemia and 69 healthy controls before and during a 1 h oral glucose tolerance test (OGTT).[39] They found that 37% of subjects had depressed serum zinc levels, which were associated with lower fasting and 1-h post-OGTT serum insulin concentrations. Their data support the hypothesis that zinc deficiency might lead to an exacerbation of the inability of the pancreas to secrete sufficient amounts of insulin in response to glucose stimulation in patients with transfusion-dependent thalassemia.

Iron: the dogma and the dilemma

Given the relationship between iron overload and organ dysfunction in Thal, counseling patients to consume a diet low in iron has been part of the standards of care for decades. Typically, a diet that is low in iron rich foods such as red and organ meats, and fortified breakfast cereals is recommended for all patients. However, there is debate regarding the effectiveness of reducing dietary iron consumption for the transfused subject. The amount of iron obtained from just one unit of packed red blood cells (200 mg) far outweighs the amount of iron obtained from a 3 oz steak (5 mg). Typical daily iron accumulation from transfusion-related iron is ~20 mg/day (2 units every 3 weeks), compared to iron accumulation from an iron rich diet: ~4 mg (assuming 30% absorption). A low iron diet may decrease the quality of life in some transfusion-dependent patients and/or create a false sense of security; that is, if they decrease their dietary iron intake, they may need to be less diligent with regard to chelator adherence.

For the nontransfusion-dependent patient with thalassemia, reducing iron in the diet is an important part of nutritional counseling as these patients have a tendency to over absorb iron from the intestinal track. Black tea has been shown in one study from 1979 ($n = 6$ subjects) to reduce the absorption of dietary iron from plant based foods up to 95%.[40]

Current nutritional guidelines

Guidelines for monitoring dietary intake and nutritional status in patients with thalassemia have been published either online or as pamphlets by many organizations involved with patients such as the Thalassaemia International Federation (www.thalassaemia.org.cy), Cooley's Anemia Foundation (www.cooleysanemia.com), and the Northern California Comprehensive Thalassemia Center (www.thalassemia.com). Most experts agree that the nutritional status of patients should be evaluated annually by the medical team, which includes a registered dietitian or nutritionist. The adequacy of dietary intake of many important nutrients including calcium, vitamin D, folate, trace minerals (zinc, copper, selenium), and antioxidant vitamins (E and C) should be considered. Annual monitoring of nutritional labs should include albumin, folate, vitamins C, E, zinc, copper, ceruloplasmin, and selenium. Because of the seasonal effects on circulating levels of vitamin D, it is recommended that it be assessed every 6 months (Table 2). Supplementation to the diet is made after investigation of dietary history, and estimated requirements and consideration of growth status, pubertal development and bone health. Typically, a daily multivitamin mineral supplement without iron is suggested for most transfused patients. For nontransfused subjects, folate supplementation is recommended (1 mg daily). Nutritional counseling should be offered to patients with special dietary needs including those with iron-induced diabetes, vegetarians or vegans, lactose intolerant, have numerous food allergies, those who are pregnant, on oral chelation therapy and/or who may be taking bisphosphonate medications.

Summary and future directions

Depressed circulating levels of key fat and water-soluble vitamins as well as important essential

Table 2. Nutrition monitoring recommendations

Growth/development	Sample type	Frequency	Adequacy
Height and weight		Monthly	[a]
Sitting height		Every 3 months	
Calculate growth velocity		Annually	
Puberty: Tanner staging		Every 6 months	
Nutritional laboratory			
Albumin		Annually	3.5–5.0 g/dL
Folate	Serum	Annually	>3 ng/mL
Vitamin D, 25-OH	Serum	Every 6 months	≥ 30 ng/mL
Vitamin C- Ascorbate	Plasma	Annually	>0.4 mg/dL
Vitamin E- α- and γ-tocopherol	Serum	Annually	Age and gender dependent
Zinc	Serum (TE, F)	Annually	≥70 μg/dL
Copper	Serum (TE)	Annually	≥70 μg/dL
Selenium	Serum (TE)	Annually	>45 μg/L
Ceruloplasmin		Annually	>17 mg/dL
Other			
Bone densitometry		Annually, starting at 8 years	*Z*-score >−2.0

[a]Adequacy of growth is dependent upon the child's genetic potential for growth determined by the mid-parental height index.
TE, All trace elements need to be collected into trace element free vacutainers; F, it is important that these are collected in the fasted state.
For transfused patients, best to draw laboratory values prior to transfusion (e.g., morning of).
May be possible to use red blood cell folate in the non-transfused patient, as it is typically a better indicator of tissue stores than serum folate.
Adapted from Standards of Care Guidelines for Thalassemia, Children's Hospital and Research Center, Oakland, December (2008).

minerals have frequently been observed in patients with thalassemia. There is a paucity of robust information on dietary intake; however, there is increasing evidence that patients with thalassemia have increased needs for certain nutrients owing to either poor nutrient absorption, elevated losses, or increased nutrient turnover. The etiology of frequently reported comorbidites in thalassemia can no longer simply be ascribed to the toxic effects of transfusion-related iron overload. However, more trials are needed to support a causal association between nutritional status and overall health in patients with thalassemia.

Suggested areas of future research for patients with thalassemia include the following:

(1) Noninvasive, potentially anabolic nutritional interventions for improvement of bone density in young patients, for whom bisphosphonate medications may be contraindicated.
(2) Thoughtful investigation of the effect of oral chelation therapy on trace element status (zinc, copper, selenium), including assessment of static as well as functional markers of trace element status and biomarkers of oxidative stress.
(3) Exploration into the role of vitamin D deficiency and risk/benefits of supplementation with vitamin D not only in bone health but also immune function and cardiac disease.
(4) Collaborative, multicenter site studies to explore relationships between circulating levels of nutrients and various comorbidities.
(5) Randomized controlled clinical trials to test the efficacy of individual nutritional therapies towards the improvement of growth, pubertal development, immune function, oxidative damage, and bone health.

Conflicts of interest

The authors declare no conflicts of interest.

References

1. American Academy of Pediatrics, Committee on Nutrition; 2008. *Pediatric Nutrition Handbook*, R.E. Kleinman, Eds., 6th ed. American Academy of Pediatrics. Elk Grove Village, IL.
2. Joint WHO/FAO Expert Committee. 2003. Diet, nutrition and the prevention of chronic diseases. WHO Technical Report Series, 916. WHO, Geneva, Switzerland.
3. Vogiatzi M., E.A. Macklin, F.L. Trachtenberg, *et al.* 2009. Differences in the prevalence of growth, endocrine and vitamin D abnormalities among the various thalassemia syndromes in North America. *Br. J. Haematol.* **146:** 546–156.
4. De Sanctis V., A. Eleftheriou, C. Malaventura, *et al.* 2004. Prevalence of endocrine complications and short stature in patients with thalassemia major: a multicenter study by the Thalassemia International Federation (TIF). *Pediatr. Endocrinol. Rev.* (Suppl 2): 249–255.
5. Kwan E.Y.W., A.C.W. Lee, A.M.C. Li, *et al.* 1995. A cross-sectional study of growth, puberty and endocrine function in patients with thalassemia major in Hong Kong. *J. Paediatr. Child Health* **31:** 83–87.
6. Fikry S.I., S.A. Saleh, N.N. Sarkis & H. Mangoud. 2003. Study of serum zinc in relation to nutritional status among thalassemia patients in Damanhour Medical National Institute. *J. Egypt. Public Health Assoc.* **78:** 73–93.
7. Filosa A., S. Di Maio, G. Esposito, *et al.* 2001. Persistence of delayed adrenarche in boys with thalassemia. *J. Pediatr. Endocrinol.* **14:** 407–414.
8. Tienboon P. 2003. Effect of nutrition support on immunity in paediatric patients with beta-thalassaemia major. *Asia-Pac. J. Clin. Nutr.* **12:** 61–65.
9. Fuchs G.J., P. Tienboon, S. Linpisarn, *et al.* 1996. Nutritional factors and thalassemia major. *Arch. Dis. Child.* **74:** 224–227.
10. Soliman A.T., W. El-Matary, M.M. Fattah, *et al.* 2004. The effect of high-calorie diet on nutritional parameters of children with beta-thalassaemia major. *Clin. Nutr.* **23:** 1153–1158.
11. Vaisman N, A. Akivis, D. Sthoeger, *et al.* 1995. Resting energy expenditure in patients with thalassemia major. *Am. J. Clin. Nutr.* **61:** 582–584.
12. Suh J.R., A.K. Herbig & P.J. Stover. 2001. New perspectives on folate catabolism. *Annu. Rev. Nutr.* **21:** 255–282.
13. Ozdem S., A. Kupesiz & A. Yesilipek. 2008. Plasma homocysteine levels in patients with b-thalassemia major. *Scand. J. Clin. Lab. Invest.* **68:** 134–139.
14. Walter P.B., E.B. Fung, Killilea D.W., *et al.* 2006. Oxidative stress and inflammation in iron-overloaded patients with β-thalassaemia or sickle cell disease. *Br. J. Haematol.* **135:** 254–263.
15. Lal A. 2010. Nutrition and Antioxidant Therapies in Thalassemia. Presented at the Ninth Cooley's Anemia Symposium, Oct. 21–24, 2009.
16. Suthutvoravut U., P. Hathirat, P. Sirichakwal, *et al.* 1993. Vitamin E status, glutathione peroxidase activity and the effect of vitamin E supplementation in children with thalassemia. *J. Med. Assoc. Thai.* **76**(Suppl 2): 146–152.
17. Kajanchumpol S., T. Tatu, W. Sasanakul, *et al.* 1997. Zinc and copper status of thalassemia children. *Southest Asian J. Trop. Med. Public Health* **28:** 877–880.
18. Claster S., J.C. Wood, L. Noetzli, *et al.* 2009. Nutritional deficiencies in iron overloaded patients with hemoglobinopathies. *Am. J. Hematol.* **84:** 344–348.
19. Vogiatzi M., E.A. Macklin, E.B. Fung, *et al.* 2009. Bone disease in thalassemia: a frequent and still unresolved problem. *J. Bone Miner. Res.* **24:** 543–557.
20. Fung E.B., Y. Xu, N. Olivieri, *et al.* 2010. Inadequate dietary intake in patients with thalassemia. Pediatric Blood & Cancer. 54, 6, 799. Abstract.
21. Holick M.F. & T.C. Chen 2008. Vitamin D deficiency: a worldwide problem with health consequences. *Am. J. Clin. Nutr.* **87:** 1080S–1086S.
22. Napoli N., E. Carmena, S. Bucchieri, *et al.* 2006. Low serum levels of 25-hydroxy vitamin D in adults affected by thalassemia major or intermedia. *Bone* **38:** 888–892.
23. Soliman A., A. Adel, M. Wagdy, *et al.* 2008. Calcium homeostasis in 40 adolescents with beta-thalassemia major: a case control study of the effects of intramuscular injection of a megadose of cholecalciferol. *Pediatr. Endocrinol. Rev.* **6**(Suppl 1): 149–154.
24. Holick M.F. 2008. Vitamin D: a D-Lightful health perspective. *Nutr. Rev.* **66**(Suppl 2): S182–S194.
25. Chung M., E.M. Balk, M. Brendel, *et al.* 2009. *Vitamin D and Calcium: A Systematic Review of Health Outcomes.* Evidence Report No 183. (Prepared by the Tufts Evidence Based Practice Center, under contract No. HHSA 290–2007-10055-I) AHRQ Publication No. 09-E015. Agency for Health Care Research and Quality, Rockville, MD.
26. Wood J.C., S. Claster, S. Carson, *et al.* 2008. Vitamin D deficiency, cardiac iron and cardiac function in thalassemia major. *Br. J. Haematol.* **141:** 891–894.
27. Dimitriadou M., A. Christoforidis, M. Economou, *et al.* 2009. Elevated serum parahormone levels are associated with myocardial iron load in patients with beta-thalassemia major. *Eur. J. Haematol.* Sept 10, Epub ahead of print.
28. El-Edel R.H., M.M. Ghonaim, O.M. Abo-Salem & F.M. El-Nemr. 2010. Bone mineral density and vitamin d receptor polymorphism in beta-thalassemia major. *Pak. J. Pharm. Sci.* **23:** 89–96.
29. Belostotsky V., Z. Mughal & N.J. Webb. 2009. A single high dose of ergocalciferol can be used to boost 25-hydroxy vitamin D levels in children with kidney disease. *Pediatr. Nephrol.* **24:** 625–626.
30. Boas S.R., J.R. Hageman, L.T. Ho & M. Liveris. 2009. Very high-dose ergocalciferol is effective for correcting vitamin D deficiency in children and young adults with cystic fibrosis *J. Cyst. Fibrosis* **8:** 270–272.
31. Arcasoy A. & A.O. Cavdar. 1975. Changes in trace minerals (serum zinc, copper and magnesium) in thalassemia. *Acta Haematol.* **53:** 341–346.
32. Bekheirnia M.R., A.A. Shamshirsaz, M. Kamgar, *et al.* 2004. Serum zinc and its relation to bone mineral density in beta-thalassemic adolescents. Biol. Trace Elem. Res. **97:** 215–224.
33. Cianciulli P., D. Sollecito, F. Sorrentino, *et al.* 1994. Early detection of nephrotoxic effects in thalassemic patients receiving desferrioxamine therapy. *Kidney Int.* **46:** 467–470.
34. Uysal Z., N. Akar, S. Kemahli, *et al.* 1993. Desferrioxamine and urinary zinc excretion in b-thalassemia major. *Pediatr. Hematol. Oncol.* **10:** 257–260.

35. Al-Refaie F.N., B. Wonke, D.C. Wickens, *et al.* 1994. Zinc concentration in patients with iron-overload receiving oral iron chelator 1,2-dimethyl-3-hydroxypyrid-4-one or desferrioxamine. *J. Clin. Pathol.* **47:** 657–660.
36. Maclean K.H., J.L. Cleveland, J.B. Porter. 2001. Cellular zinc content is a major determinant of iron chelator-induced apoptosis of thymocytes. *Blood* **98:** 3831–3839.
37. Arcasoy A., A.O. Cavdar, S. Cin, *et al.* 1987. Effects of zinc supplementation on linear growth in beta thalassemia (a new approach). *Am. J. Hematol.* **24:** 127–136.
38. Shamshirsaz A.A., M.R. Bekheirnia, M. Kamgar, *et al.* 2007. Bone mineral density in Iranian adolescents and young adults with beta-thalassemia major. *Pediatr. Hematol. Oncol.* **24:** 469–479.
39. Dehshal M.H., A.H. Hooghooghi, A. Kebryaeezadeh, *et al.* 2007. Zinc deficiency aggravates abnormal glucose metabolism in thalassemia major patients. *Med. Sci. Monit.* **13:** CR235–CR239.
40. de Alarcon P.A., M.E. Donovan, G.B. Forbes, *et al.* 1979. Iron absorption in the thalasemia syndromes and its inhibition by tea. *N. Engl. J. Med.* **300:** 5–8.

Ann. N.Y. Acad. Sci. ISSN 0077-8923

ANNALS OF THE NEW YORK ACADEMY OF SCIENCES
Issue: *Cooley's Anemia: Ninth Symposium*

Ferritin iron minerals are chelator targets, antioxidants, and coated, dietary iron

Elizabeth C. Theil

Children's Hospital Oakland Research Institute, Oakland, California and Department of Nutritional Sciences and Molecular Toxicology, University of California-Berkeley, Berkeley, California

Address for correspondence: Elizabeth C. Theil, CHORI, 5700 Martin Luther King, Jr. Way, Oakland, CA 94609. etheil@chori.org

Cellular ferritin is central for iron balance during transfusions therapies; serum ferritin is a small fraction of body ferritin, albeit a convenient reporter. Iron overload induces extra ferritin protein synthesis but the protein is overfilled with the extra iron that damages ferritin, with conversion to toxic hemosiderin. Three new approaches that manipulate ferritin to address excess iron, hemosiderin, and associated oxidative damage in Cooley's Anemia and other iron overload conditions are faster removal of ferritin iron with chelators guided to ferritin gated pores by peptides; more ferritin protein synthesis using ferritin mRNA activators, by metal complexes that target mRNA 3D structures; and determining if endocytotic absorption of iron from legumes, which is mostly ferritin, is regulated during iron overload to prevent excess iron entry while providing protein. More of a focus on ferritin features, including protein cage structure, iron mineral, regulatable mRNA, and specific gut absorption properties, will achieve the three novel experimental goals for managing iron homeostasis with transfusion therapies.

Keywords: iron; ferritin; chelator

Maintaining the proper amount of iron is a challenge for everyone, but particularly for humans with Cooley's Anemia. To treat the condition, iron, in the form of new red blood cells must be injected to combat the anemia. In between transfusions, if there is transient anemia, homeostatic mechanisms signal increased absorption of dietary iron that is in iron fortificants such as Fe-EDTA or in meat. The well-known iron overload in Cooley's Anemia results because humans excrete excess iron poorly, contrasting with other vitamins and minerals. At the center of managing body iron is ferritin, Nature's antirust protein nanocage (Fig. 1).[1] Ferritin is a unique protein found in all organisms, plant, animals, bacteria, and archaea. The amounts of ferritin inside cells vary, depending on the role of the mature cell in the body; serum ferritin represents the iron levels in macrophage cells and is used as a noninvasive marker of iron status. Generally, ferritin is in the cytoplasm of animal cells, except for a small amount in mitochondria. Serum ferritin is a very small fraction of tissue ferritin, but reflects tissue ferritin and iron under normal conditions. Serum ferritin as a reporter for body iron is less accurate during iron overload for two reasons. First, the ferritin content of selected tissues increases. Because the ferritin is not same protein sequence in all tissue and the antibody for the serum ferritin analysis is prepared against ferritin form only a few tissues, a change in the tissue source of the serum ferritin will alter the analytical results for serum ferritin. Second, because the serum ferritin assays measure ferritin protein by an immunologic assay, the actual iron content of the tissue remains only an estimate. When the iron content of tissue ferritin increases, as it does during extreme iron overload, the ferritin protein content will increase much less. Nevertheless, serum ferritin is a reasonably reliable indicator of general increases or decreases in body iron during small changes in iron homeostasis and the most accessible method currently available at many sites around the world.

What is the normal function of ferritin? Because iron is so insoluble under physiological conditions,

doi: 10.1111/j.1749-6632.2010.05575.x

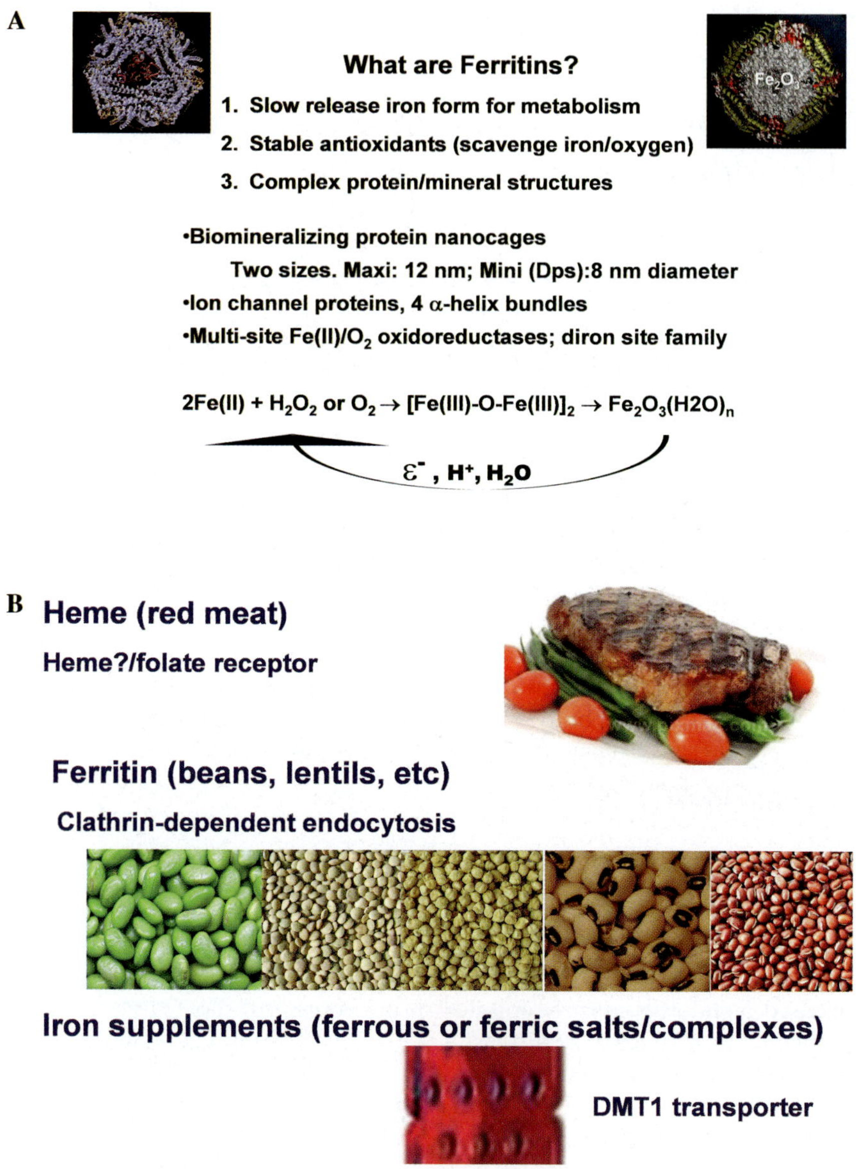

Figure 1. A. Molecular functions of ferritin protein cages and dietary ferritin iron. Functions of the ferritin protein cages in synthesizing and dissolving the iron–oxygen minerals. Ferritin protein cages have catalytic sites that oxidize and couple two iron atoms, channels that facilitate nucleation and movement to cavity entrances,[1] and gated pores that control Fe(II) entry for oxidation/mineralization and exit after mineral reduction and dissolution. Dioxygen is the oxidant but the mineral reductant *in vivo* is unknown; reductants that function in solution to reduce the mineral and allow mineral dissolution (addition of water) are $\varepsilon^- =$ NADH/FMN (also found in tissues) or diothionite. *In vivo* the reductant could be $FMNH_2$ but is currently unknown. B. Ferritin is one of three major forms of dietary iron; each has different mechanisms of iron absorption. Nonheme iron has at least two different chemical forms in terms of recognition by the gut during absorption. The classically studied bioavailable form is found in supplements such as ferrous sulfate or Fe-EDTA; small complexes of iron in plants are often poorly absorbed, for example, ferric phytate or tannate. Iron in the ferritin mineral, recently recognized as an abundant form of iron in whole legumes, is readily bioavailable.[6]

cells have to concentrate iron to have enough for synthesizing iron proteins. First, ferritins concentrate iron in a solid mineral in advance of cell need, and release the iron atoms a few at a time for synthesizing iron proteins in the cell. Iron proteins are catalysts important in critical cell functions such as; making deoxyribose (for DNA), recovering energy from foods (respiration), carrying oxygen (hemoglobin and myoglobin), using solar energy (photosynthesis), making unsaturated fatty acids, and synthesizing steroids. Second, ferritins respond to oxidant damage that releases Fe^{2+} from iron-damaged proteins to react with O_2 and produce free radicals (ROS). Mineralized iron in ferritin cannot react readily with ROS because of the protein cage (Figs. 1 and 2). In addition, the two substrates of ferritin catalytic sites are Fe^{2+} and O_2, which react to form mineral precursors and eventually the ferric oxide mineral itself. By consuming Fe^{2+} and O_2 to make the mineral, ferritin has antioxidant activity. Finally, ferritin is a source of natural, slow release dietary iron that has only been recognized recently.[2–5] The iron in many whole legume seed, such as soybeans, lentils, and chickpeas is largely ferritin iron, the natural, protein coated, iron-rich nutrient.[6]

Three approaches, reflecting properties of ferritin during iron overload will be discussed. (1) The ferritin protein cage as a target for novel chelators targeted to the protein (Fig. 2); (2) ferritin mRNA as a target for small molecules to increase ferritin protein synthesis during iron overload, to decrease ferritin iron/ferritin protein and hemosiderin formation (Fig. 4); (3) ferritin found in natural foods is a readily absorbed form of iron that might be more efficaciously regulated during iron overload. While the three topics are particularly important for transfusion-treated patients with both Cooley's Anemia and sickle cell disease,[7] some of the ideas can be useful in hemochromatosis and in iron deficiency anemias.

Ferritin protein cages as a target to increase rates of removal of iron

Ferritin protein cages have conserved structures that function as gated pores in ferritin channels between the outside of the cage and the mineral in the cavity. The mineral inside ferritin needs to be protected from reductants in the cytoplasm to prevent rapid turnover/dissolution of the mineral to minimize consumption cell reductants, and to minimize leakage of Fe^{2+}. When the amino acids that hold the pores closed are changed the iron can be reduced and chelated very quickly (Fig. 2). Very likely there are proteins in the cell that regulate ferritin pore opening and are coupled to the use of ferritin iron in the synthesis of iron proteins. The reason iron chelation therapy is so slow in Cooley's Anemia and other transfusion treated iron overload is that the ferritin pores will be "closed" when iron is in excess.

We identified five synthetic peptides that bound tightly to ferritin from a combinatorial group of 10^9 heptapeptides. Only one of the five binding peptides increased the rate of iron removal when the peptide was mixed with desferrioxamine B as the chelator (Fig. 2). The pore unfolding amino acid substitutions had a much larger effect, likely because the pores stayed open longer, allowing more iron mineral to be reduced and for the chelator to bind to the emerging Fe^{2+}. We reasoned that if the chelator were bound to the peptide that unfolded the pores, when the ferritin iron was dissolved and Fe^{2+} approached the exit pores, the chelator attached to the binding peptide would be so close that chelation would occur before the pores had a chance to close and retain the Fe^{2+}. Our hypothesis turned out to be correct.[8] When the ferritin pore-opening peptide was linked to the chelator, desferrioxamine B in this example, the rate of chelation of ferritin iron in solution was as high as for the ferritin with an amino acid replacement that forced the pores to be open continuously (Fig. 2, top panel). The experiment proves the importance of targeting chelators directly to ferritin pores. New chelators, developed in the future, could work more effectively, if they are targeted to ferritin, the main site the source of the iron to be removed. The idea is applying the well-known strategy of drug targeting, in this case to ferritin where the extra iron is, to chelators of today and the future for enhanced iron chelation therapy.

Ferritin genes as targets to increase ferritin protein synthesis

During iron overload, ferritin synthesis increases by two mechanisms. Oxidant damage from excess iron that is not stored safely in ferritin will induce ferritin gene transcription mediated by changing the antioxidant response element (ARE) interactions with the DNA transcription regulator bach 1 (Fig. 3). Even before the iron reaches toxic levels and causes oxidative damage and ferritin gene transcription,

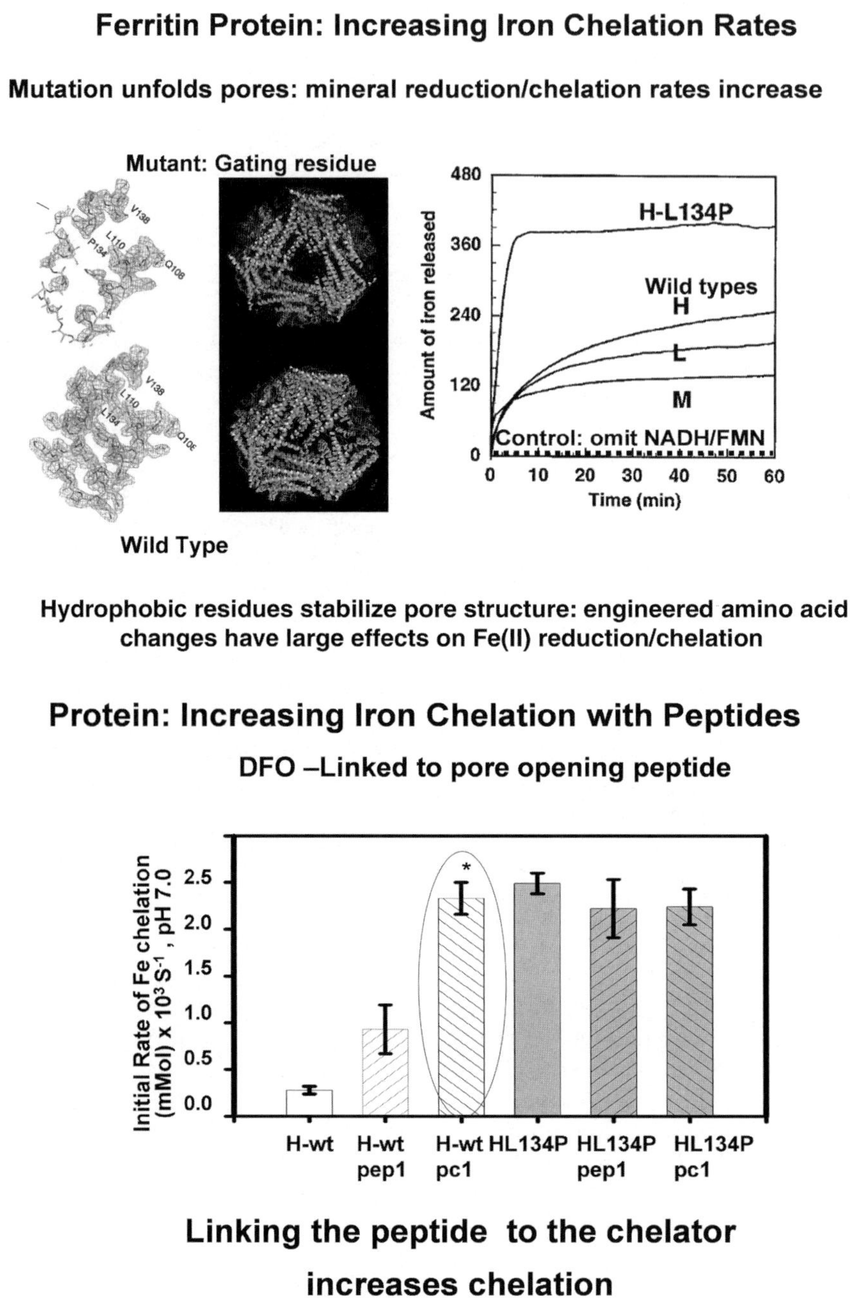

Figure 2. Pores in ferritin protein cages control rates of iron chelation. Iron chelation rates increase in solution when ferritin protein cage pores are modified (unfolded/opened). Amino acids substitution by site-directed mutagenesis unfolds ferritin pores without unfolding the protein cage, redrawn from Takagi *et al.*[23] Similar effect can be obtained in solution with physiological concentrations of urea or low heat[24] or synthetic peptides from a combinatorial library.[8] Rates determined in solution with bipyridyl chelator. Bottom panel. Chemical links between chelators to ferritin pore-modifying peptides increase iron chelation rates. Synthesizing a complex with the chelator covalently linked to desferrioxamine B increases the speed of chelating ferritin iron compared to peptide-desferrioxamine B alone; the rate with the new peptide-chelator is as fast with natural ferritin as with the engineered, unnatural, engineered ferritin. The figure is modified from Takagi *et al.*;[8] and the data are the averages of two to three protein preparations and analyses with the error as the standard deviation. *Significantly different ($P < 0.01$) from control (no peptide) or peptide mixed with chelator) or peptide DFO, deferroxamine B; Pep1, pore-opening peptide; Pc1-Pep1, deferroxamine B conjugate.

DNA: Ferritin transcription is coordinately regulated with antioxidant response (Phase II) proteins

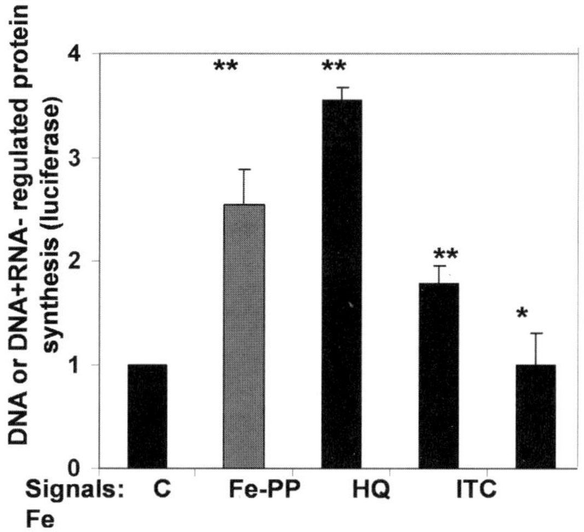

Signals:

Fe-PP:Fe-protoporphyrin (heme); HQ: t-butylhydroquinone; sulforophane (isothiocyanato-4- (methylsulphinyl)butane.

Coordinate gene regulation-ARE promoter :

thioredoxin reductase, NADPH quinone reductase; heme oxygenase, ferritin H & L

Common protein transcription repressor:

Bach 1

Ferritin DNA transcription: Oxidants > Fe

Figure 3. DNA: Ferritin transcription is coordinately regulated with antioxidant response (Phase II) proteins. Regulation of the ferritin promoter, the upstream, ARE (antioxidant response element) linked to a Luc reporter studies in HepG2 cells is similar to other ARE protein such as thioredoxin reductase and NADPH quinone oxdioreductase and shows greater sensitivity to oxidants or antioxidant inducers than to iron, contrasting with ferritin mRNA regulation which is more sensitive to iron. The figure is modified from Hintze *et al.*,[25] and represents at least three independent cultures and transfections. $^{**}P < 0.01$; $^{*}P < 0.05$.

additional ferritin protein is synthesized by allowing more ferritin mRNA to bind to ribosomes (Fig. 4, top panel); small amounts of free Fe^{2+} weaken the binding of the IRP protein repressor to the ferritin IRE mRNA structure releasing IRP,[9] which is then degraded[10,11] as the ferritin mRNA binds to ribosomes. The DNA + RNA regulation of ferritin protein synthesis is unusually complex, indicating the biological importance of ferritin. A significant feature of the regulatory pathway is the preferential targeting of ferritin DNA by oxidant/O_2 and of ferritin mRNA by Fe^{2+}, although there is some crosstalk. Because iron and O_2 are also the substrate, when the genetic system is upregulated by iron and oxygen signals, ferritin protein synthesis increases to consume the iron and oxygen signals creating a feedback loop with the iron and oxygen signals/substrates.[12]

Transfusion iron overload apparently pushes safe limits to beyond homeostatic mechanisms because the iron content of each ferritin protein cage increases abnormally.[12,13] The extra iron entering ferritin minerals damages the ferritin protein cage because hemosiderin form (damaged ferritin) during iron overload; hemosiderin is a toxic form of iron in the cell contrasting with the intact protein cage of ferritin. Not even the sophistication of ferritin DNA + mRNA regulatory targets is enough. However, for reasons that are unknown, even during iron overload some of the ferritin mRNA remains bound to the IRP repressor (Fig. 4, top panel).[14]

The protein repressor (IRP) binding site on ferritin mRNA is a folded, three-dimensional RNA structure, much like a folded, three-dimensional protein structure (Fig. 4, bottom left panel). The folded, IRE-RNA structure has metal binding sites, as do proteins. In a "proof of principle experiment," using a metal complex, $Cu(phen)_2$, which binds to two or three sites on the ferritin IRE-RNA as a reporter, we observed that $Cu(phen)_2$, cleaved ferritin mRNA in HeLa cells at the same sites as in solution.[15,16] The results proved that small, RNA-binding molecules can enter living cells and that the structure of the ferritin IRE-RNA studied in solution (NMR, nuclease probing, X-ray crystallography)[17–19] folded in the same way in living cells. Thus, a search for selectively binding molecules that can enter cells should be able to recruit any unused ferritin mRNA and decrease the hemosiderin content of cells during iron overload.

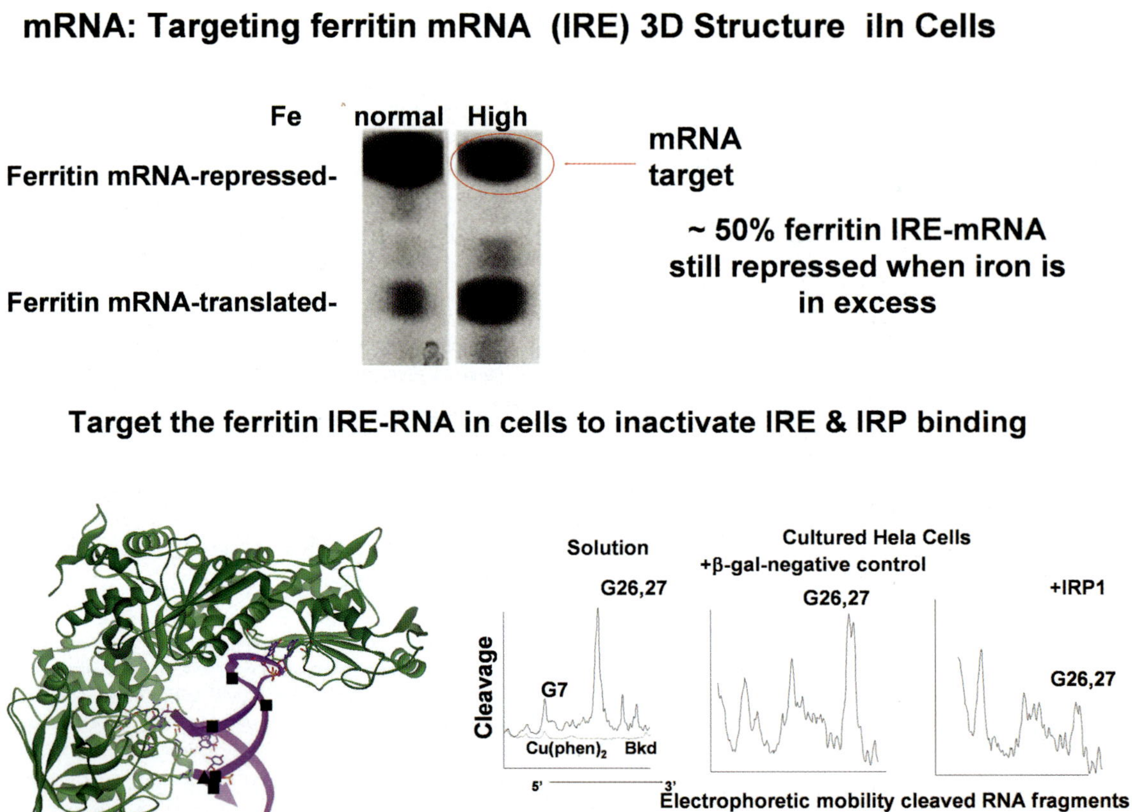

Figure 4. Recruiting unused ferritin mRNA for protein synthesis to minimize hemosiderin formation in iron overload: targeting three-dimensional properties of the IRE-RNA. During iron overload, iron increases inside each ferritin protein cage leading to ferritin damage and hemosiderin formation. Some of the mRNA remains bound to repressor[14] (top). Approximately 50% ferritin IRE-mRNA is still repressed when iron is in excess. Physical studies of the RNA show the IRE structure is a target that binds metals[9] and is recognized by small organic–metal complexes in living cells (bottom right panel). Figure taken from Ke *et al.*,[15] allowing drug design that uses the principles of protein drug discovery to exploit the smaller target size of mRNA and addition information of three-dimensional information, contrasting with the limited two-dimensional structure information of and avoiding cells responses to siRNA. Crystals: structure from Ref. 16 shows exposed IRE-RNA (*purple portion*) RNA; (*green portion*) protein; solution: ■, metal sites from chemical nuclease and NMR analyses.[17,19,26]

Ferritin iron in foods as a dietary source resistant to iron absorption changes

Current molecular information about the absorption of iron is incomplete (Fig. 1, bottom panel). Of the three chemical forms of iron known that are recognized by the gut, heme (iron-protoporphyrin), ferritin (iron-oxy mineral), and iron ions, only the transporter for ferrous ions DMT1 (also called DCT1 or nRAMP2) is extensively studied.[20,21] Mutations in DMT1, expressed both in intestine and red blood cells are associated with anemia. Before the availability of processed, iron-fortified foods in the twentieth century, little iron would have been available from natural foods as ferrous ion. Thus, transporters/receptors for other chemical forms of nonheme iron must exist.

The two natural forms of iron in the diet, consumed for millennia before food processing are heme (meat) and ferritin (whole legumes). Currently, the only heme transporter known is also a folate transporter, SLC46A1.[20,21] Given the selectivity of known carriers of heme beyond the gut[22] and the importance of heme iron in early humans, it seems unlikely that the only heme transporter is one shared with folate. Information about ferritin iron absorption is different than for heme, but is also incomplete. The presence of a high affinity receptor that binds the ferritin nanocage, followed by clathrin-dependent endocytosis of the intact protein and mineral is known; after entering the cell, the iron is released from the ferritin mineral and the protein cages is degraded.[4,22] However, the intracellular iron carriers, and the receptor itself remain unidentified.

A feature of ferritin absorption, which is different from heme or fortificant iron, is the absorption efficiency. For each single heme or iron atom that crosses the membrane, for example, on DMT1 or SLC46A transporter, more than 1,000 iron atoms will enter from ferritin. Iron excess depresses the DMT1 transport of nonheme iron salts, but whether the repression is more or less efficient for ferritin or nonheme iron is unknown. If absorption of ferritin iron via the endocytic receptor were regulated more efficiently than ferrous iron absorption via DMT1, or heme iron, dietary recommendations in transfusion-associated iron overload could be modified to increase the consumption of nonheme iron from ferritin-rich foods and eliminate the extra iron entering the body from food. The research to study iron regulation of gut receptors for iron from ferritin, especially during transfusion iron overload, remain to be performed. Because the mechanism of ferritin absorption is different than heme or ferrous salts, and more iron enters/absorption event, regulation of ferritin iron absorption might be more sensitive to body iron than heme or ferrous salts. If so, legumes rich in protein and ferritin might be more efficacious food than meat.

Summary and conclusions

Ferritin mineralized protein cages are the sites of much of the extra body iron introduced by lifetime infusions of red bloods cells to correct Cooley's Anemia. The finite capacity of the body to synthesize ferritin and the toxic effects hemosiderin, which is ferritin damaged by too much iron, require iron removal by chelators. Three novel, complementary approaches are outlined. (1) Targeting iron chelators (current or in the future) to ferritin protein pores by linking to a synthetic peptide known to modify the pores and increase iron removal and chelation ex vivo; (2) recruiting the ferritin mRNA unused during iron overload, with small, IRE-inactivating molecules to synthesize more ferritin protein and minimize hemosiderin; (3) Explore the regulation of ferritin iron absorption by the gut during iron overload with the goal of minimizing dietary iron absorption by increasing the intake of foods such as legumes that are rich in ferritin iron.

Acknowledgments

NIH (DK20251); Condycet (Project number 1050068), CHORI and Cooley's Anemia Foundations. The author gratefully acknowledges the creative contributions and thoughtful discussion made by members of the Theil Group and our many colleagues.

Conflicts of interest

The authors declare no conflicts of interest; NIH funded.

References

1. Liu, X. & E.C. Theil. 2005. Ferritin: dynamic management of biological iron and oxygen chemistry. *Acc. Chem. Res.* **38:** 167–175.
2. Murray-Kolb, L.E., R. Welch, E.C. Theil & J.L. Beard. 2003. Women with low iron stores absorb iron from soybeans. *Am. J. Clin. Nutr.* **77:** 180–184.
3. Davila-Hicks, P., E.C. Theil & B. Lonnerdal. 2004. Iron in ferritin or in salts (ferrous sulfate) is equally bioavailable in nonanemic women. *Am. J. Clin. Nutr.* **80:** 936–940.
4. San Martin, C.D., C. Garri, F. Pizarro, *et al.* 2008. Caco-2 intestinal epithelial cells absorb soybean ferritin by mu2 (AP2)-dependent endocytosis. *J. Nutr.* **138:** 659–666.
5. Kalgaonkar, S. & B. Lonnerdal. 2008. Effects of dietary factors on iron uptake from ferritin by Caco-2 cells. *J. Nutr. Biochem.* **19:** 33–39.
6. Theil, E.C. 2004. Iron, ferritin and nutrition. *Annu. Rev. Nutr.* **24:** 327–343.
7. Walter, P.B., P. Harmatz & E. Vichinsky. 2009. Iron metabolism and iron chelation in sickle cell disease. *Acta Haematol.* **122:** 174–183.
8. Liu, X.S., L.D. Patterson, M.J. Miller & E.C. Theil. 2007. Peptides selected for the protein nanocage pores change rates of iron recovery from the ferritin mineral. *J. Biol. Chem.* **282:** 31821–31825.
9. Khan, M.A., W.E. Walden, D.J. Goss & E.C. Theil. 2009. Direct Fe^{2+} sensing by iron-responsive messenger RNA × repressor complexes weakens binding. *J. Biol. Chem.* **284:** 30122–30128.
10. Wallander, M.L., E.A. Leibold & R.S. Eisenstein. 2006. Molecular control of vertebrate iron homeostasis by iron regulatory proteins. *Biochim. Biophys. Acta* **1763:** 668–689.
11. Rouault, T.A. 2006. The role of iron regulatory proteins in mammalian iron homeostasis and disease. *Nat. Chem. Biol.* **2:** 406–414.
12. Theil, E.C. & D.J. Goss. 2009. Living with iron (and oxygen): questions and answers about iron homeostasis. *Chem. Rev.* **109:** 4568–4579.
13. Treffry, A., P.J. Lee & P.M. Harrison. 1984. Iron-induced changes in rat liver isoferritins. *Biochem. J.* **220:** 717–722.

14. Melefors, O., B. Goossen, H.E. Johansson, *et al.* 1993. Translational control of 5-aminolevulinate synthase mRNA by iron-responsive elements in erythroid cells. *J. Biol. Chem.* **268:** 5974–5978.
15. Ke, Y. & E.C. Theil. 2002. An mRNA loop/bulge in the ferritin iron responsive element (IRE) formed *in vivo*, and detected by radical probing with Cu-phen and protein (IRP) footprinting. *J. Biol. Chem.* **277:** 2373–2376.
16. Walden, W.E., A.I. Selezneva, J. Dupuy, *et al.* 2006. Structure of dual function iron regulatory protein 1 complexed with ferritin IRE-RNA. *Science* **314:** 1903–1908.
17. Wang, Y.-H., S.R. Sczekan & E.C. Theil. 1990. Structure of the 5′ untranslated regulatory region of ferritin mRNA studied in solution. *Nucleic Acids Res.* **18:** 4463–4468.
18. Addess, K.J., J.P. Basilion, R.D. Klausner, *et al.* 1997. Structure and dynamics of the iron responsive element RNA: implications for binding of the RNA by iron regulatory binding proteins. *J. Mol. Biol.* **274:** 72–83.
19. Gdaniec, Z., H. Sierzputowska-Gracz & E.C. Theil. 1998. Iron regulatory element and internal loop/bulge structure for ferritin mRNA studied by cobalt(iii) hexamine binding, molecular modeling, and NMR spectroscopy. *Biochemistry* **37:** 1505–1512.
20. Laftah, A.H., G.O. Latunde-Dada, S. Fakih, *et al.* 2009. Haem and folate transport by proton-coupled folate transporter/haem carrier protein 1 (slc46a1). *Br. J. Nutr.* **101:** 1150–1156.
21. Andrews, N.C. & P.J. Schmidt. 2007. Iron homeostasis. *Annu. Rev. Physiol.* **69:** 69–85.
22. Severance, S. & I. Hamza. 2009. Trafficking of heme and porphyrins in metazoa. *Chem. Rev.* **109:** 4596–4616.
23. Takagi, H., D. Shi, Y. Hall, *et al.* 1998. Localized unfolding at the junction of three ferritin subunits. A mechanism for iron release? *J. Biol. Chem.* **273:** 18685–18688.
24. Liu, X., W. Jin & E.C. Theil. 2003. Opening protein pores with chaotropes enhances Fe reduction and chelation of Fe from the ferritin biomineral. *Proc. Natl. Acad. Sci. USA* **100:** 3653–3658.
25. Hintze, K.J., Y. Katoh, K. Igarashi & E.C. Theil. 2007. Bach1 repression of ferritin and thioredoxin reductase1 is heme-sensitive in cells and *in vitro*, and coordinates expression with heme oxygenase1, beta-globin and NADP(h) quinone (oxido)reductase1. *J. Biol. Chem.* **282:** 34365–34371.
26. Ke, Y., H. Sierzputowska-Gracz, Z. Gdaniec & E.C. Theil. 2000. Internal loop/bulge and hairpin loop of the iron-responsive element of ferritin mRNA contribute to maximal iron regulatory protein 2 binding and translational regulation in the iso-iron-responsive element/iso-iron regulatory protein family. *Biochemistry* **39:** 6235–6242.

Ann. N.Y. Acad. Sci. ISSN 0077-8923

ANNALS OF THE NEW YORK ACADEMY OF SCIENCES
Issue: *Cooley's Anemia: Ninth Symposium*

Pulmonary hypertension in thalassemia

Claudia R. Morris[1] and Elliott P. Vichinsky[2]

[1]Department of Emergency Medicine, [2]Department of Hematology/Oncology, Children's Hospital and Research Center Oakland, Oakland, California

Address for correspondence: Claudia R. Morris, M.D., Department of Emergency Medicine, Children's Hospital & Research Center Oakland, 747 52nd Street, Oakland, CA 94609. claudiamorris@comcast.net

Pulmonary hypertension (PH) is common in thalassemia and contributes to mortality. Advancing age and a history of splenectomy are major risk factors in this population. The etiology of PH is multifactorial, involving a complex interaction of platelets, the coagulation system, erythrocytes, and endothelial cells along with inflammatory and vascular mediators. The long-term effect of splenectomy, red cell membrane pathology, coagulation abnormalities, low nitric oxide (NO) bioavailability, excess arginase activity, platelet activation, oxidative stress, iron overload, and chronic hemolysis play a role. The process of hemolysis disables the arginine-NO pathway through the simultaneous release of erythrocyte arginase and cell-free hemoglobin. Both NO and its obligate substrate arginine are rapidly consumed. The biological consequences of hemolysis on NO bioavailability ultimately translate into the clinical manifestations of PH. Guidelines for the management of PH in thalassemia have not yet been established; however, clinical trials are ongoing in an effort to guide future therapy.

Keywords: thalassemia; pulmonary hypertension; hemolysis; sildenafil; arginine; nitric oxide

The thalassemia syndromes

The thalassemia syndromes are a heterogeneous group of inherited hemoglobin disorders resulting from unbalanced production of the alpha and beta globin subunits of the hemoglobin tetramer. Over 125 different genetic lesions can cause β-thalassemia, which is characterized by decreased (β^+-thalassemia) or absent (B^0-thalassemia) synthesis of the β-globin chain. Thalassemia is most common in individuals whose ancestors originated from the Mediterranean region, Africa, southern China, Southeast Asia, and India. An estimated 900,000 births with clinically significant thalassemia disorders are expected in the next 20 years.[1] The clinical spectrum is a consequence of imbalanced globin chain accumulation, resulting in impaired erythropoiesis and hemolytic anemia. The two clinically significant phenotypes of β-thalassemia have been designated thalassemia major (TM) and thalassemia intermedia (TI). TM is characterized by severe anemia starting during the first year of life, requiring life-long transfusion therapy for survival, while TI has a later clinical onset with a milder anemia, does not typically require chronic transfusions, and offers a longer life expectancy.[1] Heart failure is the most common cause of death in both forms of the disease.[2–5] Thalassemia heart disease involves mainly left ventricular dysfunction caused by transfusion-induced iron overload. However, recent studies suggest that both TM and TI patients have a unique hemodynamic pattern consistent with right ventricular cardiomyopathy and pulmonary hypertension (PH), in addition to the left ventricular abnormalities.[6] PH in β-thalassemia represents a common,[7–11] yet less well explored complication in the cardiopulmonary spectrum of the disease.

Definition of pulmonary hypertension

Secondary PH is emerging as a significant cause of mortality and morbidity in patients with hemolytic anemia.[12–14] PH is defined as a mean pulmonary artery pressure of ≥ 25 mmHg at rest or ≥ 30 mmHg during exercise, and can result from a wide range of conditions. It is a vascular disorder of the lung in which the pulmonary artery pressure rises above

doi: 10.1111/j.1749-6632.2010.05580.x

normal levels, compromises oxygenation and right-heart function, and can ultimately become life-threatening.[15] PH is a poorly understood, complex syndrome with many clinical phenotypes. The initial injury leading to PH in different disease states may vary, however they share a common pathway of vascular remodeling that result in a similar clinical and histopathologic condition. PH in thalassemia is associated with vasoconstriction, vascular smooth muscle proliferation, and irregular endothelium in pulmonary arteries with associated thrombosis. These conditions all contribute to luminal narrowing, and eventual right ventricular failure. Autopsy studies in thalassemia revealed histopathological findings that are common to all forms of PH, including plexiform and concentric medial hyperplastic pulmonary vascular lesions, and *in situ* pulmonary artery thrombosis.[16,17] However, despite multiple similarities with pulmonary artery hypertension, PH in hemolytic disease is a unique disorder that differs from other forms of PH, with lower pulmonary pressures, and higher cardiac output from anemia.

Prevalence and risk factors

PH is increasingly recognized in thalassemia and can contribute to heart failure and death.[3,4,6–8,18–22] Studies in both TI and TM demonstrate that adults frequently have undetected PH, with a prevalence of 60–75% reported.[11,23] Although the high prevalence of PH in nontransfused TI patients has now been well documented,[23,24] mild to moderate PH was diagnosed in over 50% of patients with β-thalassemia despite transfusion.[7,10,24] In another study of TM, pulmonary systolic pressure above 30 mmHg was found in all patients over 22 years of age.[7] Recent PH studies in more uniformly treated TM and TI patients have shown a lower frequency in chronically transfused TM patients[4] while in TI patients increased pulmonary pressure was more commonly detected. In one study, 60% of TI patients had a pulmonary systolic pressure greater than 30 mmHg with preserved left ventricular systolic function[3] while another study showed a pulmonary systolic pressure greater than 35 mmHg in 23% of thalassemia patients.[4]

An abnormally high tricuspid regurgitant jet velocity (TRV) $>$ 2.5 m/sec measured by Doppler echocardiography is greater than two standard deviations above normal.[12,15] Using a TRV $>$ 2.5 m/sec as a proxy for PH in patients clinically screened by echocardiography, evidence suggesting PH was found in 31% of patients with a measurable TRV, including 16% of the children evaluated in a recent analysis of the Thalassemia Clinical Research Network (TCRN) sponsored Thalassemia Longitudinal Cohort (TLC).[25] A remarkably similar prevalence was also reported in patients with hemoglobin E/β-thalassemia in Thailand. An abnormally high TRV was identified in 37% of 110 Thai patients screened for PH, and was associated with splenectomy, a high hemolytic rate, an increase in activated platelets and nucleated red blood cells, and chronic inflammation and elevated circulating adhesion molecules.[26] Although limited data have been reported in children, a recent study out of Cairo found a 37.5% prevalence of PH in children with TM.[27] Together with the observations from the TLC,[25] this suggests that even young patients with thalassemia are at risk for PH, although the long-term consequences of this observation remain unknown.

Advancing age and a history of splenectomy are major risk factors for PH in this population.[24–26,28,29] In one study of patients with TM, the degree of anemia, number of transfusions, and serum ferriten levels did not appear to correlate with risk,[10] while a more recent report found ferriten to be a strong indicator of an elevated TRV in patients with both TM and TI.[30] Larger studies are needed to reconcile these discrepancies. Since strict compliance with chronic transfusion and chelation therapy to prevent iron overload reduces the occurrence of heart failure, and prevents PH,[4,8,20] insufficiently transfused thalassemia patients may be at greater risk for the development of PH.

Etiology

The etiology of PH in thalassemia is multifactorial, involving a complex interaction of platelets, the coagulation system, erythrocytes, and endothelial cells along with inflammatory and vascular mediators (Table 1). Although overlap in mechanisms contributing to vasculopathy and PH is expected in all forms of thalassemia, the pathophysiology of PH is fundamentally different in patients with TI compared to TM. Hemolysis is likely a driving force toward PH in nontransfused TI patients, while the consequences of iron overload and oxidative stress play a more significant role in TM patients on transfusion therapy. The long-term sequelae of

Table 1. Etiology and risk factors for pulmonary hypertension in thalassemia

Advancing age
Splenectomy
Hemolysis
Oxidative stress
Iron overload
Chronic inflammation
Hypercoagulable state
Hypoxemia
Red blood cell membrane alterations
Low nitric oxide bioavailability
Arginine dysregulation
Arginase excess

splenectomy, red cell membrane pathology, coagulation abnormalities, low nitric oxide bioavailability, excess arginase activity, platelet activation, oxidative stress, iron overload, and chronic hemolysis will simultaneously contribute to various degrees.[4,6,22,24,25] Endothelial dysfunction is the result of an impaired arginine-nitric oxide pathway, oxidative stress, and tissue damage, which enhances hypercoagulability and *in situ* thrombus formation within the pulmonary artery walls, contributing to functional and structural alterations of pulmonary vessels (Fig. 1). The process of hemolysis disables the arginine-nitric oxide pathway through the simultaneous release of erythrocyte arginase[31] and cell-free hemoglobin.[12,14,22,32] Both nitric oxide and its obligate substrate arginine are rapidly consumed[17,22]. Intravascular hemolysis also has the potential to drive a procoagulant state. Nitric oxide normally has properties that inhibit platelet activation, tissue factor expression, and thrombin generation[14,33,34] that are lost in hemolytic disorders as a result of the diminished nitric oxide bioavailability. In addition, free heme induces endothelial tissue factor expression,[33] creating another avenue by which hemolysis enhances coagulation abnormalities. Oxidative stress is an additional key mechanism in the pathogenesis of PH that is exacerbated by hemolysis, the presence of iron overload and through cycles of ischemia and reperfusion. Iron overload, present in transfused thalassemia patients, also affects PH by other mechanisms. It induces interstitial pulmonary fibrosis[19] as well as left and right cardiac hemosiderosis, which subsequently results in cardiac dysfunction and affects pulmonary vascular resistance.[19] Chronic anemia and hypoxemia lead to further vasoconstriction and increase of pulmonary vascular resistance.

Finally, alterations in the glutathione buffering system in thalassemia[35] may render erythrocytes incapable of handling the increased oxidant burden, thereby predisposing them to hemolysis. The biological consequences of hemolysis and oxidative stress on nitric oxide bioavailability ultimately translate into the clinical manifestations of PH (Fig. 2).[12–14,17] We recently discovered that a depletion of erythrocyte glutamine concentration and aberrations in erythrocyte glutathione metabolism are linked to severity of PH in sickle cell disease (SCD) and biomarkers of hemolytic rate including levels of arginase activity in the plasma.[36] Glutamine, an essential precursor in nicotinamide adenine dinucleotide phosphate (NADPH) biosynthesis, is metabolized to the glutathione substrate glutamate in the process of NADPH production. Glutamine thus plays an antioxidant role through preservation of intracellular NADPH, making it an important amino acid for glutathione homeostasis. Glutamine also serves as a precursor for the *de novo* production of arginine through the citrulline-arginine pathway. Its depletion in PH may impact arginine and nitric oxide bioavailability. Glutamine therapy has shown initial promise in SCD,[22] and is currently being investigated for its ability to decrease oxidative stress in patients with thalassemia and PH.

There is growing evidence that PH is a disease process that involves altered arginine metabolism or decreased bioavailability.[17,22,36–39] As in SCD,[22,38] we found that dysregulated arginine metabolism also occurs in patients with thalassemia,[39,40] suggesting a state of decreased arginine bioavailability in both hemoglobinopathies.[38,39] Low global arginine bioavailability, associated with mortality in SCD[38] has recently been prospectively linked to increased cardiovascular risk, coronary artery disease, and adverse cardiovascular events including death, myocardial infarction, and stroke in over 1,000 patients undergoing elective cardiac catheterization.[41] This supports a more extensive role for arginine bioavailability in the pathogenesis of vasculopathy independent of genotype.

High concentrations of the arginine-consuming enzyme arginase are found in the erythrocytes

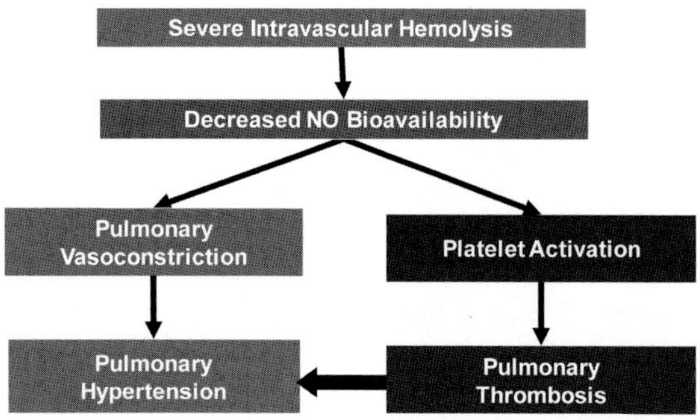

Figure 1. Intravascular hemolysis: an initiating trigger in the pathogenesis of pulmonary hypertension. Severe intravascular hemolysis leads to decreased nitric oxide bioavailability and its consequences: endothelial cell activation, upregulation of the potent vasoconstrictor endothelin-1, pulmonary vasoconstriction, platelet activation, increased tissue factor, activation of coagulation pathways, and pulmonary thrombosis, all of which ultimately translate into the clinical manifestations of pulmonary hypertension. Reproduced with permission from Dr. Gregory Kato, M.D.

of thalassemia patients.[42] Hemolysis, hypoxia, and high thrombin levels will independently contribute to the excess arginase activity found in thalassemia,[31,39,40] a relevant factor given that increased arginase activity has been implicated in the pathogenesis of PH in many disease states.[31,37,38,43] Arginase redirects the metabolism of L-arginine to L-ornithine and the formation of polyamines and L-proline, which are essential for smooth muscle cell growth and collagen synthesis.[31,43] Therefore, the induction of arginase promotes aberrant vessel wall remodeling and neointima formation,[43] contributing to the structural changes that are observed in the lungs of patients with hemoglobinopathies. By creating a shift toward ornithine metabolism, the arginases set off a process that contributes to a proliferative vasculopathy regardless of the initiating trigger.

The thalassemia syndromes have many biologic and epidemiologic factors in common with SCD, including chronic hypoxia, long-term effect of splenectomy, red cell membrane pathology,[28,29,44,45] coagulation abnormalities,[24,44,46] platelet activation,[24,44,46] oxidative stress,[47] iron overload,[5,6,8,19,23] chronic hemolysis,[22,40] and excess arginase activity.[38–40,42] In particular, analogous to SCD and other chronic hemolytic disorders,[13,14,17] hemolysis-associated PH is emerging as an important entity in thalassemia, particularly for patients with TI.[14,22,39,40] Red cell destruction, elevated free plasma hemoglobin, anemia, and abnormal nitric oxide metabolism exist in both nontransfused and transfused patients.[10] A study of 202 TM patients concluded that strict compliance with chronic transfusion and chelation therapy to prevent iron overload reduces the occurrence of heart failure, and prevents PH.[4,8,20] Although more aggressive transfusion programs may provide greater protection from the development of PH,[4,20,48] and correct hypercoagulability,[48] the occurrence of intramedullary hemolysis, thrombocytosis, iron deposits, and a resultant vasculopathy may still be able to induce PH, which likely progresses slower. Nevertheless, these findings highlight the beneficial effect of regular transfusion in either prevention or slowing down the progression of PH in thalassemia.[4,20,48]

Clinical presentation

Early stages of PH in chronic hemolytic disorders may be asymptomatic or associated with mild symptoms. Classic symptoms of PH like exertional dypsnea overlap with those of chronic anemia, often delaying clinical suspicion until late in the course of disease. In addition, the multiorgan complications of hemolytic anemia may limit exercise tolerance independent of elevations in pulmonary vascular resistance.[15] Asthma may also be a cofounding complication in hemolytic anemia[49,50] manifesting overlapping symptoms with PH that requires screening.[50] Hypoxemia, which could also be the result of restrictive lung disease, may be an early sign of PH. Although cardiac function is frequently compromised owing to iron overload, chronic anemia, hypoxemia, liver disease, and a hypercoagulable state, more specific symptoms of PH such as angina, syncope, and lower extremity edema are uncommon and are associated with severe and advanced PH. Physical findings suggestive of right ventricular dysfunction, including jugular venous distention, right ventricular S3 gallop, an accentuated pulmonary component of S2, oxygen desaturation, ascites, peripheral edema, although rare, should raise suspicion, and a high prevalence of clubbing in sickle cell and thalassemia patients with PH has been observed. Other conditions commonly found in these patients, such as left ventricular systolic or diastolic dysfunction, pulmonary fibrosis, and cirrhosis of the liver also contribute to the pathogenesis of PH.[15]

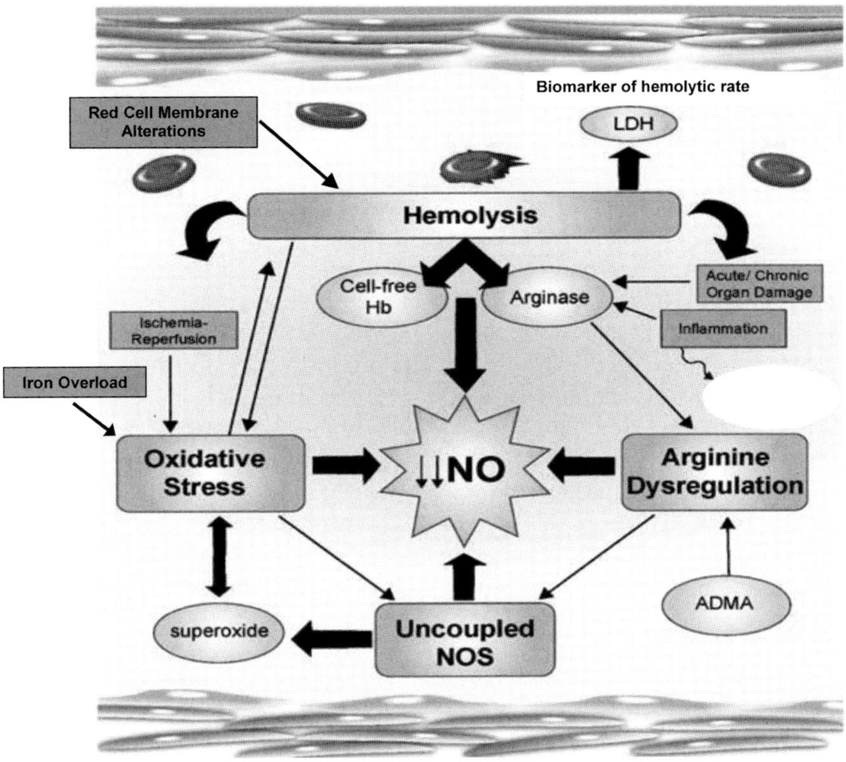

Figure 2. Mechanisms of vasculopathy leading to pulmonary hypertension. Hemolysis, arginine dysregulation, oxidative stress, and uncoupled nitric oxide synthase (NOS) are key mechanisms that contribute to the complex vascular pathophysiology of hemolytic disorders like thalassemia, resulting in a clinical scenario of pulmonary hypertension. These events limit nitric oxide (NO) bioavailability through several paths that ultimately provoke increased consumption and decreased production of the potent vasodilator, NO. Although often discussed independently, there is significant overlap closely linking these pathways of endothelial dysfunction that prohibit determining cause and effect. The contribution of inflammation coupled with antioxidant depletion, red cell membrane alterations creating a susceptibility to hemolysis, ischemia-reperfusion injury, and acute as well as chronic end organ damage obscure mechanistic boundaries further. During hemolysis, cell-free hemoglobin and arginase are simultaneously released from the erythrocyte and profoundly contribute to low NO bioavailability. Lactate dehydrogenase (LDH) is also released from the erythrocyte and represents a convenient biomarker of hemolytic rate. Reproduced with permission from the American Society of Hematology.[22]

Clinical work-up

Doppler echocardiography can identify patients at risk for PH when a detectable TRV is present, however technical diligence is needed to increase the fraction of echocardiograms with a measured TRV in order to better identify specific patients at risk. Cardiac catheterization is the gold standard for the diagnosis of PH, and can confirm a suspicion of PH based on echocardiogram and assess severity while excluding other contributors, such as left heart disease. Experts in the field recommend that hemoglobinopathy patients with a TRV $\geq$ 3.0 m/sec measured by Doppler echocardiography undergo right heart cardiac catheterization.[15]

Diagnostic evaluations for PH in patients with hemolytic disorders should follow the same guidelines established for other causes of pulmonary artery hypertension. Symptoms evaluation should include the World Health Organization classification and a Borg Dypsnea Score. Vital signs should include monitoring of systolic and diastolic blood pressure as well as oxygen saturation by pulse-oximetry. History and laboratory assessment should be performed to exclude other conditions associated with PH, including collagen vascular disorders, HIV, viral hepatitis, particularly hepatitis C, pregnancy, and stimulant use. Liver and renal function tests, biomarkers of hemolytic rate (LDH, reticulocyte count, hemoglobin/hematocrit, bilirubin),

NT-proBNP levels, and severity of iron overload should also be monitored. An electrocardiogram should be routinely performed to evaluate for a prolonged QTc commonly found in patients with TM,[51] given the association of prolonged QT interval corrected for heart rate (QTc) with sudden death, and link to PH in SCD.[52] Since abnormal pulmonary function is common in thalassemia,[53,54] a comprehensive pulmonary evaluation should also incorporate annual pulmonary function testing to include spirometry, lung volumes, and diffusion capacity (DL_{CO}) corrected for hemoglobin.

The 6-min walk test is the most commonly used exercise test in patients with PH as an index of cardiopulmonary function[15] and is helpful to follow over time as an early gauge of clinical deterioration or to monitor improvement from therapeutic interventions.

Heart failure due to iron overload remains a chief cause of death in TM and other transfusion-dependent anemia,[4,5] and contributes to the high frequency of PH in these disorders.[8,19,40] Cardiac magnetic resonance imaging (MRI) is effective in detecting iron in the heart and liver. It is routinely used in chronically transfused thalassemia patients to screen for iron cardiotoxicity.[55] Cardiac MRI is a noninvasive tool that also reliably determines other hemodynamic indices in addition to iron burden, such as right and left ventricular volume and ejection fraction, left ventricular mass, and cardiac output. Cardiac MRI can accurately qualify left ventricular function (independent of septal geometry) and measure cardiac output. Combined with a peripheral blood pressure measurement, total vascular resistance (mean blood pressure/cardiac output) can be determined. Cardiac MRI may be a helpful assessment tool in the management of PH in thalassemia.

Treatment/management

Guidelines specifically for the management of PH in thalassemia have not yet been established, however recommendations for the approach and treatment of heart complications in TM have recently been published[56] Much of what is being done clinically with PH in patients with hemoglobinopathies is based upon the pulmonary artery hypertension literature and case reports.[57,58] An unexpected absence of PH in 50 patients with TI treated with long-term hydroxyurea (HU) suggests a protective capacity of HU against the development PH that warrants further investigation.[59] A small open-label study of oral L-carnitine therapy in 12 children with TM and PH demonstrating a significant improvement in TRV also deserves additional attention.[27] Treatment with oral sildenafil improved exercise tolerance and PH in patients with thalassemia in two small studies.[57,58] Sildenafil is a selective pulmonary vasodilator, however its ability to inhibit platelet activation[34] may provide additional benefits for PH in thalassemia. Sildenafil is one of over 10 Food and Drug Administration (FDA)-approved therapies for the treatment of PH, although indications for thalassemia-associated PH have not yet been established. Given the high risk of mortality associated with this complication in other disorders, the TCRN has developed a protocol to evaluate the potential use of sildenafil in patients with thalassemia and PH. This clinical trial is now enrolling, and will also serve to characterize the cardiopulmonary and biochemical characteristics of patients with PH compared to thalassemia patients without PH in order to gain mechanistic insight. More information can be found on http://clinicaltrials.gov; http://clinicaltrials.gov/ct2/show/NCT00872170?term=sildenafil+for+thalassemia&rank=1

An open-label trial of oral L-glutamine is also currently recruiting thalassemia patients with PH, as low erythrocyte glutamine levels strongly correlated to a high TRV in patients with SCD.[36] The ability of oral L-glutamine to decrease oxidative stress and PH is being studied in both SCD and thalassemia. http://clinicaltrials.gov/ct2/results?term=glutamine+for+pulmonary+hypertension

These efforts will provide the needed data to develop randomized controlled trials, and help guide recommendations and therapy for PH in thalassemia in the future.

Currently, general recommendations for the treatment of PH include intensification of thalassemia-directed therapies, treatment of causal factors or associated diseases, general supportive measures, and use of PH-specific pharmacologic agents in patients with a diagnosis of PH confirmed by right heart cardiac catheterization.[15] Patients with an abnormally high TRV on echocardiography suggestive of PH should be referred to a cardiopulmonary specialist with expertise in the evaluation and treatment of PH. Specific therapy with selective pulmonary vasodilator and remodeling drugs should be considered in patients with PH, particularly if the patient has symptomatic dyspnea on exertion, which has progressed in recent months or years. Drugs that are FDA-approved for PH include the endothelin receptor antagonists (bosentan and ambrisentan), various forms of prostaglandin therapy (epoprostenol, treprostinol, and iloprost), and the phosphodiesterase-5 inhibitors (sildenafil, cialis, and tadalafil). No published randomized studies in the thalassemia population exist for any of these agents, although the pilot trials in the thalassemia syndromes mentioned earlier have been initiated.

Since strict compliance with chronic transfusion and chelation therapy was found to prevent PH,[4,8,20] early transfusion to keep the hemoglobin greater than 10 g/dL and iron chelation should be offered to all thalassemia patients with PH, even those with TI. Patients with low oxygen levels may benefit from oxygen therapy although this has not been specifically studied in thalassemia. Some patients may require supplemental oxygen only with exertion or sleep, while others may need continuous therapy. Given the contributory role of thromboembolism and a hypercoagulable state to PH in the thalassemia syndromes,[22,24,40,46] long-term anticoagulation and/or antiplatelet therapy, although controversial, should be considered.

Conclusion

Randomized trials evaluating the effects of specific therapies for PH in thalassemia are clearly indicated. The etiology of PH in thalassemia is complex and multifactorial, including hemolysis and its effect on the arginine-nitric oxide pathway, oxidative stress, splenic dysfunction/asplenia, thrombosis, hypoxia, chronic lung disease, and iron overload. Combination therapies targeting multiple mechanisms including hemolysis and oxidative stress may surpass benefits of any single strategy.[22] Children with hemoglobinopathies who have an human leukocyte antigen (HLA)-compatible sibling can be cured by allogeneic bone marrow transplantation before they have a chance to develop chronic organ damage and PH. However, bone marrow transplantation is an expensive option associated with significant adverse effects that calls for careful deliberation of risks versus benefits. Alternative sources of donor hematopoietic cells that include HLA-matched unrelated donor and umbilical cord blood are being pursued for hemoglobinopathies, with promising initial results.[60]

Improved longevity in patients with thalassemia is due to advances in medical management over the last decade. Since progressing age is a risk factor for PH, the number of patients experiencing this complication will only increase over time. Prospective longitudinal studies are needed to determine the natural history of PH in thalassemia, especially given the high mortality risk associated with this complication in every other disease state it arises that has been previously studied. PH is not a benign incidental occurrence. Improved awareness of PH by clinicians and annual screening by Doppler echocardiography targeting children as well as adults will help to identify patients at risk, while sustained research efforts are critical to guide best practices for PH in thalassemia in the future.

Conflicts of interest

The authors declare no conflicts of interest.

References

1. Vichinsky, E.P. 2005. Changing patterns of thalassemia worldwide. *Ann. N.Y. Acad. Sci.* **1054:** 18–24.
2. Borgna-Pignatti, C. *et al.* 1998. Survival and disease complications in thalassemia major. *Ann. N.Y. Acad. Sci.* **850:** 227–231.
3. Aessopos, A. *et al.* 1995. Pulmonary hypertension and right heart failure in patients with B-thalassemia intermedia. *Chest* **107:** 50–53.
4. Aessopos, A. *et al.* 2005. Thalassemia heart disease: a comparative evaluation of thalassemia major and thalassemia intermedia. *Chest* **127:** 1523–1530.
5. Fung, E.B. *et al.* 2007. Morbidity and mortality in chronically transfused subjects with thalassemia and sickle cell disease: a report from the multi-center study of iron overload. *Am. J. Hematol.* **82:** 255–265.
6. Hahalis, G. *et al.* 2005. Heart failure in beta-thalassemia syndromes: a decade of progress. *Am. J. Med.* **118:** 957–967.
7. Du, Z.D. *et al.* 1997. Pulmonary hypertension in patients with thalassemia major. *Am. Heart J.* **134:** 532–537.
8. Aessopos, A. & D. Farmakis. 2005. Pulmonary hypertension in beta-thalassemia. *Ann. N.Y. Acad. Sci.* **1054:** 342–349.
9. Tam, D.H. & H.W. Farber. 2006. Pulmonary hypertension and beta-thalassemia major: report of a case, its treatment, and a review of the literature. *Am. J. Hematol.* **81:** 443–447.
10. Hagar, R.W., C.R. Morris & E.P. Vichinsky. 2006. Pulmonary hypertension in thalassaemia major patients with normal left ventricular systolic function. *Br. J. Haematol.* **133:** 433–435.
11. Grisaru, D. *et al.* 1990. Cardiopulmonary assessment in beta-thalassemia major. *Chest* **98:** 1138–1142.

12. Gladwin, M. *et al.* 2004. Pulmonary hypertension as a risk factor for death in patients with sickle cell disease. *N. Engl. J. Med.* **350:** 22–31.
13. Barnett, C.F., P.Y. Hsue & R.F. Machado. 2008. Pulmonary hypertension: an increasingly recognized complication of hereditary hemolytic anemias and HIV infection. *JAMA* **299:** 324–331.
14. Rother, R.P. *et al.* 2005. The clinical sequelae of intravascular hemolysis and extracellular plasma hemoglobin: a novel mechanism of human disease. *JAMA* **293:** 1653–1662.
15. Machado, R.F. & M.T. Gladwin. 2006. Hemolytic anemia association pulmonary hypertension. In *Pulmonary Vascular Disease.* Mandel, J. & D. Taichman, Eds.: 170–187. Saunders Elsevier. Philadelphia, PA.
16. Sonakul, D., P. Pacharee & K. Thakerngpol. 1988. Pathologic findings in 76 autopsy cases of thalassemia. *Birth Defects Orig. Artic. Ser.* **23:** 157–176.
17. Morris, C.R., M.T. Gladwin & G. Kato. 2008. Nitric oxide and arginine dysregulation: a novel pathway to pulmonary hypertension in hemolytic disorders. *Curr. Mol. Med.***8:** 81–90
18. Derchi, G. *et al.* 1999. Pulmonary hypertension in patients with thalassemia major. *Am. Heart J.* **138:** 384.
19. Zakynthinos, E. *et al.* 2001. Pulmonary hypertension, interstitial lung fibrosis, and lung iron deposition in thalassaemia major. *Thorax.* **56:** 737–739.
20. Aessopos, A. *et al.* 2004. Cardiac status in well-treated patients with thalassemia major. *Eur. J. Haematol.* **73:** 359–366.
21. Wu, K.H. *et al.* 2004. Tricuspid regurgitation in patients with beta-thalassemia major. *Ann. Hematol.* **83:** 779–783.
22. Morris, C.R. 2008. Mechanisms of vasculopathy in sickle cell disease and thalassemia. *Hematology Am. Soc. Hematol. Educ. Program.* **2008:** 177–185.
23. Aessopos, A. *et al.* 2001. Cardiac involvement in thalassemia intermedia: a multicenter study. *Blood* **97:** 3411–3416.
24. Singer, S.T. *et al.* 2006. Pulmonary hypertension in thalassemia: association with platelet activation and hypercoagulable state. *Am. J. Hematol.* **81:** 670–675.
25. Morris, C.R. *et al.* 2009. Pulmonary hypertension in thalassemia assessed by echocardiography: a report from baseline data of the thalassemia clinical research network Longitudinal Cohort Study. *Blood* **114:** 796 [abst 2016].
26. Chuncharunee, S. *et al.* 2009. Prevalence and predictors of pulmonary arterial hypertension in hemoglobin E/ β-Thalassemia patients *Blood* **114:** 795 [abst 2015].
27. El-Beshlawy, A. *et al.* 2008. Pulmonary hypertension in beta-thalassemia major and the role of L-carnitine therapy. *Pediatr. Hematol. Oncol.* **25:** 734–743.
28. Atichartakarn, V. *et al.* 2003. Pulmonary arterial hypertension in previously splenectomized patients with beta-thalassemic disorders. *Int. J. Hematol.* **78:** 139–145.
29. Phrommintikul, A. *et al.* 2006. Splenectomy: a strong risk factor for pulmonary hypertension in patients with thalassaemia. *Heart* **92:** 1467–1472.
30. Mokhtar, G.M. *et al.* 2010. N-terminal natriuretic peptide and ventilation-perfusion lung scan in sickle cell disease and thalassemia patients with pulmonary hypertension. *Hemoglobin* **34:** 78–94.
31. Morris, C.R. 2010. Role of arginase in sickle cell lung disease and hemolytic anemias. *Open Nitric Oxide J.* **2:** 41–54.
32. Reiter, C. *et al.* 2002. Cell-free hemoglobin limits nitric oxide bioavailability in sickle cell disease. *Nat. Med.* **8:** 1383–1389.
33. Setty, B.N. *et al.* 2008. Heme induces endothelial tissue factor expression: potential role in hemostatic activation in patients with hemolytic anemia. *J. Thromb. Haemost.* **6:** 2202–2209.
34. Villagra, J. *et al.* 2007. Platelet activation in patients with sickle disease, hemolysis-associated pulmonary hypertension and nitric oxide scavenging by cell-free hemoglobin. *Blood* **110:** 2166–2172.
35. Chakraborty, D. & M. Bhattacharyya. 2001. Antioxidant defense status of red blood cells of patients with beta-thalassemia and Ebeta-thalassemia. *Clin. Chim. Acta.* **305:** 123–129.
36. Morris, C.R. *et al.* 2008. Erythrocyte glutamine depletion, altered redox environment, and pulmonary hypertension in sickle cell disease. *Blood* **140:** 104–112.
37. Maarsingh, H., T. Pera & H. Meurs. 2008. Arginase and pulmonary diseases. *Naunyn Schmiedebergs Arch. Pharmacol.* **378:** 171–184.
38. Morris, C.R. *et al.* 2005. Dysregulated arginine metabolism, hemolysis-associated pulmonary hypertension and mortality in sickle cell disease. *JAMA* **294:** 81–90.
39. Morris, C.R. *et al.* 2005. Hemolysis-associated pulmonary hypertension in thalassemia. *Ann. N.Y. Acad. Sci.* **1054:** 481–485.
40. Morris, C.R., E. Vichinsky & S.T. Singer. 2007. Pulmonary hypertension in thalassemia: association with hemolysis, arginine metabolism dysregulation and a hypercoaguable state. *Adv. Pulm. Hypertens.* **5:** 31–38.
41. Tang, W.H. *et al.* 2009. Diminished global arginine bioavailability and increased arginine catabolism as metabolic profile of increased cardiovascular risk. *J. Am. Coll. Cardiol.* **53:** 2061–2067.
42. Reynolds, J., J.H. Follette & W.H. Valentine. 1957. The arginase activity of erythrocytes and leukocytes with particular reference to pernicious anemia and thalassemia major. *J. Lab. Clin. Med.* **50:** 78–92.
43. Durante, W., F.K. Johnson & R.A. Johnson. 2007. Arginase: a critical regulator of nitric oxide synthesis and vascular function. *Clin. Exp. Pharmacol. Physiol.* **34:** 906–911.
44. Borenstain-Ben Yashar, V. *et al.* 1993. Phosphatidylserine in the outer leaflet of red blood cells from beta-thalassemia patients may explain the chronic hypercoagulable state and thrombotic episodes. *Am. J. Hematol.* **44:** 63–65.
45. Borgna Pignatti, C. *et al.* 1998. Thromboembolic events in beta thalassemia major: an Italian multicenter study. *Acta Haematol.* **99:** 76–79.
46. Eldor, A. & E.A. Rachmilewitz. 2002. The hypercoagulable state in thalassemia. *Blood* **99:** 36–43.
47. Walter, P.B. *et al.* 2006. Oxidative stress and inflammation in iron-overloaded patients with beta-thalassaemia or sickle cell disease. *Br. J. Haematol.* **135:** 254–263.
48. Atichartakarn, V. *et al.* 2004. Correction of hypercoagulability and amelioration of pulmonary arterial hypertension by chronic blood transfusion in an asplenic hemoglobin E/beta-thalassemia patient. *Blood* **103:** 2844–2846.

49. Palma-Carlos, A.G., M.L. Palma-Carlos & A.C. Costa. 2005. "Minor" hemoglobinopathies: a risk factor for asthma. *Allerg. Immunol. (Paris)* **37:** 177–182.
50. Morris, C.R. 2009. Asthma management: reinventing the wheel in sickle cell disease. *Am. J. Hematol.* **84:** 234–241.
51. Kocharian, A., M. Rooyfard & R. Aghanouri. 2003. Prolonged dispersion of QT and QTc in thalassemia major patients. *Acta Med. Iran.* **41:** 233–237.
52. Akgul, F. *et al.* 2007. Increased QT dispersion in sickle cell disease: effect of pulmonary hypertension. *Acta Haematol.* **118:** 1–6.
53. Piatti, G. *et al.* 2006. Lung function in beta-thalassemia patients: a longitudinal study. *Acta Haematol.* **116:** 25–29.
54. Carnelli, V. *et al.* 2003. Pulmonary dysfunction in transfusion-dependent patients with thalassemia major. *Am. J. Respir. Crit. Care Med.* **168:** 180–184.
55. Wood, J.C. & N. Ghugre. 2008. Magnetic resonance imaging assessment of excess iron in thalassemia, sickle cell disease and other iron overload diseases. *Hemoglobin* **32:** 85–96.
56. Cogliandro, T. *et al.* 2008. Guideline recommendations for heart complications in thalassemia major. *J. Cardiovasc. Med. (Hagerstown)* **9:** 515–525.
57. Derchi, G. *et al.* 2005. Efficacy and safety of sildenafil in the treatment of severe pulmonary hypertension in patients with hemoglobinopathies. *Haematologica* **90:** 452–458.
58. Littera, R. *et al.* 2002. Long-term treatment with sildenafil in a thalassemic patient with pulmonary hypertension. *Blood* **100:** 1516–1517.
59. Karimi, M. *et al.* 2009. Echocardiographic finding in beta-thalassemia intermedia and major: absence of pulmonary hypertension following hydroxyurea treatment in beta-thalassemia intermedia. *Eur. J. Haematol.* **82:** 213–218.
60. Michlitsch, J.G. & M.C. Walters. 2008. Recent advances in bone marrow transplantation in hemoglobinopathies. *Curr. Mol. Med.* **8:** 675–689.

Ann. N.Y. Acad. Sci. ISSN 0077-8923

ANNALS OF THE NEW YORK ACADEMY OF SCIENCES
Issue: *Cooley's Anemia: Ninth Symposium*

The natural history of thalassemia intermedia

Caterina Borgna-Pignatti, Maria Marsella, and Nicolò Zanforlin
Department of Clinical and Experimental Medicine, Università di Ferrara, Ferrara, Italy

Address for correspondence: Prof. C. Borgna-Pignatti, Clinica Pediatrica, Dipartimento di Medicina Clinica e Sperimentale, Università di Ferrara, Via Savonarola 9, 44100 Ferrara, Italy. bre@unife.it

The severity of thalassemia intermedia depends on the degree of imbalance between alpha and non-alpha chains as well as other genetic and environmental factors that modify the natural history of the disease. By definition, the patients spontaneously maintain hemoglobin at or above 7 g/dL, sometimes at the price of intense hyperplasia of the bone marrow that is in turn responsible for bone deformities, osteoporosis, and extramedullary erythropoietic masses that often characterize thalassemia intermedia. Transfusion may become necessary with advancing age, during infection and pregnancy, and when hypersplenism develops. Splenectomy is often needed. Iron overload in nontransfused patients is due to increased gastrointestinal absorption and involves mainly the liver. Complications affecting the lives of patients with thalassemia intermedia include pulmonary hypertension, leg ulcers, pseudoxanthoma elasticum, gallstones, hepatocellular carcinoma, and thromboembolic events.

Keywords: thalassemia intermedia; extramedullary erythropoiesis; pseudoxanthoma elasticum; iron overload; transfusion

The natural history of thalassemia intermedia is greatly variable and depends in large part on the degree of imbalance between alpha and nonalpha globin chains. In addition, several complications, both genetically and nongenetically determined, can modify the clinical picture of the disease.

In homozygous or compound heterozygous β-thalassemia, any condition able to reduce globin imbalance causes a milder form of the disease, while the worsening of the imbalance can transform the usually asymptomatic state of a heterozygous carrier in a more severe clinical picture (Table 1). An overview of the defects causing thalassemia intermedia has been recently reported.[1] In addition several other genetic and environmental characteristics contribute to modify the phenotype of patients with thalassemia intermedia (Table 2).

Clinical features

Conventionally, thalassemia is defined intermedia when the patient maintains hemoglobin at or above 7–7.5 g/dL. Transfusion, however, may become necessary with advancing age and in particular conditions, like infection, hypersplenism, and pregnancy. Thalassemia intermedia can be diagnosed at any age, but usually the diagnosis is made at an older age than in thalassemia major. In a study, the children who remained transfusion independent were diagnosed at 17.4 ± 11.8 months as compared with 8.5 ± 1.8 months for those who developed transfusion dependence.[2] In another series, 59% of patients with thalassemia intermedia were diagnosed after the second year of life.[3]

The clinical spectrum of thalassemia intermedia is wide and ranges from mild anemia and jaundice, usually associated with a palpable spleen, to severe anemia, hypersplenism, bone abnormalities, extramedullary erythropoiesis, iron overload, leg ulcers, and gallstones. In the mild form of thalassemia intermedia, growth is not impaired, at least until hypersplenism develops, causing a decrease in hemoglobin levels and, sometimes, neutropenia and thrombocytopenia. On the contrary, stunted growth is an inevitable consequence of more severe anemia and intense ineffective erythropoiesis. Bone abnormalities are frequently associated and include frontal bossing, prominence of the zygomatic

doi: 10.1111/j.1749-6632.2010.05550.x

Table 1. Genetic mechanisms of thalassemia intermedia: phenotype is correlated to the degree of globin imbalance

Heterogeneous genotypes	
Homozygous or compound heterozygous β-thalassemia	Heterozygous β-thalassemia
• Presence of mild or silent β-thalassemia alleles • Coinheritance of α-thalassemia • Coinheritance of genetic determinants increasing γ-chain production	• Coinheritance of 1 or 2 α-globin chains (ααα/αα or ααα/ααα) • Heterozygousity for β-thalassemia and structural β-chain variants • Hyperunstable hemoglobins
Correspond to heterogeneous phenotypes	

bones, depression of the base of the nose, shortening of long bones, excessive thinning of cortices and dilatation of the medullary cavities. Pain and fractures, even in the absence of severe trauma, are common. The more severe bone abnormalities develop when erythropoiesis is excessively increased to compensate for the anemia and represent an indication to transfusion inception.[4] Osteoporosis is a constant finding in thalassemia intermedia, especially after the first decade of life. An association has been proposed with specific polymorphisms in candidate genes (vitamin D receptor, estrogen receptor, calcitonin receptor, and collagen type 1 alpha 1) but the hypothesis has not been confirmed.[5] Extramedullary erythropoiesis is a frequent complication of thalassemia intermedia and it has been found in up to 65% of adult patients.[6] (Fig. 1) It is best demonstrated by magnetic resonance imaging (MRI) or by computed tomography.[7,8] The ectopic erythropoietic masses can cause variable symptoms, depending on the site where, and the rapidity at which, they develop. When fibrotic or adipose tissue predominates, they are usually asymptomatic and do not require therapy. Conversely, spinal cord compression causing paraparesis and cauda equina syndrome require urgent treatment. Hydroxyurea and transfusion are both effective, but when rapid regression is required, X-ray therapy, despite its side effects, is indicated.[9,10]

Transfusion therapy

Thalassemia intermedia, by definition, does not require transfusion therapy. However, except for the milder forms of the disease, transfusion therapy becomes often necessary at some time during the life of a patient. In a child, in addition to the level of hemoglobin, the indication to transfuse is given by stunted growth, poor general condition, and skeletal deformities. Also, the development of extramedullary erythropoiesis needs to be monitored. Aplastic crises, typically due to parvovirus B19 infection, can complicate the course of thalassemia intermedia, and cause extremely severe anemia characterized by peripheral retyculocytopenia and giant and bizarre pronormoblasts in the bone marrow. Sometimes transient pancytopenia is present.[11]

Pregnancy represents an indication to transfusion, especially in the second and third trimester. The role of transfusion in preventing the development of pulmonary hypertension is debated.

Of great importance is the size of the spleen. A large spleen can in fact be at the origin of increasing severity of the anemia and it can cause neutropenia and thrombocytopenia. Splenectomy can reestablish the equilibrium and allow a good level of activity in the absence of transfusion. An exception is represented by the newly described association of duplication of alpha genes plus heterozyogous β-thalassemia, in which splenectomy can aggravate the hemolytic process.[12] In any case, the risks of infection and thrombosis should always be kept in mind.

In older patients who have been transfusion independent for decades, transfusions can become necessary because of reduced marrow activity. This phenomenon has been attributed by some authors to a decreased production of erythropoietin, but further research is necessary to confirm this hypothesis.

The need for transfusion must be evaluated carefully because the risk of alloimmunization and autoimmunization is high in thalassemia patients who had not been transfused in the first years of life. A Greek study reported a frequency of alloimmunization of 20.9% versus 47.5% in patients transfused before and after the age of 3 years.[13] Thirty-four percent of 139 patients with thalassemia intermedia developed this complication.[14] The consequences

Table 2. Mutations external to the globin genes that can modify the phenotype of thalassemia intermedia

Cholelithiasis jaundice	• Gilbert syndrome: homozygosity [(TA)7/(TA)7] for the mutation of the A(TA)nTAA motif of the promoter of the bilirubin UDP-glucuronosyltransferase gene
Hypercoagulability	• Factor V Leiden; • Prothrombin mutations; • MTHFR mutations; • Decreased levels of Protein C and S and AT III
Osteoporosis	• Sp1 polymorphism of COLIA1, FokI, and BsmI; polymorphism of the Vit D receptor gene; • Polymorphism of ER α and β genes
Hemochromatosis	• C282Y and H63D alleles

can be dramatic when the autoimmune hemolytic anemia develops during pregnancy, causing severe anemia incompatible with the fetus survival.[15] The pathogenesis is unclear and it has been attributed to "hidden" antigens from peripheral red blood cell fragmentation.

Therapy with immune suppressants, intravenous immunoglobulins, hydroxyurea, and even splenectomy can be attempted. A few cases have been reported in whom stem cell transplantation was successfully performed. In one case allogeneic bone marrow was obtained from an HLA-matched unrelated donor.[16]

Iron overload

Untransfused or minimally transfused patients accumulate up to 2–5 g of iron per year through the digestive tract. Rarely the iron burden is significant before age 20 years. Intestinal iron absorption is triggered by chronic anemia, ineffective erythropoiesis and, as recently demonstrated, decreased serum hepcidin. In fact, the release of hepcidin, a 25-amino acid peptide produced by the hepatocytes, is increased by iron loading and inhibited by erythropoietic activity. In thalassemia intermedia, the high erythropoietic drive causes hepcidin deficiency and therefore hyperabsorption of dietary iron while the iron depletion of macrophages lowers the secretion of ferritin. As a consequence, serum ferritin levels underestimate the extent of iron overload in the thalassemia intermedia patients.[17] An aggravating effect of splenectomy on hemosiderosis has been suggested.[18]

The majority of the iron accumulates in liver parenchymal cells, while cardiac overload, the main cause of morbidity and mortality in thalassemia major, is rare or absent both in mice and in humans with thalassemia intermedia, as demonstrated by MRI.[19]

The iron accumulation in the liver, especially when associated to previous hepatitis C or B infection, exposes the patients to the risk of developing hepatocellular carcinoma. In a report, half or the patients with thalassemia who had developed the tumor were affected by thalassemia intermedia.[20] The inheritance of one of the hemochromatosis genes can, in theory, worsen the iron overload.

Cardiac disease

Despite the fact that the heart of patients with thalassemia intermedia is usually not affected by severe hemosiderosis, a large multicenter study on 110 patients of a mean age of 32.5 ± 11.4 years and with a mean hemoglobin of 9.1 ± 1.1 g/dL, found that 5.4% had congestive heart failure, 8% had a history of acute pericarditis, 34% had chronic pericardial changes, and more than half had some kind of valvular defect.[21] A smaller study of left ventricular function by two-dimensional and M-mode echocardiography in 24 asymptomatic young adults affected by β-thalassemia intermedia demonstrated significant increases in left ventricular volumes, left ventricular mass, and cardiac index, more pronounced than those found in patients affected by thalassemia major.[22]

The main cardiac problem in thalassemia intermedia, however, is pulmonary hypertension, an important cause of secondary right heart failure and the leading cause of cardiac failure in thalassemia intermedia patients.

Pulmonary hypertension

Pulmonary hypertension is defined as systolic pulmonary artery pressure >25 mmHg at rest and

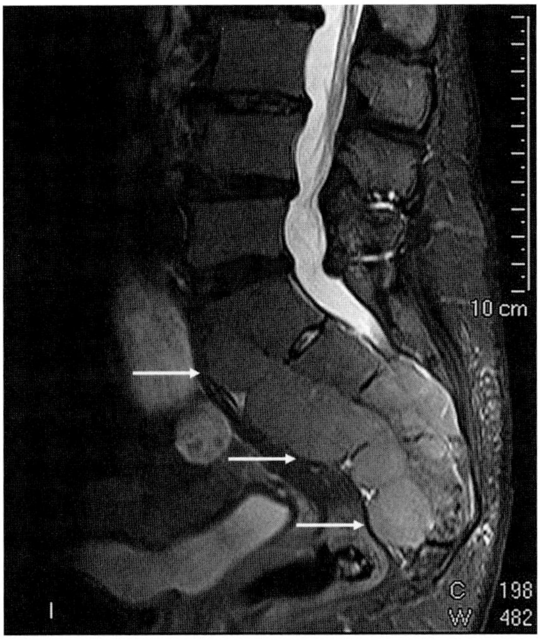

Figure 1. T2 weighted MRI showing paravertebral extramedullary erythropoiesis in a 60-year-old woman with thalassemia intermedia.

>30 mmHg during exercise with a normal pulmonary artery wedge pressure <15 mmHg and an increased pulmonary vascular resistance greater than three Wood units. It has been described in most forms of hemolytic anemias.

In the two largest cardiological studies carried out on thalassemia intermedia patients, pulmonary hypertension was encountered in nearly 60% of cases while congestive heart failure was encountered in 5.4% of 110 patients aged 32.5 years and 2.7% of 74 patients aged 28.2 years, respectively;[21,23] interestingly, all the thalassemia intermedia patients with congestive heart failure had severe pulmonary hypertension and normal systolic left ventricular function.

Therefore, the role of chronic hemolysis in the development of pulmonary hypertension through the induction of nitric oxide (NO) and arginine deficiency has received particular attention.[24] In fact, inactivation of NO correlates with hemolytic rate and is associated with the erythrocyte release of cell-free hemoglobin, which consumes NO directly, and the simultaneous release of the arginine-metabolizing enzyme arginase, which limits bioavailability of the NO synthase substrate arginine during the process of intravascular hemolysis. Then, depletion of nitric oxide, and increased arginase activity (may lead to vasoconstriction, vessel wall hypertrophy, hypercoagulability, local thrombosis, increase of thromboxane and endothelin, resulting in chronic organ damage and endothelial dysfunction. Moreover, platelets may have an important role, as pro-coagulant, by increasing platelet release of serotonin (contributing to smooth muscle vasoconstriction and proliferation), vascular endothelial growth factor and platelet-derived growth factor.[25] However, when thalassemia patients with or without pulmonary hypertension were compared, no biochemical transfusional or clinical differences were found. The role of transfusion in protecting from pulmonary hypertension is still debated.

Endocrine problems

The frequency of endocrine complications is highly variable, hypogonadism being the most frequent, followed by diabetes and hypothyroidism. Puberty is normal or delayed, but fertility is usually preserved.[26] Hundreds of children have been born to women and men with thalassemia intermedia, mostly after spontaneous conception.[27] Sometimes splenectomy can become necessary to give space to the enlarging uterus. The risk of thrombosis is severe enough to warrant antithrombotic therapy before and after delivery.[28]

In addition to this, anemia becomes more severe during pregnancy, especially during the first and second trimester and, in order to prevent fetal growth restriction due to hypoxia, blood transfusion is often required, with the consequent risk of antibodies formation in previously untransfused women.[15,29]

Leg ulcers

Trophic ulcers developing above the medial malleolus are a common and distressing problem, that has been attributed to hypoxia, to the abnormal rheology of the thalassemic red cells and to the increased hemoglobin F causing reduced oxygen release to the tissues.[30] An interesting hypothesis attributes the ulcers to the oxidative damage of nontransferring bound iron present in the tissues as a consequence of venous stasis.[31]

Treatment is difficult: it includes pressure dressing, skin grafting, blood transfusion, hydroxyurea, arginine butyrate, G-CSF, and platelet growth factor.

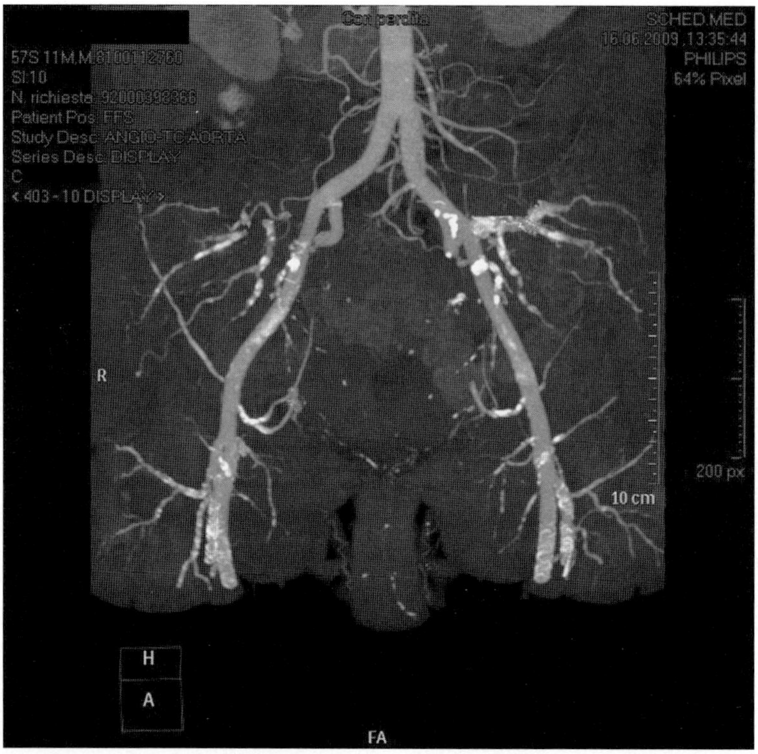

Figure 2. Angio CT scan showing multiple calcifications of abdominal arteries in a patient with thalassemia intermedia and pseudoxanthoma elasticum.

Thrombotic risk

The existence of a chronic hypercoagulable state has been demonstrated in thalassemia intermedia. In a report on 8,860 thalassaemia patients from the Mediterranean countries and Iran, thromboembolism occurred four times more frequently in thalassaemia intermedia than in thalassemia major.[32] Also, an Italian study reported a high prevalence of venous thrombotic events in patients with thalassaemia intermedia.[28]

Several authors have suggested that the presence of a chronic hypercoagulable state could be due to the procoagulant effect of the anionic phospholipids exposed on the surface of the damaged circulating red blood cells, to the increased numbers of platelets, and to abnormal plasma coagulation.[33] The co-inerithance of thrombophilic mutations increases the risk of thrombosis.

Anti-coagulant prophylaxis should be instituted before surgery and in the peripartum period, while heparin therapy, followed by long-term oral anticoagulants, is indicated after significant thrombotic episodes.

Cholelithiasis

Patients with thalassemia intermedia are often affected by mild to moderate jaundice that gives them an unpleasant old wax complexion. This is due in part to chronic hemolysis and it is made more severe by the association with the mutation of the A(TA)nTAA motif of the promoter of the bilirubin UDP-glucuronosyltransferase gene, the Gilbert mutation. Phenobarbital can decrease the bilirubin levels. Gallstones are a frequent complication of hemolytic anemias.

In a study, cholelithiasis was found in 20.3% of patients with thalassemia major and in 57% of those with thalassemia intermedia. The co-inheritance of the Gilbert mutation further increases the risk.[34]

Pseudoxanthoma elasticum

The first report of two patients affected by thalassemia and coexistent Pseudoxanthoma elasticum (PXE) was published by Aessopos and colleagues in 1989.[35] Several subsequent reports have confirmed the existence of a clinical syndrome resembling PXE in patients with thalassemia intermedia and other haemolytic conditions.[36,37]

The presence of PXE is usually suspected because of the characteristic skin lesions. The typical histopathological features of PXE both in the inherited and the acquired form are the abnormal, mineralised, and fragmented elastic fibers (elastorrhexia) in skin, eyes, and arterial blood vessels. In a study published in 1998 and including patients affected by thalassemia intermedia older than 30 years, arterial calcifications were found in 55%, skin lesions in 20%, and ocular alterations in 52%. Eighty-five percent had at least one of the three typical lesions[38] (Fig. 2).

In the PXE syndrome developing in thalassemia, the defect is believed to be acquired. A genetic study performed in these patients has not found the mutation of the inherited form.[39]

Infections

Infection represents the second cause of death in patients with thalassemia major. Patients with thalassemia intermedia are also exposed to a high risk of infection. Predisposing factors include anemia, iron overload, splenectomy, and a range of immune abnormalities. The reduced formation of nitric oxide in the presence of iron contributes to the risk of infection and iron has also an inhibitory effect on the activity of interferon gamma. As a consequence, iron-loaded macrophages lose the ability to kill intracellular pathogens via the interferon-gamma-mediated pathways.[40]

Encapsulated organisms frequently found in splenectomized patients are readily controlled by prophylactic vaccination and prophylactic antibiotic treatment. Conversely, infections due to ferrophilic organisms, such as Yersinia and Klebsiella are increasingly being reported in patients chelated with deferoxamine.

Conclusions

The molecular pathophysiology of thalassemia intermedia is variable. As a consequence, the clinical picture and the natural history of the disease can span from mild anemia with no bone abnormalities to severe anemia, intense erythropoietic activity, marked bone deformities. Numerous complications, among which pulmonary hypertension, thrombotic events, pseudoxanthoma elasticum, leg ulcers, osteoporosis, autoimmune haemolytic anemia contribute to modify the natural history of the disease. The decision of when to transfuse and whether to splenectomize are crucial. Several therapeutic approaches are possible, although none is curative.

Acknowledgments

We thank Cinzia Tonioli for secretarial assistance and Daniele Canella for expert technical support.

Conflicts of interest

The authors declare no conflicts of interest.

References

1. Borgna-Pignatti, C. & R. Galanello. 2009. Thalassemias and related disorders: quantitative disorders of hemoglobin synthesis. In *Wintrobe's Clinical Hematology*, Vol. 38. J.P. Greer, J. Foerster, G.M. Rodger, F. Paraskevas, B. Glader, D.A. Arber & R.T. Means Jr., Eds.: 1084–1090, 12th edn. Lippincott Williams & Wilkins. Philadelphia.
2. Cao, A. 1988. Diagnosis of beta-thalassemia intermedia at presentation. *Birth Defects Orig. Artic. Ser.* **23:** 219–226.
3. Modell, B. & V. Berdoukas, editors. 1984. *The Clinical Approach to Thalassemia*, p. 242. Grune & Stratton. London, 1984. p. 242.
4. Dresner Pollack, R., E. Rachmilewitz, A. Blumenfeld, *et al.* 2000. Bone mineral metabolism in adults with beta-thalassaemia major and intermedia. *Br. J. Haematol.* **111:** 902–907.
5. Origa, R., E. Fiumana, M.R. Gamberini, *et al.* 2005. Osteoporosis in beta-thalassemia: clinical and genetic aspects. *Ann. N.Y. Acad. Sci.* **1054:** 451–456.
6. Dore, F., P. Cianciulli & S. Rovasio. 1992. Incidence and clinical study of ectopic erythropoiesis in adult patients with thalassemia intermedia. *Ann. Ital. Med. Int.* **7:** 137–140.
7. Pippard, M.J., B. Rajagopalan, S.T. Callender & D.J. Weatherall. 1982. Iron loading, chronic anaemia, and erythroid hyperplasia as determinants of the clinical features of β-thalassaemia intermedia. In *Advance in Red Blood Cell Biology*. D.J. Weatherall, G. Fiorelli, S. Gorini, Eds.: 103. Raven Press. New York.
8. Chourmouzi, D., K. Pistevou-Gompaki, G. Plataniotis, *et al.* 2001. MRI findings of extramedullary haemopoiesis. *Eur. Radiol.* **11:** 1803–1806.
9. Issaragrisil, S., A. Piankigagum & P. Wasi. 1981. Spinal cord compression in thalassemia. Report of 12 cases and recommendations for treatment. *Arch. Int. Med.* **141:** 1033–1036.
10. Aliberti, B., A. Patrikiou, A. Terentiou, *et al.* 2001. Spinal cord compression due to extramedullary haematopoiesis in two patients with thalassaemia: complete regression with blood transfusion therapy. *J. Neurol.* **248:** 18.
11. Yarali, N., F. Duru, T. Sipahi, *et al.* 2000. Parvovirus B19 infection reminiscent of myelodysplastic syndrome in three children with chronic hemolytic anemia. *Pediatr. Hematol. Oncol.* **17:** 475.
12. Refaldi, C., W. Barcellini, E. Cassinerio, *et al.* 2009. Severe thalassemia intermedia resulting from coinheritance

of IVSI-110 G>A beta gene mutation and duplication of alfa-lobin gene cluster in homozygosis. *Abstract n. 35, Ninth Cooley's Anemia Symposium,* 2009 October 21–24.

13. Spanos, T., M. Karageorga, V. Ladis, *et al.* 1990. Red cell alloantibodies in patients with talassemia. *Vox Sang.* **58:** 50–55.
14. Kruatrachue, M., S. Sirisinha, P. Pacharee, *et al.* 1980. An association between thalassaemia and autoimmune haemolytic anaemia (AIHA). *Scand. J. Haematol.* **25:** 259–263.
15. Origa, R., A. Piga, G. Quarta, *et al.* 2010. Pregnancy and beta-thalassemia: an Italian multicenter experience. *Haematologica* **95:** 376–381.
16. De Stefano, P., M. Zecca, G. Giorgiani, *et al.* 1999. Resolution of immune haemolytic anaemia with allogeneic bone marrow transplantation after an unsuccessful autograft. *Br. J. Haematol.* **106:** 1063–1064.
17. Origa, R., R. Galanello, T. Ganz, *et al.* 2007. Liver iron concentrations and urinary hepcidin in ß-thalassemia. *Haematologica* **92:** 583–588.
18. Fiorelli, G., S. Fargion, A. Piperno, *et al.* 1990. Iron metabolism in thalassemia intermedia. *Haematologica* **75:** 89–95.
19. Gardenghi, S., M.F. Marongiu & P. Ramos. 2007. Ineffective erythropoiesis in beta-thalassemia is characterized by increased iron absorption mediated by down-regulation of hepcidin and up-regulation of ferroportin. *Blood* **109:** 5027–5035.
20. Borgna-Pignatti, C., G. Vergine, T. Lombardo, *et al.* 2004. Hepatocellular carcinoma in the thalassaemia syndromes. *Br. J. Haematol.* **124:** 114–117.
21. Aessopos, A., D. Farmakis, M. Karagiorga, *et al.* 2001. Cardiac involvement in thalassemia intermedia: a multicenter study. *Blood* **97:** 3411–3416.
22. Vaccari, M., R. Crepaz, M. Fortini, *et al.* 2002. Left ventricular remodeling, systolic function, and diastolic function in young adults with beta-thalassemia intermedia: a Doppler echocardiography study. *Chest* **12:** 506–512.
23. Aessopos, A., D. Farmakis, S. Deftereos, *et al.* 2005. Thalassemia heart disease: a comparative evaluation of thalassemia major and thalassemia intermedia. *Chest* **127:** 1523–1530.
24. Morris, C.R., M.T. Gladwin & G.J. Kato. 2008. Nitric oxide and arginine dysregulation: a novel pathway to pulmonary hypertension in hemolytic disorders. *Curr. Mol. Med.* **8:** 620–632.
25. Gabbay, E., J. Fraser & K. McNeil. 2007. Review of bosentan in the management of pulmonary arterial hypertension. *Vasc. Health Risk Manage.* **3:** 887–900.
26. Nassar, A.H., I.M. Usta, J.B. Rechdan & A. Taher 2006. Pregnancy in patients with beta-thalassemia intermedia: outcome of mothers and newborns. *Am. J. Hematol.* **81:** 499–502.
27. Skordis, N., S. Christou, M. Koliou, *et al.* 1998. Fertility in female patients with thalassemia. *J. Pediatr. Endocrinol. Metab.* **11:** 935–943.
28. Cappellini, M.D., L. Robbiolo, B.M. Bottasso, *et al.* 2000. Venous thromboembolism and hypercoagulability in splenectomized patients with thalassaemia intermedia. *Br. J. Haematol.* **111:** 467–473.
29. Borgna-Pignatti, C. 2007. Modern treatment of thalassaemia intermedia. *Br. J. Haematol.* **138:** 291–304.
30. Camaschella, C. & M.D. Cappellini. 1995. Thalassemia intermedia. *Haematologica* **80:** 58–68.
31. Zamboni, P., M. Izzo & V. Lanzara. 2003 Chronic venous insufficiency (CVI) and hemosiderinuria. *J. Vasc. Surg.* **37:** 132–136.
32. Taher, A., H. Isma'eel, G. Mehio, *et al.* 2006. Prevalence of thromboembolic events among 8,860 patients with thalassemia major and intermedia in the Mediterranean area and Iran. *Thromb. Haemost.* **96:** 488–491.
33. Eldor, A. & E.A. Rachmilewitz. 2002. The hypercoagulable state in thalassemia. *Blood* **99:** 36–43.
34. Galanello, R., S. Piras, S. Barella, *et al.* 2001. Cholelithiasis and Gilbert's syndrome in homozygous beta-thalassaemia. *Br. J. Haematol.* **115:** 926–928.
35. Aessopos, A., G. Stamatelos, P. Savvides, *et al.* 1989. Pseudoxanthoma elasticum and angioid streaks in two cases of beta-thalassaemia. *Clin. Rheumatol.* **8:** 522–527.
36. Tsomi, K., M. Karagiorga-Lagana, F. Karabatsos, *et al.* 2001 Arterial elastorrhexis in beta-thalassaemia intermedia, sickle cell thalassaemia and hereditary spherocytosis. *Eur. J. Haematol.* **67:** 135–141.
37. Aessopos, A., D. Farmakis, M. Karagiorga, *et al.* 2001. Cardiac involvement in thalassemia intermedia: a multicenter study. *Blood* **97:** 3411–3416.
38. Aessopos, A., M. Samarkos, E. Voskaridou, *et al.* 1998. Arterial calcifications in beta-thalassemia. *Angiology* **49:** 137–143.
39. Hamlin, N., K. Beck, B. Baccelli, *et al.* 2003. Acquired Pseudoxanthoma elasticum-like sindrome in beta-thalassemia patients. *Br. J. Haematol.* **122:** 852–854.
40. Vento, S., F. Cainelli & F. Cesario. 2006. Infections and thalassaemia. *Lancet Infect. Dis.* **6:** 226–233.

Ann. N.Y. Acad. Sci. ISSN 0077-8923

ANNALS OF THE NEW YORK ACADEMY OF SCIENCES
Issue: *Cooley's Anemia: Ninth Symposium*

Hepcidin and Hfe in iron overload in β-thalassemia

Sara Gardenghi,[1] Pedro Ramos,[1] Antonia Follenzi,[2] Niva Rao,[1] Eliezer A. Rachmilewitz,[3] Patricia J. Giardina,[1] Robert W. Grady,[1] and Stefano Rivella[1]

[1]Division of Hematology-Oncology, Department of Pediatrics, Children's Cancer and Blood Foundation Laboratories, Weill Cornell Medical College, New York, New York. [2]Albert Einstein College of Medicine, Bronx, New York. [3]Department of Hematology, The Edith Wolfson Medical Center, Holon, Israel

Address for correspondence: Stefano Rivella, Ph.D., Weill Medical College of Cornell University, 515 East 71st St. Rm. S702, Mailbox 284, New York, NY 10021. str2010@med.cornell.edu

Hepcidin (HAMP) negatively regulates iron absorption, degrading the iron exporter ferroportin at the level of enterocytes and macrophages. We showed that mice with β-thalassemia intermedia (*th3*/+) have increased anemia and iron overload. However, their hepcidin expression is relatively low compared to their iron burden. We also showed that the iron metabolism gene *Hfe* is down-regulated in concert with hepcidin in *th3*/+ mice. These observations suggest that low hepcidin levels are responsible for abnormal iron absorption in thalassemic mice and that down-regulation of *Hfe* might be involved in the pathway that controls hepcidin synthesis in β-thalassemia. Therefore, these studies suggest that increasing hepcidin and/or *Hfe* expression could be a strategy to reduces iron overload in these animals. The goal of this paper is to review recent findings that correlate hepcidin, Hfe, and iron metabolism in β-thalassemia and to discuss potential novel therapeutic approaches based on these recent discoveries.

Keywords: β-thalassemia; iron overload; hepcidin; *Hfe*; lentiviral vectors

Introduction

The liver peptide hepcidin (HAMP)[1,2] is the key regulator of iron absorption. Hepcidin triggers the degradation of ferroportin (FPN),[3] the only known iron exporter expressed by duodenal enterocytes, hepatocytes, and macrophages. Although the mechanisms that regulate this peptide are not yet fully understood, a series of interrelated factors have been shown to affect hepcidin expression. Hepcidin is down-regulated by erythropoiesis,[4] anemia, and hypoxia,[5] whereas it is up-regulated by iron overload[6] and inflammation.[5,7–9]

One of the major complications of β-thalassemia is iron overload due to the increased iron demand associated with efforts to satisfy an augmented erythropoietic activity. Iron accumulation in different organs can lead to several complications including heart and liver failure, diabetes mellitus, and hypopituitarism.[10] For this reason, a major focus of clinical management has been on chelation therapy as a means of slowing the progression of iron overload.[11] In β-thalassemia major, where no β-globin is produced, iron overload is largely due to the blood transfusions needed to sustain life. However, many studies have also indicated that iron overload in β-thalassemia is associated with increased iron uptake from the diet. Patients suffering from β-thalassemia intermedia, a milder form of the disease, do not usually require transfusion therapy but eventually develop iron overload due to increased iron absorption from the gastrointestinal tract.[10,12] Therefore, better understanding the mechanisms of increased dietary iron absorption in β-thalassemia, especially in nontransfused patients, could lead to new therapies to manage this problem.

Hepcidin, HFE, and iron overload in β-thalassemia

β-Thalassemia is characterized by ineffective erythropoiesis (IE), anemia, and iron overload. Recent studies point to the key role of hepcidin in modulating iron absorption in β-thalassemia. Hepcidin is a peptide hormone synthesized in the liver,[2,13] which has been shown to be the primary

doi: 10.1111/j.1749-6632.2010.05595.x

regulator of iron metabolism.[14] Hepcidin exerts its effect via binding to the iron exporter ferroportin and inducing its internalization and degradation.[3] Blocking iron export from cells allows this peptide to control iron flow to the blood stream, including uptake from the duodenum, recycling within macrophages, and release from the storage compartment in the liver. Regulation of hepcidin expression is a complex process requiring integration of several signals including iron, hypoxia, erythropoietic demand, and inflammatory status.[14] Iron accumulation and inflammation drive hepcidin expression higher to limit iron release into the blood stream. On the other hand, anemia and hypoxia strongly down-regulate hepcidin, increasing iron availability. In β-thalassemia patients, anemia and iron overload coexist and exert two competing signals in modulating hepcidin expression. The first evidence of hepcidin disregulation in β-thalassemia was reported in 2004, with low hepcidin expression in mouse models of this disease.[15] Using mouse models of β-thalassemia intermedia (*th3/+*) and major (*th3/th3*), it has been shown that the level of IE determines organ iron distribution and the expression level of hepcidin.[16] In *th3/+* mice, iron accumulates progressively in the spleen and, at a lower rate, in hepatic Kupffer cells, whereas in *th3/th3* animals, iron overload occurs rapidly and involves predominantly the liver parenchymal cells. Several reports also showed that the liver hepcidin mRNA level is excessively low in *th3/th3* mice,[15–17] where extreme IE is able to override an expected increase in hepcidin due to the high liver iron concentration. On the other hand, hepcidin is initially decreased in young *th3/+* mice,[15,17,18] although it increases over time, reaching the same level as that of wild-type (wt) mice. However, the up-regulation of hepcidin was not proportional to the concurrent increase of iron overload observed in the *th3/+* animals.[16] These data suggested that low expression of hepcidin could be responsible for the high iron levels in these animals.

Administration of Hamp25 peptide to thalassemic mice

Rivera and colleagues have shown that single 50-μg doses of HAMP25 are sufficient to prevent iron absorption in wt animals for up to 48 h.[19] Using a similar approach, we administered a synthetic murine version (Hamp25) of the peptide to *th3/+* and wt mice, and evaluated the effect on hematological parameters and organ iron content *in vivo*. The synthetic Hamp25 peptide was injected intravenously (i.v.). Injection of PBS was used as a negative control.[20] All studies were done with age- and weight-matched 2-month-old female mice, kept on an iron sufficient diet containing 35-ppm of iron.[20] Because *th3/+* animals might require higher doses than wt mice to prevent abnormal iron absorption, we first tested the effects of single 50- and 100-μg doses delivered i.v., and found that 100 μg decreased serum iron levels in wt mice more than 50 μg.[20] We also evaluated the effect of multiple doses of Hamp25 (50 μg) to maximize the effect on iron absorption. The Hamp25 was injected daily for 14 days, after which we monitored serum iron levels by a colorimetric assay,[19] using serum from normal mice as a standard. We also measured organ iron contents and hematological parameters.[20]

After the last injection we observed decreased serum iron levels in both wt and *th3/+* mice, compared to animals injected with PBS ($N = 3$–5 per group, Fig. 1A). However, measurement of organ iron contents did not show significant differences between Hamp25- and PBS-injected mice.[20] However, hematological parameters such as Hb, RBC levels, and reticulocyte counts were not changed in wt and *th3/+* mice treated with the peptide compared to PBS controls.[20] Interestingly, quantitative real-time PCR analysis of the liver of these mice revealed downregulation of endogenous hepcidin expression after injection of the peptide (Fig. 1B). This observation suggests that a feedback mechanism is in place to adjust the concentration of hepcidin in the circulation (exogenous + endogenous). A possible mechanism might be that administration of Hamp25, by lowering the level of serum iron and the Tf saturation, triggers a physiological response to decrease expression of endogenous hepcidin. Alternatively, but less likely, the Hamp25 peptide itself might play a role in the regulation of hepcidin expression.

There are at least two explanations for these results. First, the dose of Hamp25 used may have been insufficient to reduce iron absorption to a level that would also reduce tissue iron levels in 14 days. Second, having observed that the level of endogenous hepcidin was reduced in treated mice, we speculate that the dose and the serum half-life[4] of the Hamp25 may have been inadequate to compensate

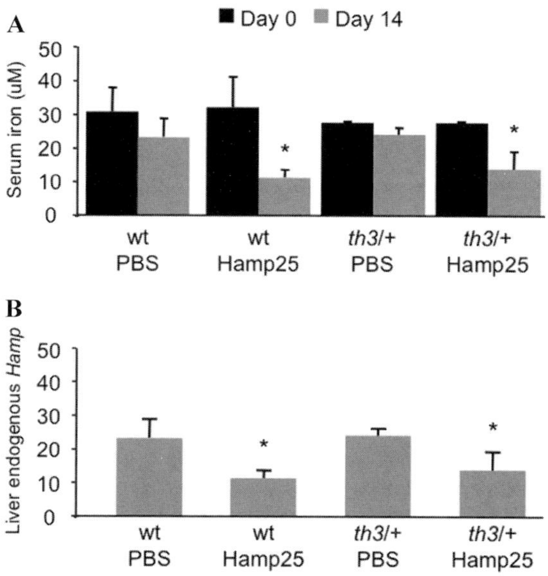

Figure 1. Administration of a synthetic Hamp25 peptide reduces serum iron levels and down-regulates endogenous hepcidin expression. Wt and *th3/+* mice ($N = 3$–5 animals/group) were injected once daily with 50 μg of Hamp25 for 14 days. Control mice were injected with PBS. (A) Serum was isolated from peripheral blood on days 0 and 14, and its iron levels measured by colorimetric assay (Thermo Electron Corporation, Melbourne, Australia), according to the manufacturer's instructions. Both wt and *th3/+* mice treated with Hamp25 showed a dramatic reduction of serum iron after 14 days of treatment, while no significant changes were detected in control mice. (B) Quantitative real-time PCR (Q-PCR) analysis on the livers from mice treated with Hamp25 and PBS showed down-regulation of endogenous *Hamp* expression after injection of the peptide. Error bars represent SDs calculated using at least three animals per group. The P values ($^*P < 0.05$) were calculated using Student's t-test.

for the decreased synthesis of endogenous hepcidin. Therefore, future studies will focus on administering increased doses of Hamp25, to determine the optimal concentration capable of reducing iron overload without impairing erythropoiesis.

Use of lentiviral vectors expressing HAMP or HFE in a liver-specific manner

We showed that *Hfe* is down-regulated in the same way as hepcidin in thalassemic mice, suggesting a correlation between the two genes.[16] Our data on wt mice have shown that the hepcidin mRNA level in the liver is 90 times higher than that of *Hfe*. In *th3/+* mice, the hepcidin level is only 20 times higher than that of *Hfe*, because of the down-regulation of hepcidin.[16] Therefore, a small increase in the expression of *Hfe* might up-regulate hepcidin to a larger extent. It is important to mention that by increasing hepcidin so as to reduce iron absorption, we could also impair erythropoiesis by reducing iron recycling through macrophages. Therefore, different strategies need to be developed to increase hepcidin levels so as to achieve a therapeutic dose of hepcidin that does not exacerbate anemia in *th3/+* mice. To investigate a different approach to achieve the up-regulation of hepcidin in thalassemic mice, we produced lentiviral vectors designed to increase the expression of hepcidin in mice either directly or indirectly through the overexpression of *Hfe*. We generated three lentiviral vectors, named pCCL.TTR.*Hamp*.IRES.GFP.WPRE (THIGW), pCCL.TTR.*Hamp*.WPRE (T*Hamp*W), and pCCL.TTR.*Hfe*.WPRE (T*Hfe*W), respectively, that carry either hepcidin or *Hfe* cDNAs and can express the proteins in a liver-specific fashion.[20,21] A similar control vector, pCCL.TTR.GFP.WPRE (TGW), expressing the enhanced green fluorescent protein (eGFP) that allows for the identification of transduced cells, was generated as well. Tissue specificity was achieved using a promoter generated by fusion of the synthetic hepatocyte-specific enhancer with the murine transthyretin (TTR) promoter.[21–23] All the vectors contain specific sequences that are able to improve lentiviral mediated gene transfer, and that are commonly inserted in HIV-derived vectors as two *cis*-acting elements. These are a polypurine tract sequence (cPPT) and a central termination sequence (CTS). They are present within the HIV polymerase (pol) gene, their function being to facilitate nuclear import of the viral preintegration complex.[24] A second sequence element, termed woodchuck hepatitis virus post-transcriptional regulatory element (WPRE)[25] was also inserted. WPRE is able to increase transgene expression in the context of plasmid DNAs or viral vectors.[25] Viral stocks were generated by transient transfection into 293T cells as previously described.[26–29] We generated two lentiviral vectors for the expression of *Hamp*, respectively named pCCL.TTR.*Hamp*.IRES.GFP.WPRE (THIGW) and pCCL.TTR.*Hamp*.WPRE (T*Hamp*W). Because of the internal ribosome entry site (IRES) element, the THIGW vector expresses hepcidin and eGFP from a bicistronic mRNA, whereas eGFP allows for the identification of transduced cells.[20] In addition, we produced a pCCL.TTR.*Hfe*.WPRE (T*Hfe*W) vector for the expression of *Hfe*, and a control vector pCCL.TTR.GFP.WPRE (TGW) expressing the

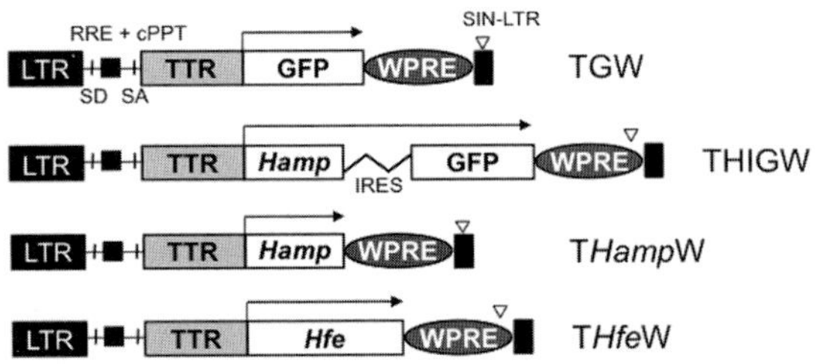

Figure 2. Schematic representation of the lentiviral vectors used during this study. The components shown are the long terminal repeat (LTR), the self-inactivating long terminal repeat (Sin-LTR), the HIV rev-response and central polypurine tract elements (RRE, cPPT), the splice donor (SD), the splice acceptor (SA), the woodchuck hepatitis virus posttranscriptional regulatory element (WPRE), the liver-specific TTR promoter (TTR), the internal ribosome entry site (IRES), the enhanced green fluorescent protein (eGFP), and the mouse *Hamp* and *Hfe* cDNA sequences.

green fluorescent protein (eGFP) (Fig. 2).[20] All the vectors were used to transduce human and mouse hepatic cell lines, such as HepG2, Hepa1–6, and Hep3B, to determine whether they were suitable for expressing hepcidin or *Hfe* in a liver-specific fashion. Flow cytometric analysis (FACS) of HepG2 cells transduced with the TGW vector showed the percentage of GFP-positive cells to be 77%. GFP levels in HepG2 cells transduced with THIGW were slightly lower, showing 41% of GFP-positive cells (Fig. 3A).[20]

To measure the VCN we used Q-PCR analysis of WPRE levels (since WPRE is present in all the vectors) on DNA extracted from transduced HepG2 cells. WPRE values were normalized to endogenous control values obtained from amplification of the human ID1 gene. We observed an average copy number of 1.2 for THIGW and T*Hamp*W, and 1.7 for T*Hfe*W.[20] The TGW vector showed a higher VCN (2.1 copies/cell). In addition, we performed Q-PCR analysis on the cDNA from transduced HepG2 cells (human), using specific primers to detect the mouse hepcidin or *Hfe* mRNA sequences expressed by the vectors. In this way we were able to discriminate between the mRNAs produced by the vectors and the endogenous mRNA synthesized by the cells. Our results confirmed the specific expression of *Hamp*, *Hfe*, GFP, and WPRE by the vectors (Fig. 3B).[20] From these analyses, the vectors appear suitable for *in vivo* experimentation. We plan to administer these vectors to thalassemic mice as a therapeutic tool to limit iron overload.

Future prospects

Developing new strategies to reduce excessive iron absorption and tissue iron overload is one of the most important goals in the treatment of β-thalassemia. The hepatic peptide hepcidin has an acknowledged primary role in regulating iron absorption and metabolism. We showed that hepcidin mRNA expression is low compared to iron burden in *th3*/+ mouse models of β-thalassemia, thus being responsible for abnormal iron absorption. Our studies aim to develop possible therapeutic strategies to up-regulate hepcidin levels in *th3*/+ mice.

Administration of a synthetic Hamp25 peptide showed effects on iron distribution in *th3*/+ mice, reducing serum iron levels but also down-regulating the expression of endogenous hepcidin. However, we did not observe significant changes in tissue iron concentrations. We hypothesized that these results might be caused by an insufficient dosage and/or length of treatment, so that only the more immediate effects on serum iron concentration were evident. In particular, it might be necessary to adjust the treatment with Hamp25 to compensate for the decreased synthesis of endogenous hepcidin.

From this perspective, the lentiviral vectors we used to transduce cells were able to express hepcidin, *Hfe*, and eGFP respectively, and to do so in a liver-specific manner due to the presence of the TTR

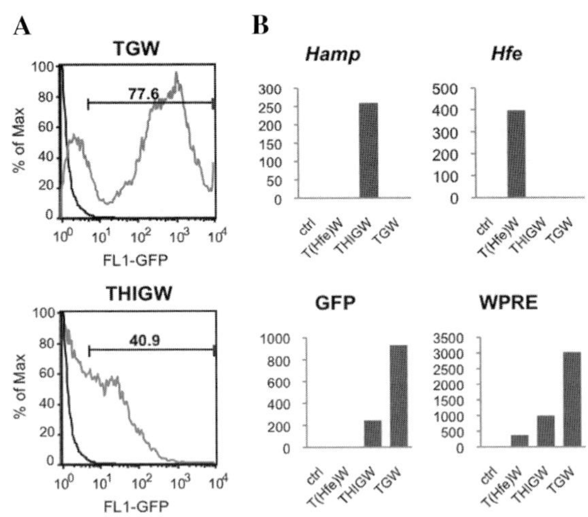

Figure 3. (A) FACS analysis of the level of GFP in HepG2 cells transduced with the TGW and THIGW vectors. (B) *Hamp*, *Hfe*, GFP, and WPRE mRNA levels expressed by the TGW, THIGW, and T*Hfe*W vectors in HepG2 cells. Because the *Hamp* and *Hfe* sequences expressed by the vectors are originated from mouse, they were easily discriminated from the endogenous *Hamp* and *Hfe* sequences of HepG2 cells that are, instead, of human origin.

promoter. We transduced common hepatic cell lines with the vectors, to assure high-transducibility, a good copy number, and high levels of expression. Moving forward, we will study the vectors *in vivo* to determine the level and stability of expression, as well as organ iron concentrations and hematological parameters.

Acknowledgments

This work was supported by the Cooley's Anemia Foundation-CAF, the Associazione Veneta Lotta alla Talassemia (AVLT) (S.G.), and by grants from the Carlo and Micol Schejola Foundation, the Children's Cancer and Blood Foundation and NIH-R21DK065169 (S.R.), R01DK55463 (R.W.G.), the American Portuguese Biomedical Fund (APBRF, USA)/Inova grant (P.R.). S.G. is a fellow of the Cooley's Anemia Foundation. P.R is a fellow from Fundação para a Ciência e Tecnologia, Portugal (SFRH/BD/24813/2005).

Conflicts of interest

The authors declare no conflicts of interest.

References

1. Krause, A. *et al.* 2000. LEAP-1, a novel highly disulfide-bonded human peptide, exhibits antimicrobial activity. *FEBS Lett.* **480:** 147–150.
2. Park, C.H. *et al.* 2001. Hepcidin, a urinary antimicrobial peptide synthesized in the liver. *J. Biol. Chem.* **276:** 7806–7810.
3. Nemeth, E. *et al.* 2004. Hepcidin regulates cellular iron efflux by binding to ferroportin and inducing its internalization. *Science* **306:** 2090–2093.
4. Pak, M. *et al.* 2006. Suppression of hepcidin during anemia requires erythropoietic activity. *Blood* **108:** 3730–3735.
5. Nicolas, G. *et al.* 2002. The gene encoding the iron regulatory peptide hepcidin is regulated by anemia, hypoxia, and inflammation. *J. Clin. Invest.* **110:** 1037–1044.
6. Pigeon, C. *et al.* 2001. A new mouse liver-specific gene, encoding a protein homologous to human antimicrobial peptide hepcidin, is overexpressed during iron overload. *J. Biol. Chem.* **276:** 7811–7819.
7. Nemeth, E. *et al.* 2003. Hepcidin, a putative mediator of anemia of inflammation, is a type II acute-phase protein. *Blood* **101:** 2461–2463.
8. Nemeth, E. *et al.* 2004. IL-6 mediates hypoferremia of inflammation by inducing the synthesis of the iron regulatory hormone hepcidin. *J. Clin. Invest.* **113:** 1271–1276.
9. Wrighting, D.M. & N.C. Andrews. 2006. Interleukin-6 induces hepcidin expression through STAT3. *Blood* **108:** 3204–3209.
10. Bannerman, R.M. *et al.* 1967. Thalassemia intermedia, with iron overload, cardiac failure, diabetes mellitus, hypopituitarism and porphyrinuria. *Am. J. Med.* **42:** 476–486.
11. Giardina, P.J. & R.W. Grady. 2001. Chelation therapy in beta-thalassemia: an optimistic update. *Semin. Hematol.* **38:** 360–366.
12. Pippard, M.J. *et al.* 1979. Iron absorption and loading in beta-thalassaemia intermedia. *Lancet* **2:** 819–821.
13. Nicolas, G. *et al.* 2001. Lack of hepcidin gene expression and severe tissue iron overload in upstream stimulatory factor 2 (USF2) knockout mice. *Proc. Natl. Acad. Sci. USA* **98:** 8780–8785.
14. Nemeth, E. & T. Ganz. 2009. The role of hepcidin in iron metabolism. *Acta Haematol.* **122:** 78–86.
15. Adamsky, K. *et al.* 2004. Decreased hepcidin mRNA expression in thalassemic mice. *Br. J. Haematol.* **124:** 123–124.
16. Gardenghi, S. *et al.* 2007. Ineffective erythropoiesis in {beta}-thalassemia is characterized by increased iron absorption mediated by down-regulation of hepcidin and up-regulation of ferroportin. *Blood* **109:** 5027–5035.
17. Weizer-Stern, O. *et al.* 2006. mRNA expression of iron regulatory genes in beta-thalassemia intermedia and beta-thalassemia major mouse models. *Am. J. Hematol.* **81:** 479–483.
18. De Franceschi, L. *et al.* 2006. Liver expression of hepcidin and other iron genes in two mouse models of beta-thalassemia. *Haematologica* **91:** 1336–1342.
19. Rivera, S. *et al.* 2005. Synthetic hepcidin causes rapid dose-dependent hypoferremia and is concentrated in ferroportin-containing organs. *Blood* **106:** 2196–2199.
20. Gardenghi, S. *et al.* 2008. Increased hepcidin expression in Mice affected by β-thalassemia reduces iron overload with no effect on Anemia. *Blood* **112:** 53.
21. Follenzi, A. *et al.* 2002. Efficient gene delivery and targeted expression to hepatocytes *in vivo* by improved lentiviral vectors. *Hum. Gene. Ther.* **13:** 243–260.
22. Costa, R.H. & D.R. Grayson. 1991. Site-directed mutagenesis of hepatocyte nuclear factor (HNF) binding sites in the mouse transthyretin (TTR) promoter reveal synergistic interactions with its enhancer region. *Nucleic Acids Res.* **19:** 4139–4145.
23. Vigna, E. *et al.* 2005. Efficient Tet-dependent expression of human factor IX *in vivo* by a new self-regulating lentiviral vector. *Mol. Ther.* **11:** 763–775.
24. Follenzi, A. *et al.* 2000. Gene transfer by lentiviral vectors is limited by nuclear translocation and rescued by HIV-1 pol sequences. *Nat. Genet.* **25:** 217–222.
25. Zufferey, R. *et al.* 1999. Woodchuck hepatitis virus post-transcriptional regulatory element enhances expression of transgenes delivered by retroviral vectors. *J. Virol.* **73:** 2886–2892.
26. Zufferey, R. *et al.* 1998. Self-inactivating lentivirus vector for safe and efficient *in vivo* gene delivery. *J. Virol.* **72:** 9873–9880.
27. Zufferey, R. *et al.* 1997. Multiply attenuated lentiviral vector achieves efficient gene delivery *in vivo. Nat. Biotechnol.* **15:** 871–875.
28. Naldini, L. *et al.* 1996. *in vivo* gene delivery and stable transduction of nondividing cells by a lentiviral vector [see comments]. *Science* **272:** 263–267.
29. Naldini, L. *et al.* 1996. Efficient transfer, integration, and sustained long-term expression of the transgene in adult rat brains injected with a lentiviral vector. *Proc. Natl. Acad. Sci. USA* **93:** 11382–11388.

Ann. N.Y. Acad. Sci. ISSN 0077-8923

ANNALS OF THE NEW YORK ACADEMY OF SCIENCES
Issue: *Cooley's Anemia: Ninth Symposium*

Fertility potential in thalassemia major women: current findings and future diagnostic tools

Sylvia T. Singer,[1] Nancy Sweeters,[2] Olivia Vega,[2] Annie Higa,[2] Elliott Vichinsky,[1] and Marcelle Cedars[3]

[1]Hematology/Oncology Department, Children's Hospital and Research Center at Oakland, California. [2]Clinical Research Center, Children's Hospital and Research Center at Oakland, California. [3]Division of Reproductive Endocrinology, UCSF Medical Center San Francisco, California

Address for correspondence: Sylvia Titi Singer, M.D., Hematology/Oncology, Children's Hospital and Research Center in Oakland, Oakland, CA 94609. tsinger@mail.cho.org

Preserving fertility, preventing early menopause, and predicting reproductive ability have become crucial for many adult thalassemia major females. Luteinizing hormone/follicle-stimulating hormone (LH/FSH) and estradiol, commonly used for assessment of fertility potential in thalassemia, have a poor predictive value. Current reproductive practice uses markers of ovarian reserve testing, which were not yet studied in thalassemia women. We explored the relationship between liver iron concentration (LIC) and fertility status in 26 females (mean 30 years old). Seventeen (65%) of them experienced primary or secondary amenorrhea. Levels of LH/FSH and estradiol were low or undetectable in 48% and 35% of patients, respectively and did not correlate with age, presence of amenorrhea, and LIC. This further addresses the need for utilization of current available methods for assessment of fertility capacity in thalassemia, which will also allow future correlation with pituitary iron measures by MRI as well as early intervention for fertility preservation.

Keywords: thalassemia major women; fertility in thalassemia women; ovarian reserve testing (ORT)

Introduction

Hypogonadotrophic hypogogonadism and impairment of fertility due to deleterious effects of iron are well documented among women with thalassemia major (TM). Progress in management of iron overload has resulted in a lower prevalence of this endocrinopathy; however, a high frequency of hypogonadotrophic hypogogonadism, diagnosed in up to 50% of adult TM patients, is still reported.[1,2] As long-term survival for this patient population has improved, attainment of reproductive capacity and formation of a family has become a major goal for many adult patients. In females with TM issues of preserving fertility, preventing premature menopause and obtaining data on fertility potential, are imperative. While significant advances in the predictive capacity for fertility and in assisted reproductive technology were made over the past decade,[3] few if any have been implemented for the care of thalassemia women.

In addition, as progress is made in the use of MRI technology for determining pituitary iron overload,[4] corresponding accurate functional studies are needed for early detection of patients who are developing hypogonadism and for a consistent correlation with these new imaging tools. Methods of ovarian reserve testing (ORT), which have become routine diagnostic procedures for women with infertility problems, can provide data on the ovarian function and pituitary-gonadal axis function.[3,5] ORT can be used for prediction of fertility potential and possibly for correlation with the extent of pituitary iron on MRI. These studies have not been applied yet in the thalassemia patient population.

Fertility and iron toxicity

It has been well established that the major effect of iron toxicity on the reproductive system is a direct damage to the hypothalamic/pituitary hormonal secretion; however, there is some controversy as to the

doi: 10.1111/j.1749-6632.2010.05583.x

ability of adequate long-term iron chelation therapy to preserve it.[1,6,7] In addition, there is no sufficient data on the direct effect of iron on the gonads and the role of compromised primary ovarian function in causing infertility problems in women.

Studies on female infertility suggest that oxidative stress has a major role in women's decline in reproduction potential.[8,9] The natural mechanism of follicle aging is also thought to result from oxidative stress due to increase in reactive oxygen species (ROS) production, mitochondrial flaws, a compromised microenvironment and lower enzymatic antioxidant defense mechanisms.[10,11] Taken together, there is a recent abundance of data linking oxidative damage and decline in fertility.

Iron-induced oxidative damage has been studied in thalassemia and is thought to cause major tissue dysfunction.[12] However, the impact of oxidative stress on the reproductive system has been only infrequently investigated. In males with TM, studies have shown sperm DNA damage which is thought to be a consequence of iron-induced oxidative injury.[13–15] In thalassemia females, one study has shown increased level of redox activity in the follicular fluid from a patient with TM suggesting that redox-active iron ions mediate free radical production, induce tissue injury, and possibly contribute to impairment of reproduction in these patients.[16] It is reasonable to assume that in thalassemia females' chronic iron-induced oxidative damage can result in earlier or accelerated follicular aging, a mechanism thought to be the primary cause for reduced fertility and menopause in women.

Pregnancies in thalassemia

Over 400 pregnancies were reported; Skordis summarized a total of 290 pregnancies published in TM women up to 2004.[17] Others have since reported additional successful pregnancies.[18–20] More than half of the reported pregnancies occurred in females with primary or secondary amenorrhea, required ovulation induction and most report term delivery of normal infants.

Despite these remarkable successes, there is lack of data on the unsuccessful attempts to conceive. There is also insufficient data on pregnancy-related complications, specifically the incidence of premature labor, cardiac complications and the change in cardiac and liver iron loading over the course of pregnancy. A recent publication reports a threefold higher incidence of premature labor and growth retardation than the normal population, and a 73% incidence of cesarean section.[21] There are no data on the baseline fertility profile and ovarian reserve in thalassemia women who succeeded or failed to become pregnant.

Ovarian aging and ORT

Ovarian reserve is the fertility potential as it relates to the total number and quality of the primordial follicles remaining in the ovaries. Measurement of ovarian reserve can increase the understanding of women's reproductive potential and predict chances for pregnancy with or without treatment. Since menstruation is a poor surrogate for fertility, and age alone has limited value in predicting fertility, other markers for ovarian reserve have been extensively evaluated: (1) Biochemical tests for basal (early follicular) hormone levels (FSH, LH, Estradiol, Inhibin A and B, and anti-Mullerian hormone). (2) Ovarian stimulation tests. (3) Biophysical, ultrasound techniques for assessing the number of remaining follicles in the ovary. Several ultrasound methods have been developed; the more commonly used include ovarian volume and antral follicle count (AFC). Both have been shown to predict reproductive status.

Inhibin B is mainly secreted by pre-antral follicles and therefore is a direct measure of ovarian reserve. Anti-Mullerian hormone (AMH) is produced by the granulose cells of the ovary and has several advantages: It is the earliest marker of change with age and it has very little intercycle and intracycle variability. It is therefore a convenient measure of ovarian reserve even when randomly obtained during the cycle.[3,22] Sonographic measurement of AFC and ovarian volume have been shown to correlate with ovarian reserve, but some cycle differences may occur.[23]

Overall a combination of basal FSH, AMH, and AFC was shown useful in assessment of chances for pregnancy in women undergoing *in vitro* fertilization (IVF) or undergoing evaluation for assisted reproductive techniques (ART). AMH levels were found to correlate well with AFC[24] and seem to emerge as the single most useful marker to estimate ovarian reserve and well reflect time to the onset of the menopausal transition (determined by the onset of menstrual irregularities).[25,26] Still, more longitudinal data and clinical outcomes to assess the

Table 1. Patients' fertility and iron overload/chelation characteristics

Thalassemia type	Age (Y)	Amenorrhea (yes/no)	Pregnancies/ live birth	Splenectomy	Average LIC (mg/gr dry wt.)	Low LH/ FSH
TM	17	Y		N	31.2	N
TM	23	Y		N	8.6	Y
TM	25	N		Y	6.9	N
TM	25	Y		Y	36.6	Y
E thal	26	Y	1/0	Y	34.5	N
TM	26	Y		Y	11.5	Y
TI/TM	26	Y		N	7.1	N
TM	26	N		Y	25.0	N
TM	26	N		N	12.7	N
TM	28	Y		Y	11.3	Y
TM	29	Y		Y	5.9	Y
TM	30	Y		Y	6.3	N
E thal	30	Y		Y	9.2	Y
E thal	30	Y	1/1	Y	5.9	Y
E thal	31	N	4/4	N	41.8	N
TM	31	N		Y	6.5	Y
TM	31	Y		Y	9.5	Y
E thal	34	Y		Y	18.3	Y
TI/TM	37	N		Y	3.2	N
TM	37	Y		Y	4.1	N
TM	37	Y		Y	6.6	Y
TM	41	Y		Y	9.1	N
E thal	42	N	2/2	Y	9.4	N
Total		Y = 16 N = 7	8/7	Y = 18 N = 5		Low = 11 nL = 12
Mean ± SD	30 ± 6.2				14 ± 11.5	

TM, thalassemia major; E Thal, E-beta thalassemia; TI/TM, thalassemia intermedia transitioned to regular transfusions/chelation treatment.

predictive value of ORT and AMH in particular are needed.

For thalassemia females where age and menstrual cycle cannot assess fertility status, these novel measures can provide important predictive information and become a useful tool for clinical application.

Assessment of fertility in TM females: preliminary data

The hypothalamic/pituitary hormonal secretion appears to be particularly sensitive to the effects of iron loading, while data on the end-organ dysfunction is less well defined. In clinical practice, the standard assessment of failure of sexual development or fertility status in thalassemia females involves measuring the concentration of LH and FSH. In some cases hormone stimulation tests (GnRH) are performed.[27]

We explored the relationships between total iron burden as measured by liver iron concentration (LIC), hormonal levels and ovarian reserve; the latter not included in this report. Iron status and chelation history was studied in 23 adult females with transfusion-dependent thalassemia; median age 29, mean 30 ± 6, range 17–42 years (Table 1). Nineteen females entered puberty spontaneously at a mean age of 14.1 years, nine of them underwent secondary amenorrhea (mean age 19.2 years). Seven experienced primary amenorrhea resulting in primary or secondary amenorrhea in a total of 16 females (69%). A total of seven women were on replacement hormone therapy at the time of this study. Patients were asked to report a self assessment of their compliance with chelation treatment in five year increments, starting at age 11 years.

LIC was available in all 23 females, as assessed by annual ferrtitometer spectoferritometry (SQUID), a noninvasive, accurate technique for measuring iron level.

LH and FSH levels were low or undetectable in 11/23 females (48%) and estradiol was low or undetectable in 8 out of these 11 females. The mean levels of FSH in patients with or without amenorrhea did not differ significantly. There was a significant difference in the LH level in the two groups; some lack of concordance has been shown before in the secretion of FSH and LH.[28]

Age and LIC could not differentiate between those with or without hormonal deficiencies and there was also no correlation between age and LIC. This poor correlation of hypogonadotrophic hypogonadism with total body iron burden as indicated by mean LIC, confirms previous findings[29] and further highlights the distinctive and early effect of iron accumulation on the reproductive system; the anterior pituitary and likely the gonads as well.

The self-reported compliance questionnaire indicated poor average compliance in 50% of the patients (use of chelation 50–75% of the time prescribed for). There was an association of the compliance level with the range of hormonal levels, suggesting that on-going iron accumulation, most likely starting earlier than what can be detected as abnormal LIC, causes the irreversible pituitary damage, and underscores the need for more sensitive markers for declining fertility potential.

In summary, our preliminary results indicate that despite improved chelation methods, hypogonadotrphic hypogonadism and probable infertility problems still occur in a significant number of females with thalassemia. Fertility status in this cohort of patients could not be predicted from age, menstrual status or average liver iron measures. Similarly, as previously noted, transfusion or chelation parameters could not predict fertility.[27] This underscores the need for use of current available methods for assessment of fertility capacity, prediction of chances for pregnancy or time of menopause. We are currently applying the most successful methods of ORT and studying the levels of AMH, Inhibin B, AFC, and ovarian volume in this group of women. We expect these markers of ovarian reserve to better determine reproductive potential. Determination of ovarian reserve with such methods will also enable thalassemia women to seek assisted reproduction technologies (ART) which are continuously improving.[30]

Recent studies attempt to correlate pituitary MRI for iron deposition with LIC and cardiac iron, and develop an ability to predict hypogonadism.[4,29] When integrated with improved measures of fertility status, it could result in improved knowledge of the reproductive status in thalassemia females. Such understanding of the relationship to iron overload and of the mechanism for declining fertility potential could result in more successful interventions for preserving fertility.

Acknowledgment

This publication was made possible through grant support from Cooley's Anemia Foundation and by grant number UL1RR024131-01 from the National Center for Research Resources.

Conflicts of interest

The authors declare no conflicts of interest.

References

1. Borgna-Pignatti, C. *et al.* 2004. Survival and complications in patients with thalassemia major treated with transfusion and deferoxamine. *Haematologica* **89:** 1187–1193.
2. Al-Rimawi, H.S. *et al.* 2005. Hypothalamic-pituitary-gonadal function in adolescent females with beta-thalassemia major. *Int. J. Gynaecol. Obstet.* **90:** 44–47.
3. Coccia, M.E. & F. Rizzello. 2008. Ovarian reserve. *Ann. N.Y. Acad. Sci.* **1127:** 27–30.
4. Christoforidis, A. *et al.* 2007. MRI for the determination of pituitary iron overload in children and young adults with beta-thalassaemia major. *Eur. J. Radiol.* **62:** 138–142.
5. Lutchman Singh, K., M. Davies & R. Chatterjee. 2005. Fertility in female cancer survivors: pathophysiology, preservation and the role of ovarian reserve testing. *Hum. Reprod. Update.* **11:** 69–89.
6. Bronspiegel-Weintrob, N. *et al.* 1990. Effect of age at the start of iron chelation therapy on gonadal function in beta-thalassemia major. *N. Engl. J. Med.* **323:** 713–719.
7. Allegra, A. *et al.* 1990. Hypogonadism in beta-thalassemic adolescents: a characteristic pituitary-gonadal impairment. The ineffectiveness of long-term iron chelation therapy. *Gynecol. Endocrinol.* **4:** 181–191.
8. Agarwal, A., S. Gupta & R.K. Sharma. 2005. Role of oxidative stress in female reproduction. *Reprod. Biol. Endocrinol.* **3:** 1–21.

9. Agarwal, A., S. Gupta & R. Sharma. 2005. Oxidative stress and its implications in female infertility—a clinician's perspective. *Reprod. Biomed. Online* **11:** 641–650.
10. Tatone, C. *et al.* 2008. Cellular and molecular aspects of ovarian follicle ageing. *Hum. Reprod. Update* **14:** 131–142.
11. Tarin, J.J. 1996. Potential effects of age-associated oxidative stress on mammalian oocytes/embryos. *Mol. Hum. Reprod.* **2:** 717–724.
12. Livrea, M.A. *et al.* 1996. Oxidative stress and antioxidant status in beta-thalassemia major: iron overload and depletion of lipid-soluble antioxidants. *Blood* **88:** 3608–3614.
13. Perera, D. *et al.* 2002. Sperm DNA damage in potentially fertile homozygous beta-thalassaemia patients with iron overload. *Hum. Reprod.* **17:** 1820–1825.
14. De Sanctis, V. *et al.* 2008. Spermatozoal DNA damage in patients with B thalassaemia syndromes. *Pediatr. Endocrinol. Rev.* **6**(Suppl 1): 185–189.
15. De Sanctis, V. *et al.* 2008. Spermatogenesis in young adult patients with beta-thalassaemia major long-term treated with desferrioxamine. *Georgian Med. News* **156:** 74–77.
16. Reubinoff, B.E. *et al.* 1996. Increased levels of redox-active iron in follicular fluid: a possible cause of free radical-mediated infertility in beta-thalassemia major. *Am. J. Obstet. Gynecol.* **174:** 914–918.
17. Skordis, N. *et al.* 2004. Update on fertility in thalassaemia major. *Pediatr. Endocrinol. Rev.* **2**(Suppl 2): 296–302.
18. Tuck, S.M. 2005. Fertility and pregnancy in thalassemia major. *Ann. N.Y. Acad. Sci.* **1054:** 300–307.
19. Ansari, S., A. Azarkeivan & A. Tabaroki. 2006. Pregnancy in patients treated for beta thalassemia major in two centers (Ali Asghar Children's Hospital and Thalassemia Clinic): outcome for mothers and newborn infants. *Pediatr. Hematol. Oncol.* **23:** 33–37.
20. Cunningham, M.J. *et al.* 2004. Complications of beta-thalassemia major in North America. *Blood* **104:** 34–39.
21. Bajoria, R. & R. Chatterjee. 2009. Current perspectives of fertility and pregnancy in thalassemia. *Hemoglobin* **33**(Suppl 1): S131–S135.
22. Sowers, M.R. *et al.* 2008. Anti-Mullerian hormone and inhibin B in the definition of ovarian aging and the menopause transition. *J. Clin. Endocrinol. Metab.* **93:** 3478–3483.
23. Pavlik, E.J. *et al.* 2000. Ovarian volume related to age. *Gynecol. Oncol.* **77:** 410–412.
24. van Rooij, I.A. *et al.* 2005. Serum anti-Mullerian hormone levels best reflect the reproductive decline with age in normal women with proven fertility: a longitudinal study. *Fertil. Steril.* **83:** 979–987.
25. Knauff, E.A. *et al.* 2009. Anti-Mullerian hormone, inhibin B, and antral follicle count in young women with ovarian failure. *J. Clin. Endocrinol. Metab.* **94:** 786–792.
26. Broekmans, F.J. *et al.* 2008. Anti-Mullerian hormone and ovarian dysfunction. *Trends Endocrinol. Metab.* **19:** 340–347.
27. Papadimas, J. *et al.* 2002. β-thalassemia and gonadal axis: a cross-sectional, clinical study in a Greek population. *Hormones (Athens)* **1:** 179–187.
28. Genazzani, A.D. *et al.* 1993. FSH secretory pattern and degree of concordance with LH in amenorrheic, fertile, and postmenopausal women. *Am. J. Physiol.* **264:** E776–E781.
29. Argyropoulou, M.I., D.N. Kiortsis & S.C. Efremidis. 2003. MRI of the liver and the pituitary gland in patients with beta-thalassemia major: does hepatic siderosis predict pituitary iron deposition? *Eur. Radiol.* **13:** 12–16.
30. Miao, Y.L. *et al.* 2009. Oocyte aging: cellular and molecular changes, developmental potential and reversal possibility. *Hum. Reprod. Update.* **15:** 573–585.

Ann. N.Y. Acad. Sci. ISSN 0077-8923

ANNALS OF THE NEW YORK ACADEMY OF SCIENCES
Issue: *Cooley's Anemia: Ninth Symposium*

Redefining thalassemia as a hypercoagulable state

M. Domenica Cappellini,[1] Irene Motta,[1] Khaled M. Musallam,[2] and Ali T. Taher[2]

[1]Universitá di Milano, Policlinico Foundation IRCCS, Milan, Italy. [2]Hematology-Oncology Division, Department of Internal Medicine, American University of Beirut Medical Center, Beirut, Lebanon

Address for correspondence: Maria Domenica Cappellini, M.D., Professor of Medicine, Universitá di Milano, Fondazione Ospedale Maggiore Policlinico, Mangiagalli, Regina Elena IRCCS, Milan, Italy. maria.cappellini@unimi.it

As the life expectancy of β-thalassemia patients has markedly improved over the last decade, several new complications are being recognized. The presence of a high incidence of thromboembolic events, mainly in thalassemia intermedia patients, has led to the identification of a hypercoagulable state in thalassemia. In this review, the molecular and cellular mechanisms leading to hypercoagulability in thalassemia are highlighted, and the current clinical experience is summarized. Recommendations for thrombosis prophylaxis are also discussed.

Keywords: thalassemia; hypercoagulability; thromboembolism; stroke

Introduction

Extremely diverse phenotypes exist within the homozygous and compound heterozygote states for β-thalassemia. The terms thalassemia major (TM) and intermedia (TI) lack specific molecular correlates, but encompass a wide spectrum of clinical, as well as laboratory abnormalities.[1] Although once considered a fatal disease, the life expectancy of TM patients has markedly improved over the last few years, as a result of regular blood transfusions and compliance with tight iron chelation therapies.[2] However, TM patients still suffer from many complications of their chronic disease, and a series of serious previously undescribed complications are now being acknowledged, including thrombosis.[3] Patients with TI have, in general, a milder clinical phenotype than those with TM and remain largely transfusion independent.[4] The pathophysiology of TI is characterized by extravascular hemolysis, with the release into the peripheral circulation of damaged red blood cells (RBCs) and erythroid precursors because of a high degree of ineffective erythropoiesis.[3] This has also been recently attributed to severe complications such as pulmonary hypertension (PHT) and thromboembolic phenomena.[3] This review summarizes current knowledge of the clinical and pathophysiological characteristics of hypercoagulability in thalassemia patients and highlights available strategies to prevent the associated thromboemoblic events (TEE).

Hypercoagulability

Diverse factors contributing to the hypercoagulable state in patients with β-thalassemia have been identified (Fig. 1). In most cases, a combination of these abnormalities leads to clinical thrombosis.

Platelets

The medical literature is rich in evidence suggesting that patients with β-thalassemia have activated platelets. Moreover, flow cytometric studies have also confirmed the chronic platelet activation status. In β-thalassemia, there is evidence of increased platelet aggregation,[5] an increased proportion of platelets expressing CD62P (P-selectin) and CD63,[6,7] and a shortened platelet survival due to enhanced platelet consumption (especially in splenectomized patients).[8] Further, evidence of chronic platelet activation in patients with thalassemia was provided by the measurement of urinary metabolites of prostacyclin (PGI2) and thromboxane A2 (TXA2). A study comparing splenectomized patients with TM, nonsplenectomized patients with TI, and healthy individuals found a significant increase (4- to 10-fold) in the urinary excretion of the stable hydrolysis products of TXA2 and PGI2 in thalassemic patients compared to controls. No

doi: 10.1111/j.1749-6632.2010.05548.x

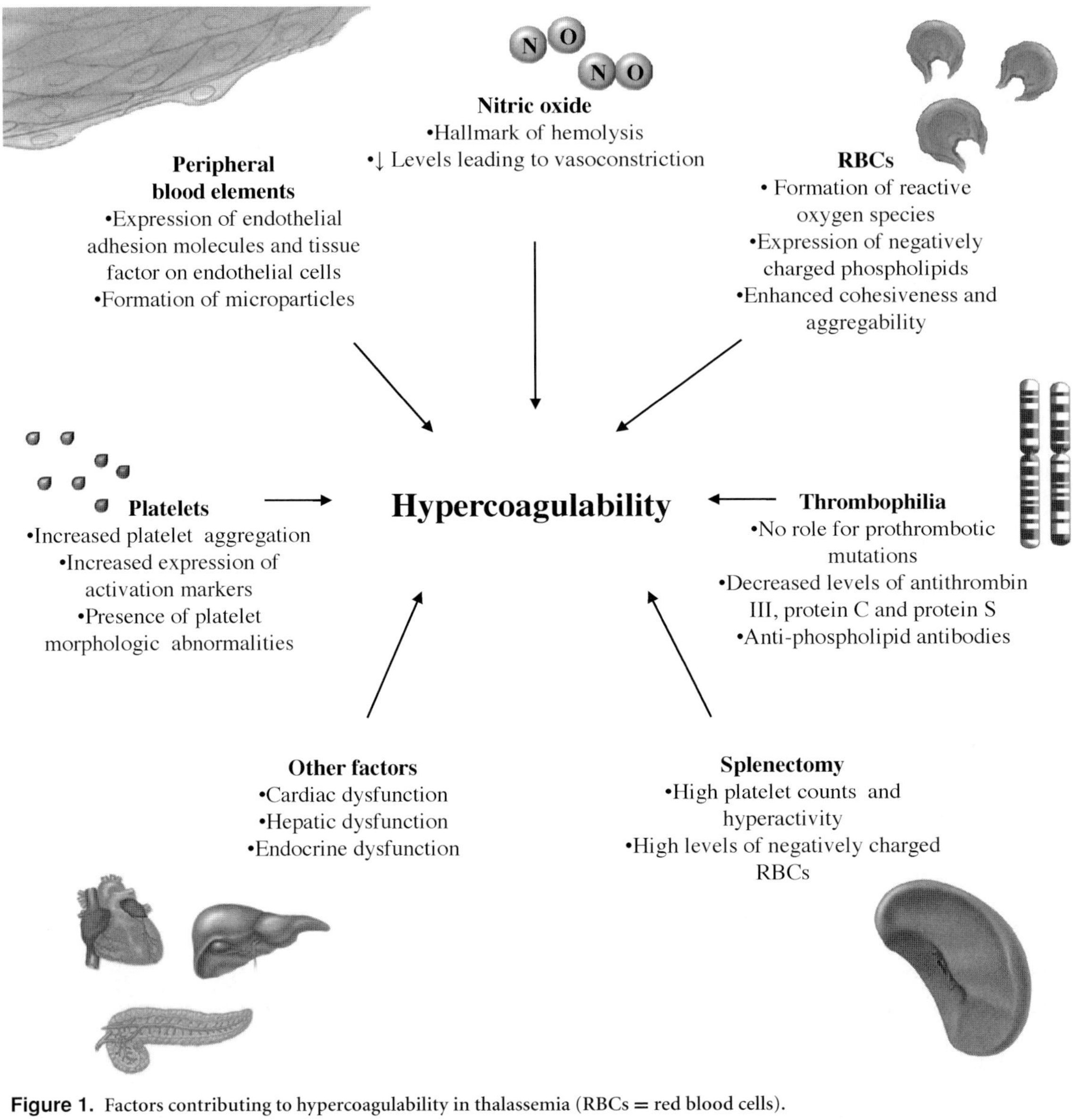

Figure 1. Factors contributing to hypercoagulability in thalassemia (RBCs = red blood cells).

significant differences were found in the concentrations of these metabolites between TM and TI patients.[9]

Red blood cells

Alteration in RBCs, namely the oxidation of globin subunits in thalassemia erythroid cells, leads to the formation of hemichromes.[10] Hemichromes bind to or modify various components of the mature RBC membrane, such as protein band 3, ankyrin, and spectrin.[11] After the precipitation of hemichromes, heme disintegrates, and toxic nontransferrin-bound iron species are released from the heme disintegration.[12] The resulting free iron catalyzes the formation of reactive oxygen species. Iron-dependent oxidation of membrane proteins and formation of red-cell "senescence" antigens such as phosphatidylserine[13] cause thalassemic red cells to become rigid and deformed and to aggregate, resulting in premature cell removal.[14] Studies have shown that thalassemic RBCs may be a source of negatively charged phospholipids, which can eventually increase thrombin generation.[15,16] This was verified by experiments that showed that annexin V, a protein with high affinity and specificity for anionic phospholipids, could block the procoagulant effect of isolated thalassemic RBCs.[16] An even higher number of circulating RBCS with negatively charged phospholipids was found in splenectomized patients.[17] Several studies have also demonstrated that RBCs from thalassemic patients show enhanced cohesiveness and aggregability. These abnormalities have been reduced to normal range after the patients have received a blood transfusion.[18]

Other peripheral blood elements

The finding of elevated levels of endothelial adhesion proteins (E-selectin [ELAM-1], intercellular adhesion molecule-1 [ICAM-1] and von Willebrand factor [VWF]), and vascular cell adhesion molecule-1 [VCAM-1] in thalassemic patients suggests that endothelial injury or activation may be a feature of the disease.[19,20] RBCs from patients with TM and TI also show increased adhesion to cultured endothelial cells (EC).[21] In addition, circulating EC expressing adhesion molecules and tissue factor have been recognized in patients with thalassemia.[22] This plays an important role in the recruitment of white blood cells (WBCs) and RBCs and promotes thrombosis at vascular inflammation sites, vessel obstruction, tissue hypoxia, and death.[23,24] More recently, it was shown that microparticles of RBC origin were elevated in patients with TI versus controls; these have a potential to aggravate thrombotic events.[25]

Splenectomy

Clinical observations have suggested that splenectomy in patients with TI can contribute to an increased susceptibility to thrombosis.[26,27] This has been ascribed to the presence of high platelet counts and aggregation following splenectomy[28,29] and/or to increased number of damaged RBCs.[17] In splenectomized TI patients, thrombin generation is significantly higher than in control subjects and patients who had not undergone splenectomy.[27]

Inherited and acquired coagulation defects

From the available data, DNA mutations do not appear to play an important role in the pathogenesis of thrombosis observed in β-thalassemia. In two studies from the Eastern Mediterranean region the presence of factor V Leiden, prothrombin, and methylene tetrahydrofolate reductase gene mutations was not significantly correlated with the thrombotic risk.[30,31] However, many investigators have reported changes in the levels of coagulation factors and inhibitors in thalassemic patients. Prothrombin fragment 1.2, a marker of thrombin generation, is elevated in TI patients. The status of protein C and protein S was investigated in β-thalassemia in many studies and they were generally found to be decreased.[27] The presence of anti-phospholipid antibodies has been reported in the serum of β-thalassemia patients. However, the exact nature of these antibodies and their relation to coexistent hepatitis C virus infection is still under investigation.[32] Other pathological mechanisms have been correlated with hypercoagulability in thalassemia and these include cardiac dysfunction, hormonal deficiencies, and liver dysfunction.[3]

Nitric oxide

The pathophysiological roles of hemolysis and the dysregulation of nitric oxide (NO) homeostasis are correlated with PHT in sickle cell disease (SCD) and in thalassemia. Nitric oxide binds soluble guanylate cyclase, which converts GTP to cGMP, relaxing vascular smooth muscle and causing vasodilatation. When plasma hemoglobin liberated from intravascularly hemolyzed sickle erythrocytes consumes NO, the balance is shifted toward vasoconstriction. PHT is aggravated and in SCD, it is linked to the intensity of hemolysis. Whether the same mechanism contributes to hypercoagulability in thalassemia is not yet known and needs to be investigated.[3]

Clinical experience

Epidemiological data on the overall frequency of TEE in patients with β-thalassemia is limited. A study on survival and causes of death in TM, carried out in Italy at the end of the 1980s, indicated TEE as the primary cause of death in four of 159 (2.5%) transfusion-dependent thalassemic patients.[33] Even more recently, in data from seven Italian centers on 720 patients with TM, 1.1% of patients had thrombosis.[34] In a recent survey involving nine Italian pediatric thalassemia centers, TEE was observed in 4% of 683 patients with TM and in 9.6% of 52 patients with TI.[35] In another series of TI patients, 24 patients (29%) developed either deep vein thrombosis, pulmonary embolism, or portal vein thrombosis during a 10-year follow up.[27] All patients except one had undergone splenectomy. The largest clinical study to date analyzed data from 8,860 thalassemia patients (6,670 TM and 2,190 TI).[26] The authors demonstrated that TEE occurred 4.38 times more frequently in TI than TM ($P < 0.001$), with more venous events occurring in TI and more arterial events occurring in TM. Moreover, patients with TI who developed a TEE were mostly splenectomized, nontransfused, and had a hemoglobin level below 9 g/dl; which may justify a higher thrombotic drive as abnormal RBCs are expected to remain longer in the circulation. The study described age beyond 20 years, splenectomy, family history of TEE and previous TEE as the main risk factors for developing thrombosis in the study group.[26]

Logothetis and colleagues described a "stroke syndrome" and neurological deficits compatible with transient ischemic attacks (TIAs) in about 20% of 138 cases of TM in Greece.[36] Similarly, Borgna Pignatti and colleagues described TIAs accompanied by a clinical picture of headache, seizures, and hemiparesis in 2.2% of TM patients in Italy.[35] Although the incidence of overt stroke in TM was usually described as higher than TI,[26] a study done to assess the rate of silent brain damage in patients with benign hemoglobinopathies reported that 37.5% of patients with TI showed asymptomatic brain damage on brain magnetic resonance imaging (MRI).[37] More recently, a brain MRI study on adult, splenectomized TI patients showed a rate of silent white matter lesions as high as 60%.[38] Older age and transfusion naivety were associated with a higher incidence and multiplicity of lesions.[38]

Autopsy series in patients with TM and TI describe the presence of DVT, pulmonary embolism and recurrent arterial occlusion, with thrombi in small and large pulmonary vessels.[33,39–41] Autopsies of a large series of patients with β-thalassemia/hemoglobin E disease revealed thrombotic lesions in the pulmonary arteries.[42] These pulmonary arterial thromboembolism may have been due to circulating platelet aggregates. Similar findings of multiple microthrombi, which were composed mainly of platelets, were seen in the pulmonary arterioles and microcirculation in autopsies of two splenectomized patients with thalassaemia.[43]

An ounce of prevention

The higher rate of thrombosis in transfusion-independent TI compared to polytransused TM patients suggests a potential role for transfusions in decreasing the rate of TEE.[26,27,35,38] The reduction of TEE in adequately transfused patients may be the result of decreased numbers of pathological RBC exhibiting indices of membrane damage.[18] It should be noted that the benefit of regular blood transfusions is appreciated in the more frequent thromboembolic manifestations in less developed countries with inadequate transfusion resources. Moreover, the higher rate of TEE in splenectomized patients may alter the risk-benefit assessment of splenectomy as a procedure of choice. The available data on the use of anticoagulants, antiplatelet, or other agents in β-thalassemia are either lacking or involve small, poorly controlled and/or relatively low-quality studies.[3] However, TI patients who experienced a TEE and received aspirin afterwards had a lower recurrence of TEE compared with those who were not taking aspirin, although these differences were not statistically significant.[26]

Treatment with the fetal hemoglobin-inducing agents, hydroxycarbmide and decitabine, results decreased plasma markers of thrombin generation. Hydroxycarbamide, specifically approved for the treatment of SCD, may decrease coagulation activation by reducing phospholipid expression on the surface of both RBC and platelets and decreasing RBC adhesion to thrombospondin. In addition to being a NO donor, hydroxycarbamide may also decrease hemostatic activation by its effect in decreasing the white blood cell count and particularly monocytes that express transcription factor.[44] Hydroxycarbamide is only rarely used in thalassemia,[45] these patients may experience the benefits because of similar mechanisms described in SCD. Another approach would be to correct the reactive oxygen species-induced RBC membrane damage using antioxidants, although this approach has not yet been verified in clinical trials.

It may also be possible to design a thalassemia-tailored thrombosis risk-assessment model (RAM) to estimate thrombotic risk as a function of intrinsic (e.g., thalassemia type and number of circulating RBC) and extrinsic (e.g., infection, surgery, and splenectomy) factors. Moreover, tests for predisposing factors could also be performed, particularly in high-risk patients. If clinically verified, this type of model could serve as a guideline for possible preventative treatment to decrease the incidence of TEE, which can cause significant morbidity and mortality.[3] In fact, attempts to identify diagnostic tests that will help identify patients at risk are emerging,[46] with results that are promising toward establishing an evidence based preventive approach.

In conclusion, there are diverse factors contributing to the hypercoagulable state observed in patients with β-thalassemia. In most cases, a combination of these abnormalities leads to clinical thrombosis. The higher incidence of thrombotic events in TI compared to TM patients is mainly attributed to transfusion naivety and splenectomy, both of which promote an underlying procoagulant activity. Although no clear guidelines exist to establish a prophylactic strategy, an individualized approach that takes into consideration all associated risk factors is advisable.

Conflicts of interest

The authors report no conflicts of interest. The authors alone are responsible for the content and writing of the paper. This study did not receive external funding.

References

1. Weatherall, D.J. & J.B. Clegg. 2001. *The Thalassaemia Syndromes*, 4th edn. Blackwell Science. Oxford.
2. Borgna-Pignatti, C., S. Rugolotto, P. De Stefano, *et al.* 2004. Survival and complications in patients with thalassemia major treated with transfusion and deferoxamine. *Haematologica* **89:** 1187–1193.
3. Taher, A.T., Z.K. Otrock, I. Uthman & M.D. Cappellini. 2008. Thalassemia and hypercoagulability. *Blood Rev.* **22:** 283–292.
4. Taher, A., H. Ismaeel & M.D. Cappellini. 2006. Thalassaemia intermedia: revisited. *Blood Cells Mol. Dis.* **37:** 12–20.
5. Winichagoon, P., S. Fucharoen & P. Wasi. 1981. Increased circulating platelet aggregates in thalassaemia. *Southeast Asian J. Trop. Med. Public Health* **12:** 556–560.
6. Del Principe, D., A. Menichelli, S. Di Giulio, *et al.* 1993. PADGEM/GMP-140 expression on platelet membranes from homozygous beta thalassaemic patients. *Br. J. Haematol.* **84:** 111–117.
7. Ruf, A., M. Pick, V. Deutsch, *et al.* 1997. *In vivo* platelet activation correlates with red cell anionic phospholipid exposure in patients with beta-thalassaemia major. *Br. J. Haematol.* **98:** 51–56.
8. Eldor, A., Y. Krausz, H. Atlan, *et al.* 1989. Platelet survival in patients with beta-thalassemia. *Am. J. Hematol.* **32:** 94–99.
9. Eldor, A., F. Lellouche, A. Goldfarb, *et al.* 1991. *In vivo* platelet activation in beta-thalassemia major reflected by increased platelet-thromboxane urinary metabolites. *Blood* **77:** 1749–1753.
10. Rund, D. & E. Rachmilewitz. 2005. Beta-thalassemia. *N. Engl. J. Med.* **353:** 1135–1146.
11. Shinar, E, E.A. Rachmilewitz & S.E. Lux. 1989. Differing erythrocyte membrane skeletal protein defects in alpha and beta thalassemia. *J. Clin. Invest.* **83:** 404–410.
12. Hershko, C., G. Graham, G.W. Bates & E.A. Rachmilewitz. 1978. Nonspecific serum iron in thalassaemia: an abnormal serum iron fraction of potential toxicity. *Br. J. Haematol.* **40:** 255–263.
13. Kuypers, F.A. & K. de Jong. 2004. The role of phosphatidylserine in recognition and removal of erythrocytes. *Cell. Mol. Biol.* **50:** 147–158.
14. Tavazzi, D., L. Duca, G. Graziadei, *et al.* 2001. Membrane-bound iron contributes to oxidative damage of beta-thalassaemia intermedia erythrocytes. *Br. J. Haematol.* **112:** 48–50.
15. Borenstain-Ben Yashar, V., Y. Barenholz, *et al.* 1993. Phosphatidylserine in the outer leaflet of red blood cells from beta-thalassemia patients may explain the chronic hypercoagulable state and thrombotic episodes. *Am. J. Hematol.* **44:** 63–65.
16. Helley, D., A. Eldor, R. Girot, *et al.* 1996. Increased procoagulant activity of red blood cells from patients with homozygous sickle cell disease and beta-thalassemia. *Thromb. Haemost.* **76:** 322–327.
17. Atichartakarn, V., P. Angchaisuksiri, K. Aryurachai, *et al.* 2002. Relationship between hypercoagulable state and erythrocyte phosphatidylserine exposure in splenectomized haemoglobin E/beta-thalassaemic patients. *Br. J. Haematol.* **118:** 893–898.
18. Chen, S., A. Eldor, G. Barshtein, *et al.* 1996. Enhanced aggregability of red blood cells of beta-thalassemia major patients. *Am. J. Physiol.* **270:** H1951–H1956.
19. Butthep, P., A. Bunyaratvej, Y. Funahara, *et al.* 1995. Alterations in vascular endothelial cell related plasma proteins in thalassaemic patients and their correlation with clinical symptoms. *Thromb. Haemost.* **74:** 1045–1049.
20. Butthep, P., A. Bunyaratvej, Y. Funahara, *et al.* 1997. Possible evidence of endothelial cell activation and disturbance in thalassemia: an *in vitro* study. *Southeast Asian J. Trop. Med. Public Health* **28:** 141A–148A.
21. Hovav, T., A. Goldfarb, G. Artmann, *et al.* 1999. Enhanced adherence of beta-thalassaemic erythrocytes to endothelial cells. *Br. J. Haematol.* **106:** 178–181.
22. Butthep, P., S. Rummavas, R. Wisedpanichkij, *et al.* 2002. Increased circulating activated endothelial cells, vascular endothelial growth factor, and tumor necrosis factor in thalassemia. *Am. J. Hematol.* **70:** 100–106.
23. Carlos, T.M. & J.M. Harlan. 1994. Leukocyte-endothelial adhesion molecules. *Blood* **84:** 2068–2101.
24. Mann, K.G., C. van't Veer, K. Cawthern & S. Butenas. 1998. The role of the tissue factor pathway in initiation of coagulation. *Blood Coagul. Fibrinolysis* **9:** S3–S7.
25. Habib, A., C. Kunzelmann, W. Shamseddeen, *et al.* 2008. Elevated levels of circulating procoagulant microparticles in patients with β-thalassemia intermedia. *Haematologica* **93:** 941–942.

26. Taher, A., H. Isma'eel, G. Mehio, *et al.* 2006. Prevalence of thromboembolic events among 8,860 patients with thalassaemia major and intermedia in the Mediterranean area and Iran. *Thromb. Haemost.* **96:** 488–491.
27. Cappellini, M.D., L. Robbiolo, B.M. Bottasso, *et al.* 2000. Venous thromboembolism and hypercoagulability in splenectomized patients with thalassaemia intermedia. *Br. J. Haematol.* **111:** 467–473.
28. Cappellini, M.D., E. Grespi, E. Cassinerio, *et al.* 2005. Coagulation and splenectomy: an overview. *Ann. N.Y. Acad. Sci.* **1054:** 317–324.
29. Atichartakarn, V., P. Angchaisuksiri, K. Aryurachai, *et al.* 2003. *In vivo* platelet activation and hyperaggregation in hemoglobin E/beta-thalassemia: a consequence of splenectomy. *Int. J. Hematol.* **77:** 299–303.
30. Zalloua, P.A., H. Shbaklo, Y.A. Mourad, *et al.* 2003. Incidence of thromboembolic events in Lebanese thalassemia intermedia patients. *Thromb. Haemost.* **89:** 767–768.
31. Iolascon, A., P. Giordano, S. Storelli, *et al.* 2001. Thrombophilia in thalassemia major patients: analysis of genetic predisposing factors. *Haematologica* **86:** 1112–1113.
32. Giordano, P., M. Galli, G.C. Del Vecchio, *et al.* 1998. Lupus anticoagulant, anticardiolipin antibodies and hepatitis C virus infection in thalassaemia. *Br. J. Haematol.* **102:** 903–906.
33. Zurlo, M.G., P. De Stefano, C. Borgna-Pignatti, *et al.* 1989. Survival and causes of death in thalassaemia major. *Lancet* **2:** 27–30.
34. Borgna-Pignatti, C., S. Rugolotto, P. De Stefano, *et al.* 2004. Survival and complications in patients with thalassemia major treated with transfusion and deferoxamine. *Haematologica* **89:** 1187–1193.
35. Borgna Pignatti, C., V. Carnelli, V. Caruso, *et al.* 1998. Thromboembolic events in beta thalassemia major: an Italian multicenter study. *Acta Haematol.* **99:** 76–79.
36. Logothetis, J., Constantoulakis M, Economidou J, *et al.* 1972. Thalassemia major (homozygous beta-thalassemia). A survey of 138 cases with emphasis on neurologic and muscular aspects. *Neurology* **22:** 294–304.
37. Manfre, L., E. Giarratano, A. Maggio, *et al.* 1999. MR imaging of the brain: findings in asymptomatic patients with thalassemia intermedia and sickle cell-thalassemia disease. *AJR Am. J. Roentgenol.* **173:** 1477–1480.
38. Taher, A.T., K.M. Musallam, W. Nasreddine, *et al.* 2009. Asymptomatic brain magnetic resonance imaging abnormalities in splenectomized adults with thalassemia intermedia. *J. Thromb. Haemost.* doi: 10.1111/j.1538-7836.2009.03651.x [Epub ahead of print]
39. Michaeli J, M. Mittelman, D. Grisaru & E.A. Rachmilewitz. 1992. Thromboembolic complications in beta thalassemia major. *Acta Haematol.* **87:** 71–74.
40. Gillis, S, M.D. Cappellini, A. Goldfarb, *et al.* 1999. Pulmonary thromboembolism in thalassemia intermedia patients. *Haematologica* **84:** 959–960.
41. van Teunenbroek, A., F.A. Wijburg, J.W. ten Cate, *et al.* 1989. Thromboembolic complications in an asplenic HbE-β-thalassaemia patient. *Neth. J. Med.* **35:** 123–127.
42. Sonakul, D., P. Pacharee, T. Laohapand, *et al.* 1980. Pulmonary artery obstruction in thalassaemia. *Southeast Asian J. Trop. Med. Public Health* **11:** 516–523.
43. Sumiyoshi, A., K. Thakerngpol & D. Sonakul. 1992. Pulmonary microthromboemboli in thalassemic cases. *Southeast Asian J. Trop. Med. Public Health* **23**(Suppl. 2): 29–31.
44. Ataga, K.I., M.D. Cappellini & E.A. Rachmilewitz. 2007. Beta-thalassaemia and sickle cell anaemia as paradigms of hypercoagulability. *Br. J. Haematol.* **139:** 3–13.
45. Karimi, M., H. Darzi & M. Yavarian. 2005. Haematologic and clinical responses of thalassemia intermedia patients to hydroxyurea during 6 years of therapy in Iran. *J. Pediatr. Hematol. Oncol.* **27:** 380–385.
46. Tripodi A., M.D. Cappellini, V. Chantarangkul, *et al.* 2009. Hypercoagulability in splenectomized thalassemic patients detected by whole-blood thromboelastometry, but not by thrombin generation in platelet-poor plasma. *Haematologica* **94:** 1520–1527.

Ann. N.Y. Acad. Sci. ISSN 0077-8923

ANNALS OF THE NEW YORK ACADEMY OF SCIENCES
Issue: *Cooley's Anemia: Ninth Symposium*

Treatment options for thalassemia patients with osteoporosis

Evangelos Terpos[1] and Ersi Voskaridou[2]

[1]Department of Clinical Therapeutics, University of Athens School of Medicine, Athens, Greece. [2]Thalassemia Center, Laikon General Hospital, Athens, Greece

Address for correspondence: Evangelos Terpos, Department of Clinical Therapeutics, University of Athens School of Medicine, Alexandra General Hospital, 80 Vas. Sofias Avenue, 11528 Athens, Greece. eterpos@hotmail.com

Osteoporosis represents a prominent cause of morbidity in patients with thalassemia. The delay in sexual maturation, the presence of diabetes and hypothyroidism, the parathyroid gland dysfunction, the progressive marrow expansion, the iron toxicity on osteoblasts, the iron chelators, and the deficiency of growth hormone or insulin growth factors have been identified as major causes of osteoporosis in thalassemia. Adequate hormonal replacement, effective iron chelation, improvement of hemoglobin levels, calcium and vitamin D administration, physical activity, and smoking cessation are the main to-date measures for the management of the disease. During the last decade, novel pathogenetic data suggest that the reduced osteoblastic activity, which is believed to be the basic mechanism of bone loss in thalassemia, is accompanied by a comparable or even greater increase in bone resorption. Therefore, the role of bisphosphonates, potent inhibitors of osteoclast activation, arises as a major factor in the management of osteoporosis in thalassemia patients.

Keywords: thalassemia; osteoporosis; bisphosphonates; therapy; pathogenesis

Introduction

Thalassemia major (TM) is a hereditary hemolytic anemia caused by a defect in the ability of erythroblasts to synthesize the β chain of adult hemoglobin. Several bone abnormalities are present in patients with TM, including the enlargement of the cranial and facial bones, spinal deformities, scoliosis, nerve compression, spontaneous fractures, and bone loss. The incidence of osteopenia or osteoporosis in well-treated TM patients has been found to be approximately 40–50%, and therefore osteoporosis represents a prominent cause of morbidity in TM patients of both genders.[1] The pathogenesis of osteoporosis in TM is very complicated and differs from the pathogenesis of bone deformities characteristically found in nontransfused patients (thalassemia intermedia; TI), who develop bone distortion mainly due to accelerated hemopoiesis and progressive marrow expansion. Several genetic and acquired factors are implicated in bone destruction in TM. The typical delay in sexual maturation, the presence of diabetes and hypothyroidism, the parathyroid gland dysfunction, the accelerated hemopoiesis with progressive marrow expansion, the direct iron toxicity on osteoblasts and the deficiency of growth hormone (GH) or insulin growth factor I (IGF-I) have been indicated as possible causes for thalassemia-induced osteoporosis.[1–3] Furthermore, iron chelation has correlated with growth failure and bone abnormalities, and high desferrioxamine dosage has been associated with cartilage alterations.[4,5] More puzzling, however, is the observation that, despite the normalization of hemoglobin levels, adequate hormone replacement, and effective iron chelation, patients continue to show an unbalanced bone turnover with an increased resorptive phase resulting in seriously diminished bone mineral density (BMD).[6,7]

Pathogenesis of osteoporosis in thalassemia

According to the Word Health Organization, osteoporosis is a disease characterized by low bone mass and microarchitectural deterioration of bone

doi: 10.1111/j.1749-6632.2010.05542.x

tissue, leading to enhanced bone fragility and a consequential increase in fracture risk.[8] The cut-off of 2.5 standard deviations below the normal mean in BMD for the respective age is used for the definition of osteoporosis, whereas the decrease of BMD between 1.5 and 2.5 standard deviations below the normal mean for the respective age is defined as osteopenia.[9] The most important factors that are implicated in the pathogenesis of bone loss in thalassemia patients are described later.

Genetic factors

Genetic factors seem to play a role in the development of low bone mass and osteoporotic fractures. These factors have been implicated in the pathogenesis of postmenopausal osteoporosis, as regulator genes of BMD, but have not been studied thoroughly in thalassemia-induced osteoporosis. The polymorphism at the Sp1 site of the collagen type Ia1 (COLIA 1) gene (collagen type I is the major bone matrix protein) was studied by Wonke and colleagues,[10] who found that approximately 30% of the TM patients were heterozygotes (Ss) and 4% were homozygotes (SS) for the Sp1 polymorphism. The authors have concluded that male patients with TM carrying the Sp1 mutation may develop severe osteoporosis of the spine and the hip more frequently than patients who do not carry this mutation. The COLIA 1 polymorphism has been associated with reduced BMD in postmenopausal osteoporosis, and predisposes women to osteoporotic fractures.[11] The genes encoding collagen types Ia1 and Ia2 (COLIA 1 and COLIA 2, respectively) are also important candidates for the genetic regulation of BMD, as mutations that affect the coding regimens of these genes are implicated in the pathogenesis of osteogenesis imperfecta and osteoarthritis.[12] The study of COLIA 1 polymorphism may help in identifying thalassemia patients who are at higher risk to develop osteoporosis and pathologic fractures.[13]

Other genetic factors that have been reported to correlate with bone mineral damage in adult patients with β-thalassemia include the vitamin D receptor (VDR) Bsml BB polymorphism, the loss-of-function mutations in the gene of the vitamin D receptor, the sequence variation of 713-8delC of transforming growth factor-β1, the presence of restriction fragment length polymorphisms for the calcitonin (CT) receptor gene, estrogen receptor and interleukin-6 gene loci.[1,13] Although further studies are needed to exact final conclusion for the association between gene polymorphisms and bone mass in TM patients, COLIA 1 gene polymorphisms seem to be of importance in the pathogenesis of thalassemia-induced osteoporosis.

Acquired factors

Endocrine complications. Hypothyroidism, hypoparathyroidism, diabetes mellitus, and mainly hypogonadism (as delayed puberty and/or secondary hypogonadism) are considered as major causes of osteopenia/osteoporosis in TM.[1–3,5] Hemosiderosis of the pituitary gonadotrophic cells and iron deposition in the testes and ovaries are involved in the pathogenesis of endocrine complications in TM.[14] Hypogonadism is a well-recognized cause of osteoporosis and osteopenia not only in patients with TM but also in the general population and is characterized by high bone turnover with enhanced resorptive phase.[15] Estrogen and progesterone appear to inhibit osteoclast activity and promote bone formation, whereas testosterone has a direct stimulatory effect on osteoblast proliferation and differentiation.[3] IGFs play also an important role in bone remodeling. Low-serum IGF levels decrease osteoblast proliferation and bone matrix formation and reduce the activation of osteoclasts.[16] Several studies have demonstrated a positive correlation between the BMD of the lumbar spine and the IGF-I concentration.[17] It is well documented that the GH–IGF axis is defective in TM. Thalassemia patients have significantly lower circulating levels of IGF-I and the corresponding binding protein (IGFBP-III) than normal individuals; thus, leading to increased bone resorption, decreased bone formation, and finally to bone loss.[18,19]

Iron overload and desferrioxamine. Iron deposition in the bone impairs osteoid maturation and inhibits mineralization locally, resulting in focal osteomalakia. The mechanism by which iron overload interferes in osteoid maturation and mineralization includes the incorporation of iron into crystals of calcium hydroxyapatite, which consequently affects the growth of hydroxyapatite crystals and reduces the bone metabolism unit tensile strength.[20] Furthermore, desferrioxamine inhibits DNA synthesis, osteoblast, and fibroblast proliferation, osteoblast precursors differentiation, and collagen formation, although enhances osteoblast apoptosis, especially in patients who receive inappropriately high doses of desferrioxamine.[21]

Bone marrow expansion. Bone marrow expansion, which is a typical finding in patients with TM, has been considered as a major cause of bone destruction.[20] Transferrin receptor studies have demonstrated increased bone marrow activity even in patients with low reticulocyte count or marrow hypoplasia.[22] However, there was found no direct correlation between serum levels of soluble transferrin receptor and the severity of osteoporosis.[10]

Vitamin deficiencies. Vitamin C deficiency in iron-overload patients with low levels of serum ascorbic acid induces the risk of osteoporotic fractures.[23] Vitamin D deficiency is also implicated in the pathogenesis of osteoporosis in TM patients due to the regulatory effect of vitamin D in both osteoclasts and osteoblasts. Adequate calcium intake and small amounts of vitamin D administration during skeleton development can increase bone mass in adolescents and decrease bone loss in adult life. However, most studies have failed to show reduced serum levels of 25-hydroxyvitamin D in TM patients.

Physical activity. Patients with TM have reduced physical activity due to the complications of the disease and the overprotection by their parents who do not encourage muscle activity. Thus, the lack of physical activity is another predisposing factor for osteoporosis in TM patients and muscle activity has to be encouraged in these patients.[1–3]

These factors can lead to the destruction of bone in thalassemia patients by increasing the osteoclast function and/or reducing the osteoblast activity.

Increased osteoclast function in thalassemic patients with osteoporosis. During the last decade, there was sufficient data supporting that increased osteoclast activation is present in TM patients. Patients with TM and osteoporosis have elevated markers of bone resorption, such as N-terminal cross-linking telopeptide of collagen type-I (NTX) and tartrate-resistant acid phosphatase type 5b (TRACP-5b)[24,25] that correlated with BMD of the lumbar spine in these patients.[25,26] This increased osteoclast activity seems to be at least partially due to an imbalance in the receptor–activator of nuclear factor-kappa B ligand (RANKL)/osteoprotegerin (OPG) system and the overproduction of cytokines that are involved in the osteoclast differentiation and function.[26] The RANK/RANKL/OPG pathway is of great importance for the activation and proliferation of osteoclast precursors. We and others have shown that the ratio of sRANKL/OPG in the serum was increased in thalassemia patients with osteopenia/osteoporosis, providing evidence for the role of RANKL/OPG system in the pathogenesis of osteoporosis in thalassemia.[26–28] Serum levels of IL-1α, TNF-α, IL-6, and TGF-β, that are able to increase osteoclast function, were elevated in TM and correlated with bone resorption and lumbar BMD,[29] suggesting their involvement in the pathogenesis of TM osteoporosis and supporting the role of the immune system in the bone loss of TM.

Reduced osteoblast function in thalassemic patients with osteoporosis. There is evidence of reduced osteoblast function in TM. Histomorphometry studies have revealed that increased osteoid thickness, increased osteoid maturation and mineralization lag time, which indicate impaired bone matrix maturation, and defective mineralization is present in children and adolescents with TM.[20] In addition, iron deposits appeared along mineralization fronts and osteoid surfaces, whereas focal thickened osteoid seams were found together with focal iron deposits.[20,30] Finally, dynamic bone formation histomorphometry studies established reduced bone formation rate in TM patients.[20] This reduced bone formation is thought to-date to be mainly the result of iron poisoning in osteoblasts and/or the result of reduced function of GH and IGF-1 axis in TM patients.[1] However, novel molecules seem to be implicated in osteoblast dysfunction in TM. Dickkopf-1 (Dkk-1) is a Wnt signaling inhibitor, which inhibits the osteoblast differentiation and function. We have recently shown that serum levels of Dkk-1 were increased in TM patients with osteoporosis and correlated with lumbar spine and wrist BMD. Interestingly, when zoledronic acid (ZA) was given in these patients there was a reduction in Dkk-1 levels, which was not observed in the placebo group of this randomized trial.[31]

Management of thalassemia-associated osteoporosis

Prevention and general principles. Prevention and treatment of early bone loss make the best policy. Annual checking of BMD starting in adolescence is considered indispensable. Physical activity must always be encouraged. Moderate and high impact activities are to be supported. Exercise has additional benefits: it improves cardiovascular system, reduces the risk of diabetes, and prevents depression. Smoking should be discouraged. Adequate calcium intake during skeleton development can increase bone mass in adult life and in combination with administration of low doses of vitamin D may prevent bone loss and fractures.[32] Early diagnosis and treatment of diabetes mellitus is also important, as the association between diabetes and low bone mass in TM patients has been well documented.[1] Furthermore, adequate iron chelation may prevent iron toxicity in the bone and sufficient blood transfusions may inhibit uncontrolled bone marrow expansion.

Hormonal replacement. Prevention of hypogonadism seems to be the most effective way for preventing osteoporosis and other bone deformities in thalassemia patients.[1–3,5,32] Anapliotou and colleagues recommended that continuous hormonal replacement therapy with transdermal estrogen for females or human chorionic gonadotrophin for males improves bone density parameters.[33] However, despite hormonal replacement, calcium and vitamin D administration, effective iron chelation, and normalization of hemoglobin levels, patients with TM continue to lose bone mass.[6,7]

Calcitonin. Canatan and colleagues have evaluated the effect of calcitonin (CT), a potent inhibitor of osteoclasts, on bone mass in 14 patients with TM. One hundred IU of CT were administered, three times a week, for 1 year in combination with daily administration of 250 mg of calcium. At the end of treatment period, bone pain had disappeared, radiological findings of osteoporosis had been improved, and the number of fractures had been decreased in the treatment group but not in controls. CT had no important side effects.[34] Both parenteral and intranasal instillations are available.

Hydroxyurea. Ten patients with TM were given hydroxyurea (HU), at a dose of 1.5 g p.o. daily, in an attempt to reduce marrow hyperplasia diagnosed by MRI. HU improved bone pain and MRI findings.[35] However, in another study, the administration of HU for at least 2 years did not manage to show any improvement of the BMD compared with patients who did not receive HU.[36]

Bisphosphonates. The increased bone resorption observed in patients with thalassemia-induced osteoporosis has led to the use of bisphosphonates in the management of osteoporosis in this cohort of patients. Bisphosphonates are potent inhibitors of osteoclastic bone resorption. They act by inhibiting osteoclastic recruitment and maturation, preventing the development of monocyte precursors into osteoclasts, inducing osteoclast apoptosis and interrupting their attachment to the bone. In thalassemia osteoporosis, almost all generations of bisphosphonates have been used in an attempt to increase the BMD and improve the abnormal bone remodeling. Morabito and colleagues scheduled a randomized, placebo-controlled study to investigate the effects of 2 years daily oral administration of alendronate or intramascular administration of clodronate on BMD, bone turnover markers, safety, and tolerability in 25 thalassemia patients with osteoporosis.[37] Patients were randomized to receive placebo (eight patients) or 100 mg of clodronate, i.m., every 10 days (eight patients) or 10 mg of alendronate per os daily (nine patients). All patients also received 500 mg of elemental calcium and 400 IU cholecalciferol daily. After 2 years of follow-up, the lumbar spine and femoral neck BMD had decreased significantly in the placebo group. Clodronate reduced bone resorption markers, deoxypyrydinoline, and pyrydinoline, and inhibited bone loss but it was unable to increase BMD at all studied sites. Daily treatment with alendronate normalized the rate of bone turnover, and resulted in a rise in BMD of the spine and the hip. This increment was statistically significant at the femoral neck, whereas at the lumbar spine the gain was less marked. Alendronate caused few adverse effects, including upper gastrointestinal symptoms, but no patient discontinued the study.[37] The ineffectiveness of clodronate was established in another randomized, placebo-controlled trial.[38]

Pamidronate, a second-generation aminobisphosphonate, has been given intravenously in patients with TM and osteoporosis. First, Wonke evaluated the effect of 15 mg of pamidronate on BMD. Pamidronate was given in a 40 min infusion, at monthly intervals. A significant improvement in BMD was observed in most patients.[10] Our group compared the effects of two different doses of pamidronate, 30 mg versus 60 mg, on BMD of the lumbar spine, femoral neck, and forearm and on markers of bone remodeling and osteoclast function in 26 patients with thalassemia and osteoporosis. Thirteen patients with TM and five patients with TI were given pamidronate at a dose of 30 mg in a 2 h i.v. infusion, once a month for 12 months; another eight patients (four with TM and four with TI) received a dose of 60 mg/month, in an attempt to explore whether increasing the dose of pamidronate might have any additional effect. Both groups included patients with comparable degrees of osteoporosis and hypogonadism. All patients were also receiving calcium and vitamin D supplement prior and during the 12-month follow-up period of the study. Administration of 30 mg of pamidronate resulted in a significant increase of the BMD of the lumbar spine in all patients, but not the BMD of the femoral neck and the forearm. The 60 mg of pamidronate group showed a similarly significant increase in the BMD of the lumbar spine in both transfusion-dependent and transfusion-independent patients. Administration of both doses of pamidronate was also followed by a clear decrease of markers of bone resorption (NTX and TRACP-5b), OPG, and osteocalcin that was similar in patients of both treatment groups. Furthermore, most patients complaining for severe bone pain at the onset of the study had a significant reduction of pain after treatment period. No severe adverse-events were reported in this study.[25]

Zoledronic acid is the most potent third generation bisphosphonate to-date and has been found to be extremely efficacious in increasing BMD in TM patients. We reported the results of a randomized, placebo-controlled trial of ZA in 66 thalassemia patients with osteoporosis. The patients were randomized to receive 4 mg ZA intravenously every 6 months (23 patients; group A) or every 3 months (21 patients; group B), or to receive placebo every 3 months (22 patients; group C), for a period of 1 year. Patients of group B had a significant increase in their lumbar spine BMD, which was accompanied by dramatic reductions in bone pain, and bone markers. Patients in placebo group showed no alteration in BMD of any studied site or in bone pain scores; on the contrary, they had an aggravation in bone resorption. Therefore, this study confirmed that ZA is an effective treatment for increasing BMD and reducing bone resorption in thalassemia-induced osteoporosis with no serious side effects.[28] As the duration of ZA therapy had not been evaluated in any trial, we followed-up our patients for 24 months after discontinuation of ZA for groups A and B and for 12 months for group C (patients of group C received ZA, 4 mg every 3 months, i.v., for 12 months after their placebo 12-month administration). We found, interestingly, that at the 36th month, patients of group B continued to show an increase in the BMD of all studied sites despite the discontinuation of ZA. Furthermore, patients of groups A and C showed a dramatic increase in BMD of all studied sites compared with baseline values ($P < 0.01$) The increase of BMD observed in groups A and C was accompanied by a comparable reduction in bone resorption marker CTX at the 36th month, which had not reported at the 12th month; on the contrary in group C there was an increase in CTX at the 12th month. These observations suggest that ZA continues to act after its discontinuation.[39]

In another recent study, we confirmed that the increase of erythropoietic activity in TI, which continues irrespectively of the improvement of BMD produced by ZA, seems to be a major cause of bone loss in this hemoglobinopathy. Soluble transferrin receptor (sTfR) and erythropoietin (Epo) serum levels are increased in TI but we showed for the first time in the literature that this elevation was further increased by time, although BMD was improved by ZA.[40]

All described studies confirm the effectiveness of bisphosphonates in the treatment of thalassemia-induced osteoporosis. Alendronate, pamidronate, and ZA seem to have the greater efficacy. However, more trials must be conducted to clarify the exact role of each biphosphonate, the long-term benefit and side effects as well as the effects of the combination of bisphosphonates with other effective agents, such as hormonal replacement, in thalassemia-induced osteoporosis.

Conclusion and future perspectives

Thalassemia-associated osteoporosis is multifactorial and, therefore, very difficult in its management. Osteoporosis is a progressive disease; thus, prevention and early diagnosis are very important. Adequate hormonal replacement, effective iron chelation, improvement of hemoglobin levels, calcium and vitamin D administration, physical activity, and smoking cessation are the main to-date measures for the management of the disease. However, novel pathogenetic data suggest that the reduced osteoblastic activity, which is believed to be the basic mechanism of bone loss in TM, is accompanied by a comparable or even greater increase in bone resorption. Therefore, the role of bisphosphonates arises as major in the management of osteoporosis in these patients. However, many aspects have to be clarified before the broad use of bisphosphonates in TM-induced osteoporosis: which one? how long? and at what dose? The combination of bisphosphonates with other effective agents has also to be evaluated in randomized trials. Other novel agents that stimulate bone formation such as teriparatide, a recombinant peptide fragment of parathyroid hormone, strontium ranelate, a second anabolic agent, that seem to prevent osteoporotic fractures in postmenopausal women, are being studied but their effects in TM-induced osteoporosis remains to be proven. Finally, antibodies against RANKL, such as denosumab, which has just been licensed by FDA for the treatment of postmenopausal osteoporosis, and antibodies against Dkk-1 or against sclerostin may be future agents for the effective management of this difficult complication of thalassemia.

Conflicts of interest

The authors have received research support and honoraria from NOVARTIS.

References

1. Voskaridou, E. & E. Terpos. 2004. New insights into the pathophysiology and management of osteoporosis in patients with beta thalassaemia. *Br. J. Haematol.* **127:** 127–139.
2. Garofalo, F., A. Piga, R. Lala, *et al.* 1998. Bone metabolism in thalassemia. *Ann. N.Y. Acad. Sci.* **850:** 475–478.
3. Voskaridou, E. & E. Terpos. 2008. Pathogenesis and management of osteoporosis in thalassemia. *Pediatr. Endocrinol. Rev.* **6**(Suppl. 1): 86–93.
4. Hatori, M., J. Sparkman, C.C. Teixeira, *et al.* 1995. Effects of deferoximine on chondrocyte alkaline phosphatase activity: proxidant role of deferoximine in thalassemia. *Calcif. Tissue Int.* **57:** 229–236.
5. Olivieri, N.F. 1999. The beta-thalassemias. *N. Engl. J. Med.* **341:** 99–109.
6. Lasco, A., N. Morabito, A. Gaudio, *et al.* 2001. Effects of hormonal replacement therapy on bone metabolism in young adults with beta-thalassemia major. *Osteoporos. Int.* **12:** 570–575.
7. Carmina, E., G. Di Fede, N. Napoli, *et al.* 2004. Hypogonadism and hormone replacement therapy on bone mass of adult women with thalassemia major. *Calcif. Tissue Int.* **74:** 68–71.
8. World Health Organization. 1994. Assessment of fracture risks and its application to screening for post-menopausal osteoporosis. Report of a WHO Study Group. *World Health Organ. Tech. Rep. Ser.* **843:** 1–129.
9. Binkley, N.C., P. Schmeer, R.D. Wasnich & L. Lenchik. 2002. What are the criteria by which a densitometric diagnosis of osteoporosis can be made in males and non-Caucasians? *J. Clin. Densitom.* **5**(Suppl.): 19–27.
10. Wonke, B., C. Jensen, J.J. Hanslip, *et al.* 1998. Genetic and acquired predisposing factors and treatment of osteoporosis in thalassaemia major. *J. Pediatr. Endocrinol. Metab.* **11**(Suppl. 3): 795–801.
11. Uitterlinden, A.G., A.E. Weel, H. Burger, *et al.* 2001. Interaction between the vitamin D receptor gene and collagen type I alpha 1 gene in susceptibility for fracture. *J. Bone Miner. Res.* **16:** 379–385.
12. Uitterlinden, A.G., H. Burger, C.M. van Duijn, *et al.* 2000. Adjacent genes, for COL2A1 and the vitamin D receptor, are associated with separate features of radiographic osteoarthritis of the knee. *Arthritis Rheum.* **43:** 1456–1464.
13. Perrotta, S., M.D. Cappellini, F. Bertoldo, *et al.* 2000. Osteoporosis in beta-thalassaemia major patients: analysis of the genetic background. *Br. J. Haematol.* **111:** 461–466.
14. Berkovitch, M., T. Bistritzer, S.D. Milone, *et al.* 2000. Iron deposition in the anterior pituitary in homozygous beta-thalassemia: MRI evaluation and correlation with gonadal function. *J. Pediatr. Endocrinol. Metab.* **13:** 179–184.
15. Riggs, B.L., S. Khosla & L.J. Melton III. 1998. A unitary model for involutional osteoporosis: estrogen deficiency causes both type I and type II osteoporosis in postmenopausal women and contributes to bone loss in aging men. *J. Bone Miner. Res.* **13:** 763–773.
16. Geusens, P.P. & S. Boonen. 2002. Osteoporosis and the growth hormone-insulin-like growth factor axis. *Horm. Res.* **58**(Suppl. 3): 49–55.
17. Rucker, D., S. Ezzat, A. Diamandi, *et al.* 2004. IGF-I and testosterone levels as predictors of bone mineral density in healthy, community-dwelling men. *Clin. Endocrinol.* **60:** 491–499.
18. Soliman, A.T., N. El Banna, M. Abdel Fattah, *et al.* 1998. Bone mineral density in prepubertal children with beta-thalassemia: correlation with growth and hormonal data. *Metabolism* **47:** 541–548.
19. Morabito, N., A. Gaudio, A. Lasco, *et al.* 2004. Osteoprotegerin and RANKL in the pathogenesis of thalassemia-induced osteoporosis: new pieces of the puzzle. *J. Bone Miner. Res.* **19:** 722–727.
20. Mahachoklertwattana, P., V. Srikulchayanonta, A. Chuansumrit, *et al.* 2003. Bone histomorphometry in children and adolescents with beta-thalassemia disease: iron-associated focal osteomalacia. *J. Clin. Endocrinol. Metab.* **88:** 3966–3972.
21. De Sanctis, V., A. Pinamonti, A. Di Palma, *et al.* 1996. Growth and development in thalassaemia major patients with severe bone lesions due to desferrioxamine. *Eur. J. Pediatr.* **155:** 368–372.
22. Ma, E.S., K.K. Lam, A.Y. Chan, *et al.* 2003. Transferrin receptor-2 polymorphisms and iron overload in transfusion independent β-thalassemia intermedia. *Haematologica* **88:** 345–346 [letter].
23. Michelson, J. & A. Cohen. 1988. Incidence and treatment of fractures in thalassemia. *J. Orthop. Trauma* **2:** 29–32.
24. Voskaridou, E., M.C. Kyrtsonis, E. Terpos, *et al.* 2001. Bone resorption is increased in young adults with thalassaemia major. *Br. J. Haematol.* **112:** 36–41.

25. Voskaridou, E., E. Terpos, G. Spina, *et al.* 2003. Pamidronate is an effective treatment for osteoporosis in patients with beta-thalassaemia. *Br. J. Haematol.* **123:** 730–737.
26. Dresner Pollack, R., E. Rachmilewitz, A. Blumenfeld, *et al.* 2000. Bone mineral metabolism in adults with beta-thalassaemia major and intermedia. *Br. J. Haematol.* **111:** 902–907.
27. Voskaridou, E. & E. Terpos. 2005. Osteoprotegerin to soluble receptor activator of nuclear factor kappa-B ligand ratio is reduced in patients with thalassaemia-related osteoporosis who receive vitamin D3. *Eur. J. Haematol.* **74:** 359–361.
28. Voskaridou, E., A. Anagnostopoulos, K. Konstantopoulos, *et al.* 2006. Zoledronic acid for the treatment of osteoporosis in patients with beta-thalassemia: results from a single-center, randomized, placebo-controlled trial. *Haematologica* **91:** 1193–1202.
29. Morabito, N., G.T. Russo, A. Gaudio, *et al.* 2007. The "lively" cytokines network in beta-Thalassemia Major-related osteoporosis. *Bone* **40:** 1588–1594.
30. Domrongkitchaiporn, S., V. Sirikulchayanonta, P. Angchaisuksiri, *et al.* 2003. Abnormalities in bone mineral density and bone histology in thalassemia. *J. Bone Miner. Res.* **18:** 1682–1688.
31. Voskaridou, E., D. Christoulas, C. Xirakia, *et al.* 2009. Serum Dickkopf-1 is increased and correlates with reduced bone mineral density in patients with thalassemia-induced osteoporosis. Reduction post-zoledronic acid administration. *Haematologica* **94:** 725–728.
32. Lindsay, R. 1993. Prevention and treatment of osteoporosis. *Lancet* **341:** 801–805.
33. Anapliotou, M.L., I.T. Kastanias, P. Psara, *et al.* 1995. The contribution of hypogonadism to the development of osteoporosis in thalassaemia major: new therapeutic approaches. *Clin. Endocrinol.* **42:** 279–287.
34. Canatan, D., N. Akar & A. Arcasoy. 1995. Effects of calcitonin therapy on osteoporosis in patients with thalassemia. *Acta Haematol.* **93:** 20–24.
35. Angastiniotis, M., N. Pavlides, K. Aristidou, *et al.* 1998. Bone pain in thalassaemia: assessment of DEXA and MRI findings. *J. Pediatr. Endocrinol. Metab.* **11**(Suppl. 3): 779–784.
36. Kosaryan, M., M.F. Zadeh & V.K. Shahi. 2004. The bone density of thalassemic patients of Boo Ali Sina hospital, Sari, Iran in 2002; does hydroxyurea help? *Pediatr. Endocrinol. Rev.* **2**(Suppl. 2): 303–306.
37. Morabito, N., A. Lasco, A. Gaudio, *et al.* 2002. Bisphosphonates in the treatment of thalassemia-induced osteoporosis. *Osteoporos. Int.* **13:** 644–649.
38. Pennisi, P., G. Pizzarelli, M. Spina, *et al.* 2003. Quantitative ultrasound of bone and clodronate effects in thalassemia-induced osteoporosis. *J. Bone Miner. Metab.* **21:** 402–408.
39. Voskaridou, E., D. Christoulas, M. Konstantinidou, *et al.* 2008. Continuous improvement of bone mineral density two years post zoledronic acid discontinuation in patients with thalassemia-induced osteoporosis: long term follow up a randomized, placebo-controlled trial. *Haematologica* **93:** 1588–1590.
40. Voskaridou, E., D. Christoulas, E. Antoniadou & E. Terpos. 2008. Continuous increase in erythropoietic activity despite the improvement in bone mineral density by zoledronic acid in patients with thalassemia induced osteoporosis. *Acta Haematol.* **119:** 40–44.

Ann. N.Y. Acad. Sci. ISSN 0077-8923

ANNALS OF THE NEW YORK ACADEMY OF SCIENCES
Issue: *Cooley's Anemia: Ninth Symposium*

Health care transition in thalassemia: pediatric to adult-oriented care

Laurice Levine[1] and Matthew Levine[2]

[1]Department of Hematology/Oncology, Children's Hospital and Research Center Oakland, Oakland, California. [2]Author and editor, Kingston, Washington

Address for correspondence: Laurice Levine, M.A., C.C.L.S., Thalassemia Outreach Coordinator, Children's Hospital and Research Center Oakland, 747 52nd Street Oakland, CA 94609–1809. LLevine@mail.cho.org

Improved technology and medical advances have increased the lifespan for people with thalassemia. As thalassemia is no longer exclusively a pediatric blood disorder, consideration must now be given to transition planning from pediatric to adult care. The complexity of thalassemia disease, coupled with the changing face of U.S. health care, creates barriers to transitional planning. Additional barriers develop because this chronic disease is less common in adults, leaving caregivers unprepared to facilitate proper adult treatment. This paper will discuss two common U.S. health care settings where care is provided to adults with thalassemia. It will also offer health care administrators, providers, policy makers, and the thalassemia community at large some recommendations on the provision of comprehensive, quality care to assure the best possible outcomes no matter what setting is available to adult patients living with thalassemia.

Keywords: thalassemia; pediatric care; adult care; transition

Thalassemia and transition

Thalassemia is a genetic blood disorder which causes severe anemia due to little or no hemoglobin production. Complications for patients, mostly due to their treatments, are frequent, and therefore, it is vital for patients to be seen by a thalassemia specialist at least once a year and for comprehensive care to be implemented as part of the treatment plan.

Advancements in medical technology, research, and treatment are credited with an increase in lifespan and quality of life for those who have thalassemia. The increase in lifespan necessitates a transition from pediatric care to adult care, which was unwarranted in previous generations, when patients' survival into adulthood was rarely seen. Transition occurs throughout all stages of development. Hence, people with lifelong chronic illness such as thalassemia evolve throughout each transition in life, and in various stages of their health care, as well.

A consensus statement from the American Academy of Pediatrics, the American Academy of Family Physicians, and the American College of Physicians–American Society of Internal Medicine in 2002 illustrates health care transition for young adults with special health care needs: "Transition in health care for young adults with special needs is a dynamic, lifelong process that seeks to meet their individual needs as they move from childhood to adulthood. The goal is to maximize lifelong functioning and potential through the provision of high-quality, developmentally appropriate health care services that continue uninterrupted as the individual moves from adolescence to adulthood."[1]

Pediatric settings

Children's hospitals are the prime delivery systems for the treatment of adult thalassemia patients. Because transition is a relatively new concept for thalassemia patients, transition often remains

doi: 10.1111/j.1749-6632.2010.05598.x

within the walls of pediatric hospitals, with pediatric providers becoming adult specialists, as well. Although there are some advantages to adults being treated in pediatric centers, there are also negative effects. Some pros include the following: There is interdisciplinary, comprehensive specialty care in a family- and patient-centered setting. The approach is more psychosocial and supportive, it retains a developmental focus, and long-established relationships with care providers since infancy build trust over time. Also, pain treatment is not questioned as much as in an adult facility, and patients have more access to research and new treatments. Despite these positive points, there are several cons, as well. For example, doctors and medical staff have less knowledge of adult issues, such as sexuality and reproductive health. Consequently, care is decentralized, because patients must seek specialists outside of the children's hospital. The permission of heavy family involvement and the more nurturing environment may foster patient dependence, rather than allowing patients to take charge of their own care. In addition, adults are often not afforded the same rights as younger patients in a children's hospital.

Adult settings

Ideally, one would think that adult patients with thalassemia would benefit from being in an adult care setting, and in the future, that will most likely be the case. However, because transition to an adult facility is a relatively new occurrence, there are both advantages and disadvantages to this setting, as well. One advantage is that caregivers are trained in adult medicine and are prepared to deal with adult health issues. Also, internists communicate directly with patients, allowing for more privacy and self-reliance. In-patient admissions are easier, care is more centralized, and the medical staff is less tolerant of noncompliance with the necessary treatment regimen. But along with these come several disadvantages. Staff members are less familiar with childhood illness, and care is more disease-centered than patient-centered. Families may become more peripheral than they should be, and the environment and/or doctor may be perceived as cold, resulting in difficulty establishing a relationship of trust. Finally, the adult care staff may pay too little attention to developmental issues and may also not be up to date on the latest research and any new therapies that might be provided to patients.

Barriers to transition

Many barriers to transition are most likely the result of the novelty of transition, and the hope is that many of these barriers will fall as pediatric transition to adult care settings becomes more commonplace. Nevertheless, formidable barriers remain in place for the present and near future, and it is only through discussion and implementation of suggestions that these barriers will eventually come down. One of the most challenging issues in transition is the difficulty in identifying adult primary care providers, as so few have the necessary knowledge, training, and experience to treat pediatric-onset illnesses. A related issue is the difficulty in identifying adult subspecialists. Patients' families may also be resistant to transition to adult care facilities due to fear of the unknown quantity that they represent. In addition, medical insurance issues create barriers as patients try to switch their care providers. There may be a lack of institutional support if an adult facility is unwilling or unable to devote the necessary time for planning and addressing important transition issues, as well as resources and personnel to care for pediatric-onset illness. Lack of communication between pediatric and adult care facilities can be a problem, and this, as well as many of the aforementioned barriers, also creates further communication problems between patients and their adult care providers. Other issues may include transitions based on age, rather than maturity, leading to patients who are not yet ready to move from pediatric to adult care; the abrupt end of pediatric treatment services without a transition process or pathway in place to facilitate movement from one care provider to another; and differences in basic orientation, philosophy, and practice between pediatric and adult care centers.

Recommendations for facilitating transition

"...we estimate that every year, more than 500,000 children with special health care needs turn 18 years of age."[2] A successful transition is critical for a patient's health and well-being. As technology progresses, there will be a greater number of patients undergoing this challenging process. Keeping in mind all stages of development, the following are suggestions for a smooth transition from birth to 5 years of age, from 6 to 11 years of age, and for adolescents.

Birth to 5 years of age:

- Facilitate trusting relationships with parents and caregivers
- Foster personal and medical independence and creative problem-solving from the beginning; the child should be a responsible member of the treatment team early in the process
- Encourage parents to document the child's medical history
- Encourage the child's decision-making skills by offering choices
- Encourage peer relationships
- Have knowledge of and recommend community support agencies
- Ask the child, "What do you want to do when you grow up?"
- Teach the child about his or her health care needs

Six to eleven years of age:

- Facilitate interactions with health care providers
- Assess the child's perception of his or her condition and build on the child's understanding
- Encourage age and developmentally appropriate play and outlet activities both in and outside of the hospital
- Encourage decision-making skills
- Discuss consequences of behaviors and choices
- Discuss future goals and plans

Adolescents:

- Develop therapeutic relationships
- Provide emotional support and foster constructive acceptance
- Facilitate the understanding of diagnosis and treatment, development of mastery, and normalization
- Encourage the patient's involvement in his or her own care
- Allow for the provision of schooling while hospitalized; aid in the pursuit of interests; discuss goals for the future; and help in the identification of family and community resources
- Advocate for teen programs in hospitals that are staffed with a dedicated child life specialist
- Celebrate transitions; develop rites of passage that mark health care transitions, such as graduation from high school
- Participate in the development of a transition plan with an interdisciplinary team; discuss closure and the appropriate and sensitive termination of pediatric care
- Have an orientation that is focused on the future
- Anticipate changes and develop a flexible plan for the future

Conclusions

We suggest potential improvements for adult care in pediatric and adult settings and ideas for both patients and families to consider as aids to improving this care.

The following are further suggestions for improved adult care in a pediatric setting:

- Centralize care
- Buy in with management
- Make sure of the commitment of everyone involved
- Install a team of adult specialists and provide psychosocial support on site
- Work better with insurance companies
- Educate all staff
- Add evening and weekend clinics
- Streamline and computerize the registration system for efficiency

The following are further suggestions for improved adult care in an adult setting:

- Add a comprehensive clinic that includes all specialties
- Set up routine meetings and collaboration
- Add education on pediatric-onset illnesses for adult doctors in medical school

The following are further suggestions for patient and family responsibilities:

- Be informed and proactive
- Seek a specialty center for annual evaluations
- Be involved in the medical team
- Vote for legislation that improves health care for patients with chronic illness
- Seek support from thalassemia organizations, i.e., the Cooley's Anemia Foundation (CAF); the Thalassemia Action Group (TAG); the

Thalassemia International Federation (TIF); and the Thalassemia Support Foundation (TSF)

- Support medical research for thalassemia treatment and actively participate in research trials

"Transition is not an event, it is a process."[3] It takes time.

Acknowledgment

The authors would like to acknowledge contributions made by Dawn Adler.

Conflicts of interest

The authors declare no conflicts of interest.

References

1. American Academy of Pediatrics, American Academy of Family Physicians, and American College of Physicians–American Society of Internal Medicine. 2002. A consensus statement on health care transition for young adults with special health care needs. *Pediatrics* **110:** 1304.
2. Reiss, J. & R. Gibson. 2002. Health care transition: destinations unknown. *Pediatrics* **110:** 1308.
3. Society for Adolescent Medicine. 1995. Summary of conference recommendations. *J. Adolesc. Health* **17:** 6–9.

Ann. N.Y. Acad. Sci. ISSN 0077-8923

ANNALS OF THE NEW YORK ACADEMY OF SCIENCES
Issue: *Cooley's Anemia: Ninth Symposium*

Ninth Cooley's Anemia Symposium: summary and perspective

Arthur W. Nienhuis

Department of Hematology, St. Jude Children's Research Hospital, Memphis, Tennessee

Addresses for correspondence: Arthur W. Nienhuis, M.D., Department of Hematology, St. Jude Children's Research Hospital, 262 Danny Thomas Place, MS 341, Memphis, TN 38105. arthur.nienhuis@stjude.org

The Ninth Cooley's Symposium provided an outstanding summary of progress in the field. Highlights of the conference included the report of clinical benefit in one of two patients treated in a gene therapy trial. Another major breakthrough was the report that the transcriptional factor, BCL11A, is a key molecular component of the γ-globin silencing mechanism that results in the fetal to adult perinatal switch. The ability to evaluate tissue iron is becoming increasingly more sophisticated, with results presented at this conference indicating that independent measurement of cardiac ferritin and hemosiderin can be achieved with specific MRI sequences. The three available iron chelators, deferoxamine, deferiprone, and deferasirox, provide a potent therapeutic armamentarium so that effective chelation regimens can be devised for most individual patients. Unfortunately, compliance remains a significant issue despite the availability of oral chelators. Modification of conditioning regimens and the use of alternative donor sources have made stem cell transplantation available to an increasing number of patients with progressive improvement in outcome. Despite many advances, the global burden of disease for the thalassemias remains very high, with many challenges that still need to be addressed in order to optimize treatment for the majority of patients.

Keywords: thalassemia; gene therapy; fetal hemoglobin; iron metabolism; iron chelators; stem cell transplantation

Introduction

I very much enjoyed attending the 9th Symposium dedicated to Cooley's Anemia and wish to congratulate Drs. Vichinsky, Neufeld, and Granger for organizing an interesting and successful meeting. As usual, the meeting was multidisciplinary with sessions covering a broad spectrum of topics ranging from basic science to clinical application. Despite being multidisciplinary, each of the symposia has a few dominant themes reflecting areas where significant progress has been made in the years following the preceding Symposium. I recall the first Symposium that I attended which was held in the Barbizon Plaza Hotel in New York in 1973. In the years leading up to this 3rd Cooley's Symposium, biologically active messenger RNA had been isolated from normal and thalassemic reticulocytes and the characteristic imbalance in chain synthesis reproduced in a cell-free system.[1,2] Discussion of these molecular advances was one of the dominant themes of that Symposium. Retroviral reverse transcriptase had been discovered in 1970[3,4] and the ability of this enzyme to transcribe any RNA molecule into DNA made possible the synthesis of complementary DNA copies of messenger RNA. Serious consideration regarding the development of gene therapy was already underway in 1973[5,6] but more than 35 years of work were required[7] before the first patients were treated. At this conference, Philippe LeBoulch reported in detail on the outcome in one of the patients. Several other presentations related to the development of gene therapy for the hemoglobin disorders making this one of the dominant themes of the 9th Symposium.

Gene therapy

At the 8th Symposium held in Orlando in 2005, Arthur Bank described a planned clinical trial of gene therapy that was soon to open in France.[8] Although some of us were skeptical because of

doi: 10.1111/j.1749-6632.2010.05549.x

uncertainty regarding whether the efficiency of stem cell targeted gene transfer was potentially adequate to achieve a therapeutic benefit, the trial opened as planned and two participants have been enrolled as described by Phiippe LeBoulch at this Symposium with very interesting results. The protocol calls for enrollment of a total of 10 participants, 5 with thalassemia and 5 with sickle cell anemia. The participants may range in age from 5 to 35 years, although the protocol stipulates that the first three participants be 15 years or older. Either bone marrow or peripheral blood may be used as a source of stem cells and cryopreserved mobilized peripheral blood $CD34^+$ cells are retained in the event they are needed because of delayed reconstitution. Participants receive 16 mg/kg of Bulsulfex over 4 days, resulting in profound myelosuppression. The first participant to be enrolled was a 30-year-old man with HbE/β° thalassemia. The transduced cells failed to engraft and the backup stem cells were given on day 27 after which the patient recovered uneventfully. The second participant was enrolled at age 17. He too had HbE/β° thalassemia and had been transfusion dependent with baseline hemoglobins of between 4 and 6 gm/dL. Now 2 years posttransplantation of transduced cells, the patient is transfusion independent with a hemoglobin of approximately 10 gm/dL. Approximately, one-third of the total hemoglobin contains the transgene-encoded globin with the remainder being approximately equal mixtures of HbE and HbF from the patient's globin genes. The clinical improvement was attributed primarily to a 10-fold increase in red cell lifespan. Approximately, 10–20% of the erythroid and myeloid cells contain the integrated vector sequences. Molecular analysis detected fewer than 300 distinct integration sites with 24 being common to both myeloid and lymphoid lineages. Sixty-five percent of the transduced cells had an integration site in HMGA2, a gene thought to be a regulator of chromatin structure and potency in stem cells; it is not expressed in normal somatic cells, although it is often expressed in both benign and malignant neoplasms.[9] Expression of a mutated version of the HMGA2 was detected in erythroid cells of the gene therapy patient. The upstream exons were spliced into a cryptic splice site in the chromatin insulator within the vector and the transcript was polyadenylated by the control elements in the long terminal repeat (LTR). The vector contains tandem copies of the 250 base pair (bp) insulator element from the chicken globin HS4 although, the integrated form of the proviral genome has a single 250 bp element in most LTRs. Mathematical analysis suggests that the HGMA2 insertion would have to confer an approximately twofold proliferative advantage in primitive, multipotent cells to account for the partial clonal dominance within the transduced cell population.

This well-studied participant in a gene therapy trial provides proof of concept with respect to the potential efficacy of lentiviral vector mediated globin gene transfer for thalassemia. A recent report of the successful use of a lentiviral vector for treatment of X-linked adrenoleukodystrophy[10] provides additional support for the use of lentiviral vectors for therapeutic gene transfer. However, experience in the hemoglobinopathy trial highlights several issues that remain to be fully addressed before broad application of gene transfer for the treatment of thalassemia becomes feasible. Engraftment of limited numbers of stem cells, marginal transduction efficiencies, insulator failure, proto-oncogene activation, and partial clonal dominance remain as significant challenges.

Reported at this meeting were on-going efforts to address these challenges. The use of alternative envelope proteins to generate vector particles has been proposed as one strategy for improving transduction efficiency.[11] However, recent work in my laboratory has indicated that the vesicular stomatitis virus-G (VSV-G) envelope protein used by LeBoulch and colleagues yields vector particles, which transduce primitive human hematopoietic cells more efficiently than other envelope proteins derived from γ-retroviruses, which have been proposed as alternates.[12,13] Dr. Yannaki and colleagues reported on their studies employing a combination of Hydroxyurea treatment to suppress hematopoiesis followed by granulocyte-colony stimulation factor mobilization (G-CSF) to recover stem cells. Results obtained to date suggest that an optimal regimen has not yet been defined. Consideration is being given to hypertransfusion as an alternative to suppress hematopoiesis. The use of AMD3100 (Perixator)[14] rather than G-CSF for mobilization is also being considered. Michel Sadelain reported on three patients successfully mobilized with G-CSF at Memorial Sloan-Kettering; recovery of $CD34^+$ cells appeared to be adequate although larger numbers may be required to insure adequate engraftment following transduction. Vector modifications developed in the Sadelain lab have resulted in a 20-fold increase in titer allowing scale-up to produce a clinical lot adequate for treatment of 10 participants. At this point, there is not a consensus on the appropriate preparative regimen. As noted earlier, the French trial uses 16 mg/kg of Busulfex whereas the trial proposed by Michel Sadelain, which is partially through regulatory review, proposes the use of half that amount. Similarly, there is not a consensus as to whether the vector should include insulator elements in the LTR to improve expression per vector copy as reported by Malik at the Symposium and potentially to enhance safety.[15] The trial at Sloan-Kettering will use an optimized vector without insulator elements. Trials proposed by Malik and Persons utilizing a vector encoding γ-globin with insulator elements are at earlier stages of development. The Bodine laboratory continues to explore the use of regulatory elements from red cell cytoskeletal protein genes as alternates to the globin regulatory elements. They have identified a barrier element from the Ankyrin-1E promoter, which has been shown by the Rivella lab to enhance β-globin gene expression in both mouse and human cells when placed in the LTR.

Fetal hemoglobin

Clinical observations indicating that higher levels of fetal hemoglobin production ameliorate the phenotype in both sickle cell anemia and thalassemia have fostered extensive efforts to understand the developmental mechanisms of hemoglobin switching. Over the past three decades since molecular characterization of the globin loci was initiated, much has been learned regarding gene organization, distant regulatory elements, the locus control region, chromatin structure, epigenetic modification, and various transcriptional activators and repressors and the sequences within the locus with which they interact. Despite this extensive fund of general knowledge regarding globin gene expression, the specific mechanism that controls HbF production during fetal and adult life remained obscure. Now work in the Orkin lab reported at the Symposium has identified BCL11A as a key factor in perinatal silencing of the γ-globin gene.[16,17] Attention had been drawn to this zinc finger protein because of genetic linkage studies, indicating that certain polymorphisms within the locus were associated with elevated HbF production in adults.[18,19] BCL11A is required for normal B-cell development but animals lacking BCL11A exhibit no erythroid phenotype. Reported by Dr. Orkin at the Symposium were recent results indicating that BCL11A knockout animals that are transgenic for the human β-globin locus have persistent expression of the γ-globin gene postnatally. Inhibition of BCL11A production by RNAi mechanisms enhances HbF in adult human erythroid cells as originally shown in the Orkin laboratory and now reproduced by Andrew Wilber and Derek Persons as reported by Dr. Persons during the Symposium. Dr. Persons also reported that an engineered zinc finger transactivator designed to interact with the proximal γ-globin gene promoter[20] enhances HbF production in erythroblasts developed from normal and thalassemic $CD34^+$ cells in culture.

Although BCL11A is clearly a major player in developmental switching and in modulating HbF levels in adult erythroid cells, substantial prior work had implicated the proximal γ-promoters as being involved in the silencing mechanism. Multiple binding sites for BCL11A are found throughout the globin locus but it does not appear to interact directly with either the γ- or β-globin gene promoters. Using engineered mouse strains, the Grosveld laboratory has developed a protocol for purification of proteins that interact with the γ-promoters in murine erythroid cells in which it has been silenced. Mass spectroscopy suggests that many proteins interact with the promoters presumably as multiprotein complexes. Dr. Grosveld reported that reduced expression of two candidate repressors by RNAi enhanced HbF production in human adult erythroid cells. Initial data suggests that BCL11A may enhance expression of one of these repressors thereby indirectly contributing to silencing in addition to its direct effect.

There is continued interest in developing agents that enhance fetal hemoglobin production in adult patients. Although the past decade has witnessed the development and approval of Hydroxyurea for this purpose, progress in the study of other agents has been slower. Dr. Perrine summarized work done with other agents, including short chain fatty acids, erythropoietin, and demethylating agents that have been studied in limited clinical trials. The combination of erythropoietin and butyrate has been used to eliminate the transfusion requirement in a small number of thalassemic patients. Newer agents are entering clinical trials. Some have argued that demethylating agents particularly should be revisited because of their potency and the fact that the fear of mutagenic effects that inhibited their use in the 80s have not been realized. Indeed, Decitabine has been approved by the FDA for use in myelodysplastic syndrome, which is often a premalignant state. A small clinical trial in patients with thalassemia is underway with NHLBI support in the Thalassemia Clinical Trials Network, which should yield interesting results.

Iron metabolism

The central role of hepcidin in iron metabolism and in the pathogenesis and management of iron toxicity and thalassemia was reviewed by Chaim Hershko in a keynote lecture. Hepcidin is 25-amino acid peptide that is produced primarily by the liver in response to a variety of stimuli known to modulate tissue iron stores and serum iron availability. Hepcidin interacts with ferroportin 1, a 12 transmembrane domain protein expressed on intracellular membranes, the basolateral surface of epithelium, and on the surface of nonpolarized cells.[21] Interaction of hepcidin with ferroportin 1 results in endocytosis and degradation of both proteins. Thus, hepcidin inhibits expression of ferroportin 1, which is the effector of cellular iron export. Diminished hepcidin expression is associated with increased iron absorption and release from macrophages, whereas excessive hepcidin results in diminished absorption and retention of iron in the phagocytic compartment. The role of hepcidin in thalassemia was described by Dr. Nemeth. Ineffective erythropoiesis is associated with release of substances from dying erythroid cells, including growth differentiation factor 15 (GDF15)[22] and twisted gastrulation (TWSG1)[23], which inhibit hepcidin production accounting for excessive iron absorption. Dr. Nemeth described efforts to derive truncated versions of hepcidin that act nevertheless to downregulate ferroportin 1. The use of such agents is compromised by their short half-life in the circulation, which may be overcome by utilization of D-amino acids for synthesis. One of the key regulators of hepcidin synthesis is TMPRSS6, a transmembrane serum protease expressed primarily in liver. As reported by Mark Fleming, mutations in this protein have been implicated in congenital and acquired iron refractory iron deficiency anemia.[24] The protease apparently cleaves hemojuvelin, which is part of a multiprotein complex that modulates hepcidin synthesis in the liver and the mutations are associated with increased hepcidin production.

The Rivella lab has explored the role of ineffective erythropoiesis in the pathophysiology of iron overload in thalassemic mouse models. Reasoning that the ineffective erythroid expansion that occurs within the thalassemic bone marrow reflects the action of erythropoietin, they treated thalassemic mice with an inhibitor of the protein kinase, Jak2, the immediate downstream effector molecule that interacts with the EPO receptor. Administration of the Jak2 inhibitor was associated with a marked decrease in ineffective erythropoiesis, a decrease in splenomegaly, and a minimal reduction in red cell production. The dramatic decrease in splenomegaly was shown to be due to a reduction of extramedullary hematopoiesis in the spleen and its complete elimination in the liver.

Iron uptake by ferritin damages the protein subunits and accelerates its conversion to toxic hemosiderin. Dr. Thiel described three general strategies to manipulate ferritin with the goal of minimizing the effects of excess iron. Ferritin is a gated pore protein and, using phage screening methodology, peptides have been identified that increase release of iron by ferritin. Most ferritin mRNA is not translated because it is in complex with a protein that blocks translation. The crystal structure of the mRNA protein complex has been determined with a goal of developing small molecules that release the mRNA to allow higher levels of ferritin synthesis. In principle, these peptides could be linked to an iron chelator to either trigger or accelerate iron release by ferritin and its removal from the cell. In the third approach, strategies are being sought to decrease nutritional iron uptake with dietary manipulation.

Tissue iron measurement

Measurement of tissue iron by magnetic resonance imaging is becoming increasingly sophisticated. Dr. Brittingham reported on a new, fast, spin-echo sequence that permits calculation of a parameter, RR2, that measures ferritin iron independently of hemosiderin. This parameter changes relatively rapidly with initiation of chelation in contrast to myocardial R2*, which predominantly reflects hemosiderin iron. Dr. Wood described the imperfect relationship between hepatic and cardiac iron. Loading of the liver as well as the pancreas occurs progressively well before iron begins to accumulate in heart. Similarly, successful chelation therapy removes substantial amounts of liver iron before myocardial iron reduction begins to occur. A low cardiac T2*, reflecting relatively high iron content, is predictive of impending cardiac failure and has rapidly become a clinical standard of care where the methodology is available. Unfortunately, as described by Dr. Walker, the availability of MRI is limited in areas of the world where thalassemia is the most common and echocardiography is being explored to provide more available assessment of cardiac function. Overall, the methodology for evaluating cardiac iron and cardiac function has become increasingly sophisticated concurrent with development of chelation regimens to prevent or reverse cardiac iron deposition.

MRI provides additional information regarding liver iron and the relative rate of accumulation of liver iron and myocardial iron over time as reported by Dr. St. Pierre. MRI also provides a means to evaluate liver pathology in that the coefficient of variation of liver iron concentration reflects the degree of fibrosis. Another remarkable application of MRI is to assess iron deposition in endocrine tissues, particularly the pituitary gland and the pancreas as reported by Dr. Wood. Iron deposition into the anterior pituitary begins early in life and later loss of volume of the gland is associated with development of hypogonadism.

A novel, fluorescence-based determination of nontransferrin bound iron in blood, reported by Phillip Hider, may provide methodology to monitor this form of iron in the context of iron overload and chelation therapy. The addition of this tool to those already available for assessing iron status is likely to provide new insights into pathophysiology as well as the effects of various chelation regimens.

Treatment of iron overload

Substantial clinical experience and many well-designed clinical trials have documented that iron overload can be prevented and reversed. Deferoxamine, deferasirox, and deferiprone have unique advantages and disadvantages in the treatment of iron overload but singularly or in combination can provide effective therapy. Recent work indicates that the individual chelators have different mechanisms for extracting iron from ferritin and inducing its degradation with deferoxamine being taken up by the endocytic pathway with lysosomal degradation of hemosiderin and ferritin, whereas deferasirox and deferiprone enter the cytoplasm and extract iron from ferritin and induce its degradation by autophagy.[25,26] Dr. Galanello reported on studies involving the combination of deferiprone and deferoxamine and Dr. Telfer described ongoing efforts to combine the two drugs either in combination or sequentially to improve cardiac outcome with optimal chelation therapy.

Despite these advances, adherence to chelation continues to be problematic as highlighted by Dr. Alan Cohen during his keynote address. Daily self-administration of subcutaneous deferoxamine by an infusion pump imposes a substantial burden, which compromises adherence. However, data has accumulated indicating a significant incidence of nonadherence to oral iron chelators. Adherence is particularly problematic in older adolescents and young adults as they transition into independence. This transition often coincides with the transition from pediatric to adult care providers, which may result in fragmentation and lack of coordination of care among multiple providers. Thus, despite the advances in evaluation of iron overload and in the use of chelation agents, many challenges remain to be overcome in on-going efforts to optimize care for children and adults with Cooley's Anemia.

Drs. Fung and Lai reported on the occurrence of nutritional deficiency in thalassemic patients, particularly those with iron overload. They also described the metabolic changes that occur as a consequence of these deficiencies and the oxidative damage imposed by iron overload. Certainly, comprehensive attention to these factors is essential for overall management of the thalassemic patient. In considering replacement of vitamin C in the context of its deficiency, the potential of high doses of vitamin C to precipitate myocardial dysfunction in the context of significant iron overload should not be forgotten.[27]

Stem cell transplantation

The potential of stem cell transplantation to cure thalassemic individuals has been well established over the past two decades. Dr. Walters provided an overview of current efforts to minimize toxicity by modifying the preparative regimen without compromising the potential for stem cell engraftment thereby making transplantation available for patients with more advanced disease. A second challenge is to make stem cell transplantation available to a larger proportion of thalassemic patients through the use of alternative donors. Significant progress has been made in the use of umbilical cord blood transplants with the use of multiple cords for transplantation improving the rate of engraftment and ultimate outcome. Progress has also been made in using stem cells from matched unrelated donors as well as from haploidentical family members. Work in the laboratory of Ryan has resulted in the development of novel mouse models of Cooley's Anemia. Animals can be rescued with regular blood transfusions and can readily be cured with postnatal injection of allogeneic bone marrow in the absence of any cytoreductive conditioning. These new models of Cooley's Anemia will provide an opportunity to explore strategies for curative stem cell transplantation while minimizing toxicity.

Global burden of disease

In his keynote lecture, Dr. Weatherall described how inclusion of the genetic disorders of hemoglobin in the Global Burden of Disease Program has allowed a more comprehensive picture of the enormous global health problem that these diseases impose on mankind. Detailed studies in several countries have documented that disease incidence may vary from region to region so that very comprehensive studies are necessary to truly understand the burden of disease in individual countries.

Only a very small proportion of patients with severe thalassemia syndromes have benefited from the curative potential of stem cell transplantation. Paradoxically, many of these have come from developing countries where the overall resources for comprehensive treatment of thalassemia are limited. This occurs when individual families have the resources to travel to a sophisticated transplant center thereby eliminating disease burden for these families without significantly affecting the disease burden in the country.

The HbE/β-thalassemias have a highly variable phenotype with individuals having an identical genotype at the β-globin locus also having variable manifestations. Dr. Weatherall described efforts to identify patients who have been transfused for extended periods but nonetheless can tolerate termination of regular transfusions with maintenance of an adequate hemoglobin concentration. Paradoxically, such efforts to conserve resources in developing countries are accompanied by reports of pulmonary hypertension, the occurrence of thrombosis and stroke as well as subclinical neurological damage by Dr. Cappelline and the occurrence of osteoporosis, which is also exacerbated in untransfused patients by Dr. Terpos. In developed countries, exacerbation of these complications in the untransfused state has prompted more liberal indications for transfusion in individuals with thalassemia intermedia. Thus, disparity in health care delivery in addition to the global burden of disease remain as an extraordinary challenge to those interested in optimizing care and treatment of the many patients with thalassemia throughout the world.

Conflicts of interest

The author declares no conflicts of interest.

References

1. Nienhuis, A.W. & W.F. Anderson. 1971. Isolation and translation of hemoglobin messenger RNA from thalassemia, sickle cell anemia, and normal human reticulocytes. *J. Clin. Invest.* **50:** 2458–2460.
2. Benz, E.J. Jr. & B.G. Forget. 1971. Defect in messenger RNA for human hemoglobin synthesis in beta thalassemia. *J. Clin. Invest.* **50:** 2755–2760.
3. Baltimore, D. 1970. RNA-dependent DNA polymerase in virions of RNA tumour viruses. *Nature* **226:** 1209–1211.
4. Temin, H.M. & S. Mizutan. 1970. RNA-dependent DNA polymerase in virions of Rous sarcoma virus. *Nature* **226:** 1211–1213.
5. Anderson, W.F. 1972. Genetic therapy. In *The New Genetics and the Future of Man.* Hamilton M., Ed.: 109–124. Eerdmans. Grand Rapids, MI.
6. Friedmann, T. & R. Robbin. 1972. Gene therapy for human genetic disease? *Science* **175:** 949–955.
7. Nienhuis, A.W. 2008. Development of gene therapy for blood disorders. *Blood* **111:** 4431–4444.
8. Bank, A., R. Dorazio & P. Leboulch. 2005. A phase I/II clinical trial of beta-globin gene therapy for beta-thalassemia. *Ann. N.Y. Acad. Sci.* **1054:** 308–316.
9. Pfannkuche, K., H. Summer, O. Li, *et al.* 2009. The high mobility group protein HMGA2: a co-regulator of chromatin structure and pluripotency in stem cells? *Stem Cell Rev. Rep.* **5:** 224–230.
10. Cartier, N., S. Hacein-Bey-Abina, C. Bartholomae, *et al.* 2009. Hematopoietic stem cell gene therapy with a lentiviral vector in X-linked adrenoleukodystrophy. *Science* **326:** 818–823.
11. Frecha, C., J. Szecsi, F.L. Cosset & E. Vethoeyen. 2008. Strategies for targeting lentiviral vectors. *Curr. Gene. Ther.* **8:** 449–460.

12. Lucas, M.L., N.E. Seidel, C.D. Porada, *et al.* 2005. Improved transduction of human sheep repopulating cells by retrovirus vectors pseudotyped with feline leukemia virus type C or RD114 envelopes. *Blood* **106:** 51–58.
13. Hanawa, H., P. Hematti, K. Keyvanfar, *et al.* 2004. Efficient gene transfer into rhesus repopulating hematopoietic stem cells using a simian immunodeficiency virus-based lentiviral vector system. *Blood* **103:** 4062–4069.
14. DiPersio, J.F., G.L. Uy, U. Yasothan & P. Kirkpatrick. 2009. Plerixafor. *Nat. Rev. Drug. Discov.* **8:** 105–106.
15. Ryu, B.Y., M.V. Evans-Galea, J.T. Gray, *et al.* 2008. An experimental system for the evaluation of retroviral vector design to diminish the risk for proto-oncogene activation. *Blood* **111:** 1866–1875.
16. Sankaran, V.G., J. Xu, T. Ragoczy, *et al.* 2009. Developmental and species-divergent globin switching are driven by BCL11A. *Nature* **460:** 1093–1097.
17. Sankaran, V.G., T.F. Menne, J. Xu, *et al.* 2008. Human fetal hemoglobin expression is regulated by the developmental stage-specific repressor BCL11A. *Science* **322:** 1839–1842.
18. Lettre, G., V.G. Sankaran, M.A. Bezerra, *et al.* 2008. DNA polymorphisms at the BCL11A, HBS1L-MYB and beta-globin loci associate with fetal hemoglobin levels and pain crises in sickle cell disease. *Proc. Natl. Acad. Sci. USA* **105:** 11869–11874.
19. Uda, M., R. Galanello, S. Sanna, *et al.* 2008. Genome-wide association study shows BCL11A associated with persistent fetal hemoglobin and amelioration of the phenotype of beta-thalassemia. *Proc. Natl. Acad. Sci. USA* **105:** 1620–1625.
20. Graslund, T., X. Li, L. Magnenat, *et al.* 2005. Exploring strategies for the design of artificial transcription factors. *J. Bio. Chem.* **280:** 3707–3714.
21. Fleming, M.D. 2008. The regulation of hepcidin and its effects on systemic and cellular iron metabolism. *Am. Soc. Hematol. Educ. Program* **1:** 151–158.
22. Tanno, T., N.V. Bhanu, P.A. Oneal, *et al.* 2007. High levels of GDF15 in thalassemia suppress expression of the iron regulatory protein hepcidin. *Nat. Med.* **13:** 1096–1101.
23. Tanno, T., P. Porayette, O. Sripichai, *et al.* 2009. Identification of TWSG1 as a second novel erythroid regulator of hepcidin expression in murine and human cells. *Blood* **114:** 181–186.
24. Finberg, K.E., M.H. Heeney, D.R. Campagna, *et al.* 2008. Mutations in TMPRSS6 cause iron-refractory iron deficiency anemia (IRIDA). *Nat. Genet.* **40:** 569–571.
25. De Domenico, I., D.M. Ward, & J. Kaplan. 2009. Specific iron chelators determine the route of ferritin degradation. *Blood* **114:** 4546–4551.
26. Theil, E.C. 2009. Mining ferritin iron: 2 pathways. *Blood* **114:** 4325–4326.
27. Nienhuis, A.W. 1981. Vitamin C and iron. *N. Engl. J. Med.* **304:** 170–171.

 Ann. N.Y. Acad. Sci. 1202 (2010) 248–254